SURVIVING GRIEF

365 Days a Year

A Daily Companion

Gary Sturgis

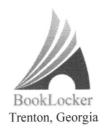

BookLocker
Trenton, Georgia

Published by BookLocker.com, Inc., Trenton, Georgia.

Printed on acid-free paper.

BookLocker.com, Inc.
2022

First Edition

Cover Images:
© Dawna Moore_123rf.com (dunes)
© AdobeStock.com_fergregory (life saver)

i

DISCLAIMER

This book details the author's personal experiences with and opinions about grief and loss. The author is not a licensed social worker.

The author and publisher are providing this book and its contents on an "as is" basis and make no representations or warranties of any kind with respect to this book or its contents. The author and publisher disclaim all such representations and warranties, including for example warranties of merchantability and professional counseling for a particular purpose. In addition, the author and publisher do not represent or warrant that the information accessible via this book is accurate, complete or current.

The statements made about products and services have not been evaluated by the U.S. government. Please consult with your own legal, accounting, medical, or other licensed professional regarding the suggestions and recommendations made in this book.

Except as specifically stated in this book, neither the author or publisher, nor any authors, contributors, or other representatives will be liable for damages arising out of or in connection with the use of this book. This is a comprehensive limitation of liability that applies to all damages of any kind, including (without limitation) compensatory; direct, indirect or consequential damages; loss of data, income or profit; loss of or damage to property and claims of third parties.

You understand that this book is not intended as a substitute for consultation with a licensed medical, legal or accounting professional. Before you begin any change your lifestyle in any way, you will consult a licensed professional to ensure that you are doing what's best for your situation.

This book provides content related to grief and loss topics. As such, use of this book implies your acceptance of this disclaimer.

Also by Gary Sturgis

NONFICTION

SURVIVING – Finding Your Way from Grief to Healing

GRIEF – Hope in the Aftermath

Dedication

In loving memory of my father

You will always be one of the voices in my heart

Introduction

If you're reading this book, you've probably experienced a loss in your life, or maybe several losses. The loss of someone you love can throw you into the darkest place of grief. The pain can seem overwhelming. The last thing you want to do is sit down and read a long book that's going to force you to concentrate and think too much about the characters and the plot.

Grief is best handled in small increments and often the best way to do that is to take it day by day. In this book I share with you one reflection of loss and hope for each day of the year. This allows you to process your grief at a gentle pace.

There's nothing worse than losing someone you love, and grieving is a painful experience. You feel the loss of a loved one acutely in your daily life. Every day you're aware of their absence. I know because I lost my spouse after a courageous battle with cancer eight years ago. The grief journey I began continues to this day, but I've found the key to my survival was to grieve at my own speed.

There will be good days and bad days. Days where you feel like doing something, and days you feel like doing nothing. Days when you feel strong and days when you don't have any energy at all.

Grief is a process that happens one day at a time, if not one moment at a time. It can make you feel alone, but I want to remind you that you're not alone. It's my own experiences, and those of many others I have encountered as a grief specialist and bereavement facilitator, that I share with you within the pages of this book.

One page at a time.

This book is a companion to *Surviving – Finding Your Way from Grief to Healing.* In that book I share with you my own personal journey through the loss of my spouse and the ways in which I was able to process my grief. Whether you read that book or not, this book stands on its own and can be read in any way you find works for you. You can read each page of the calendar year or skip around to the pages that best resonate for you.

I know from my own experience of loss how hard it is to go on living when so much has changed. I also know that no one, including myself, can utterly understand how you feel because all relationships are so unique. Only you know how intense your pain is, how much you miss your loved ones, and the heaviness of the grief you're experiencing.

I truly hope this book will give you some comfort on your own personal grief journey. Not many of us walk this journey without losing something. But I don't think we're ever capable of understanding the sudden loss of a loved one. Never being able to touch, see or speak to them again is unbearable.

If you lost someone you love, it's okay to be broken and take all the time you need to heal. In some ways you may never stop feeling the sadness associated with your loss. But the important thing I want you to know, is that it's also okay to find joy and hope again. It's normal to feel guilty as you move forward on through your life without your loved one, but they would want you to do that. They would want you to be happy. You love them and they love you.

I know that with the passage of time, an open heart, and a choice to embrace hope you will survive. When that happens, you may even find a way to become more than you were before, stronger, more aware of human frailty, more appreciative of the simple things in life, more loving, caring, and compassionate towards all things, including yourself. I have been in a similar place as you, and I know that it's possible to find peace and grace after a major loss.

I hope that you never give up and continue to find beauty in the memories of your loved ones. You may feel alone on this journey but you're not.

I hope that in some small way this book will bring you comfort. We're all just walking each other home, and I believe surviving grief is easier when it's done one day at a time.

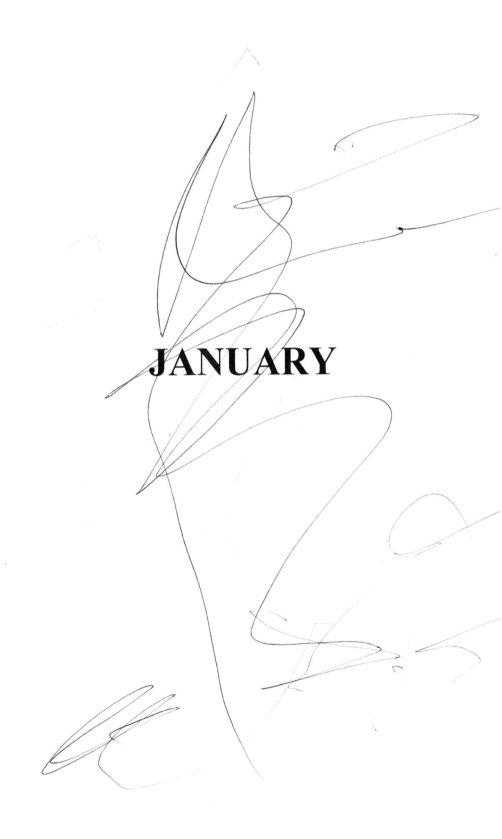

JANUARY

JANUARY 1

It's a 'New' Year

Time waits for no one. When your loved one died, life as you knew it stopped, but the world around you, and the clock, continues ticking, it moves forward without your loved one. Sometimes it seems to move on without you as well, leaving you feeling suspended in a type of time warp, unsure of how to escape it to move forward into some sort of a life without them.

It's a 'new' year, so now you reluctantly add one more year to the list of years spent without your loved one. Whether you lost your loved one last year, or many years ago, it's important to remember that where there was great love, there will also be deep grief, and no matter how long it has been since the death of your loved one, that grief will continue to surface when you least expect it.

For every special moment you shared with your loved one, there will be just as many moments of emptiness and longing for them. Nostalgia is a part of grief that is a double-edged sword, remembering the love and happiness you shared ultimately brings the sharp pain of the void that is left in your life, and in your heart, without them.

But no matter how painful it is remembering what you have lost, it's this love you shared that will eventually help you heal enough to find the life that is out there waiting for you to live. This may not be the life you had planned, but there is still some happiness that can be found.

Give yourself permission to grieve regardless of how long it's been since your loved one died.

By honoring your loss, the unsettled emotions that are involved in your grief will become more manageable. Allow yourself to feel your loss and the emotion it brings. Remember the love you shared and know that it's always with you. This love will always belong to you. This love can never be lost.

The reality is that grief will drag you through a huge range of emotions, from guilt to fear to despair to anger. The scope of possible emotions is almost endless. You'll experience different emotions as you grieve, at different intensities and lengths.

You should be aware that the emotional ups and downs that you're experiencing are normal. Healing your grief is a process. Don't feel guilty that you're experiencing all of these emotions. These emotions are what you need to experience to eventually heal your broken heart.

Remember, on this first day of a 'new' year, there's always hope to heal your broken heart enough to find some joy again.

JANUARY 2

There's No Sugarcoating Grief

There's just no way to sugarcoat the feeling of losing a loved one, there's just no sugarcoating grief.

It's one of the hardest experiences imaginable. There's so much loneliness, sadness, blame, confusion, and anger that comes with it. It's crying yourself to sleep, pushing people away, feeling depressed, detaching from the world, and not wanting to go on. It's crippling anxiety, and not getting enough sleep, or getting too much. It's questioning everything or being so numb that you stop caring about anything.

The death of a loved one is brutal and cruel, and it will beat you down and kick your butt, until you have no fight left. How can I possibly sugarcoat that? Grief sucks!

There's just no way to make it sound like walking on sunshine. I know it's not, because I've lived it. Only if you've suffered a significant loss can you understand that by not acknowledging the pain, you're not allowing yourself to move forward in the way you deserve, in the way all of us who have faced loss deserve.

I know all too well that grief is a downer. It's sad. I've come to realize that the only way to truly turn that pain into something positive is to allow yourself to be vulnerable and to just 'feel'. Forget about putting on a brave face. Cry it out because there's healing power in vulnerability. There's strength in sadness.

But I still refuse to sugarcoat grief. Instead, I write the truth about it, but I also try to share what I've discovered. That by embracing the pain, you gain strength. You love harder and care deeper. Pain in life is inevitable. But pain is power. Pain allows you to understand yourself in ways you never knew.

So, yeah, losing a loved one is hard. I don't know about you, but it's without a doubt the hardest thing I've ever been through.

JANUARY 3

Man's Best Friend

I've loved and lost pets. I now have a mini dachshund named Zoe. She's the love of my life. She was the best therapy I had after my loss. Her unconditional love helped heal my broken heart. She's almost 11 years old now and I know someday, she too, will have to leave me.

If you've ever loved and lost a pet, you'll likely understand and agree that our losing them is better than the alternative, them having to live without us. Their shorter life spans generally spare them this possibility. But I still don't see the outpouring of support and understanding around pet loss that accompanies the loss of other family members; I think that's a shame.

I know that when it comes to losing a pet, everyone's grief will run a different course, but I know that certain aspects of grieving a pet are crucial.

Surround yourself with people who "get it," people who love animals, who recognize them as important family members, and who may have experienced pet loss themselves. They might be able to provide useful navigation.

Focus on what works for you. Some people who lose a pet rush out to adopt a new one. Others take time to grieve before they open their homes and hearts to a new pet.

Realize the normalcy of pet loss grief. Losing a pet is a significant event. Plus, our animals can be such vital parts of our day-to-day experience. Pet loss involves saying goodbye to a loved one as well as radically altering your routines. Eliminating these routine behaviors can complicate your loss.

Consider if there are any actions that will help. Sometimes, you can be comforted by "doing something" with your grief and loss. That might mean donating to an animal charity, hosting a memorial service or creating a physical memorial, or having a print made of the pet you've lost.

Most of all allow yourself to grieve. Avoiding feelings doesn't make them go away. Acceptance of your loss and of all the feelings (despite how painful) is crucial to your healing. At the same time, taking breaks from mourning and utilizing coping resources can be helpful.

This is a process. There's no road map or timeline for grieving the loss. When you lose a beloved pet, allow yourself to recover in your own way and to take the time you need. In time, it's likely your distress will diminish, and memories of your pet will bring more consistent joy and peace.

One day all the pets we loved and lost will come running to us, and that's going to be a great day!

JANUARY 4

A Better Place

I know all about grief, chances are you do too. If you've loved, you know loss, and with loss, comes grief.

Grief is tough. It makes you feel like your heart is being torn from your chest. It makes you angry at the unfairness of it all. It's all-consuming, this thing that wraps itself around you and refuses to let go.

I've always been told, "They're in a better place."

I think about that a lot, the idea of a better place, and what that would look like. I don't know. Nobody does, at least no one living.

But we can still hope, right? I for one hope this isn't all there is.

I often wonder what it means to be a good person, and what kind of mark I'll leave behind on the world when I close my eyes for the last time. I guess I just always figured if I was a good person I'd go to that better place.

So, what did I do to deserve this? Why did this have to happen to me? Why didn't I get a happy ending?

I don't know the answers to these questions. I don't know if I believe in fate or if the universe is just a collection of random occurrences. I don't know why some people die way before it should be their time to do that. Good people. I don't know any of that.

But what I do know is that I've done the most I could with what I have, and if I didn't, maybe when I get to that better place, I can try to be the person I should've been in this life.

I really hope the one I love is in a better place, that's exactly where I would want him to be, and one day I hope to be there with him.

JANUARY 5

Living Single

If you've lost a spouse, I feel your pain. The road you're traveling is full of potholes and it's long.

The first year for me was all about navigating life alone. The second year was trying to learn how to redefine and recreate a purposeful meaningful life for myself. It was about living single. I was a part of a couple for 20 years. I loved being married. I loved being a husband. I loved all the great and small things about being a 'team'. Then, suddenly, it was down to me, myself, and I.

I felt cheated that we weren't given the chance to grow old together. We were happy, and that didn't seem fair, not by a long shot. I wanted more time, but that isn't the life that was given to me. So, I had to figure out how to be happy without him. I had to learn all about living single. I had to learn new social skills. I had to learn how to fit in. I had to learn how to go out without being afraid. I had to find a purpose and a reason to live.

That all takes a lot of work. It's scary trying to figure out a new direction. It's hard to move forward alone. But I had to because I was given no other choice. I eventually got tired of trying to make sense of the senseless.

So, I started working on new things, like new dreams, and I gave myself space and grace if some things worked out and some things didn't. It was a long road, with lots of potholes, but I just kept going. Grief is work. It's ongoing. It doesn't end at the one-year mark, and not the second or third, because grief is a reaction to loss, and it's personal.

I've learned there's no such thing as closure with the loss of someone you love. One thing I know for certain as I continue to move forward with my life, is that I'll always miss him. Grief isn't about moving on, it's about moving forward, one small step at a time, and grief isn't only about mourning your loss, but getting to know yourself as a different person.

JANUARY 6

Knocking On Heaven's Door

If there were a door to Heaven, I'd knock on it.

I'd be the first one waiting in line to see you again. I want to talk just one more time, and listen to you speak, so I could remember the sound of your voice. It hurts that as time passes, it's fading in my memory.

When the door opened, I'd run to you to tell you I love you, for all those times I didn't say it enough. I'd tell you I miss you just in case you didn't know. Even though you live in my heart, I miss being able to touch you.

As I enter, you'll see that even though I've tried to move on, there's still a hole in my heart, it's something that will never be filled or replaced.

If there were a door to Heaven, I'd knock on it. I know it would be you that will answer.

Your death had a way of creating a very strong bond that keeps us connected forever. I know that nothing would have changed between us. We'd pick up right where we left off. I want you to know I'm happy, but it still hurts some days. I'd ask if you're proud of the person I am now, and I'd thank you for the lessons you continue to teach me.

If there were a door to Heaven, I'd knock on it. If I were allowed in even just for one quick visit, I'd hug you, not wanting to let go. I'd thank you for the time we had together, and I'd let you know I'd rather live with the pain, than to never have known you at all.

JANUARY 7

Messages in a Bottle

Wouldn't it be nice to walk along the beach and find a message in a bottle from someone you love and lost? I often wonder what those messages would be, but I don't really know what they would say. I'm not a psychic, but what I have is my faith, particularly what I think those we've lost want us to know.

Here's what I think some of the messages would be;

"You're doing great!"

I believe our loved ones are supporting us, reassuring us, and even cheering us on. They want us to know that we're going to be fine, even without them.

"Don't be sad."

I think those who love us don't want us to mourn them forever. Instead, they want us to celebrate life. They hope we laugh again, enjoy what we can, and remember them in life, not in death.

"I'm not mad about anything."

I don't believe that resentment, anger, or pettiness is possible in death. Unlike love and the wonderful memories, we shared, our loved ones aren't holding onto any negative feelings, and they want us to know that.

"I'm with you all the time."

They may be gone, but what they leave behind are the memories and the lessons they conveyed and the impact they had on us while they lived. They still live on in the stories we tell. Faith is a personal choice. How much we want to believe about the connection with our loved one is something we all get to decide. If we were to get messages in a bottle, I think they would be positive and encouraging, and full of love.

JANUARY 8

Widower

One night I went to bed a happily married man. The next morning, I woke up, and I was alone. Widower.

It's a word I hate. Just saying it sticks to my tongue. Hearing it makes me want to knock on wood to prevent it. It makes people avoid eye contact with you. It undermines your entire identity, forcing you into a new existence filled with the brutal realities of a life you didn't sign up for, and would never want.

That night I went to bed I was me. The next day I was somebody else. I remember closing my eyes and thinking maybe it wasn't real. If I didn't open my eyes, maybe it wouldn't be true. Maybe it would all be a dream. But it wasn't. I was nowhere near prepared for the devastation. I don't know if advanced warning would have helped, but something about the unexpectedness felt even more unfair. In the blink of an eye my life was ripped in half, torn to shreds, and floating away. I'll never forget the pain. A deep intense physical pain, like feeling my heart explode in my chest.

Then came the choices. Decisions nobody wants to think about, especially when your world just got shattered. Where do you want the funeral? Burial or cremation? Who should be called? Sad choices. Too many choices. Too much to think about with a brain that suddenly just shut down. I was only used to making decisions as a team, with another person. Grief was making me confused, scared, unsure, forgetful, sad......empty. I didn't ask for this and it hurt. Bad!

Nobody escapes this life without suffering, and that morning I became a widower, it was my turn. Today may be somebody else's turn.

Tomorrow it might be someone else's. I've learned something along the way; I acknowledge I don't control anything. Life is at the wheel, and I'm just a widower along for the ride.

JANUARY 9

Why?

If you've lost someone you love you've probably asked, "Why me?" "Why the person I love?" "How could this happen" "Why now?"

I struggle with those same questions myself, and I certainly don't claim to have the answers. I also don't want to get in a debate on the subject either, but I'll be the first one to totally support your right to ask the questions.

Here's what I do know, the explosive emotions of grief like crying out in anguish, "It isn't fair!" or "I hate this!", are normal and necessary reactions that need be expressed, not repressed.

Give yourself permission to feel whatever you feel, and to express those feelings, even if they're not logical. The thinking part of you knows that illness, pain, suffering and death are all a part of being human, but when the person you love is taken from you, you see it as a sign that something has gone terribly wrong.

It's only human to rail against the horrible injustice, to feel overwhelming feelings of pain, helplessness, frustration, hurt and fear, and to scream, "Why?!" These feelings aren't right or wrong, good or bad, they just are. They let you know that you've sustained an injury that needs attention.

I know right now you're struggling with all those 'why' questions, but that's an important part of the mourning process, as you search for the meaning in your loss.

I think that life is a mystery to be lived, not a problem to be solved.

You're certainly not alone in your search. We all struggle with these questions, and we're all looking for meaning as we help each other come to terms with our own losses. We really are all just walking each other home.

You deserve to have a good life, a happy life, but the death of someone you love can change all of that in an instant. When you're grieving, you're overwhelmed as you struggle to make some sense of your suffering, and you may find it difficult, if not impossible, to continue believing that you could ever live a happy life again.

In my own struggle to make sense of the pain and suffering, and in my own search for meaning, I have hope and faith that somehow, I'll find the answers to all the 'why' questions, but I also believe that the most important question is, "What do I do now that it's happened?"

I'll never know why the people I love had to die, and I'm okay with that now, because even if I had the answer, the reason would never be good enough for me, ever!

JANUARY 10

The White Feathers

The white feathers started appearing soon after my spouse slipped away.

The first time it occurred, I was getting out of the car at the cemetery, and a white feather came floating from seemingly nowhere and dropped on the ground in front of me. My niece asked where the feather came from, and my response was, "maybe from an angel's wing."

The feathers still appear today. They've shown up in my garden, on my windowsill in the morning, on my doorstep, at my feet at a concert, just about everywhere. I smile when I see them and often say a quiet, "thank you".

One time I was driving to work and having a 'gray day', you know, those days when all you do is cry, and a feather floated in my driver's side window, right by my face, and out of the passenger side window.

Awesome, right!?

A white feather is typically seen as a sign from an angel or spirit of a loved one who has passed on. White feathers symbolize faith and protection and are most significant when found in a spot where they're not likely to be, such as inside of a home or an automobile.

So, what does it mean?

I'm a person of faith, and I'm always comforted knowing, and believing, that my loved one is on the other side waiting for me. I think these feathers are his gentle and harmless way of showing me that he's still with me, that he's here protecting and watching over me.

To some people, thinking all this might make me seem a bit strange but seeing the white feathers brings me comfort. It certainly won't bring him back, but it's a nice feeling when it happens.

JANUARY 11

Man Overboard!

Why is it when you suffer the loss of somebody you love, some people just disappear?

They abandon ship.

When death strikes, it turns your world upside down. It upsets the rhythm of your life. It rocks the foundation of your relationships. It rocks the boat.

Friendships are affected, and sometimes even families. Many people have told me how supportive their family is after their loss, but just as many have told me how some family members just walk away or completely disappear.

After a loss it feels like you're in a boat, in that boat are all your family and friends. When the person you love dies, it rocks the boat. When the boat rocks, some people stay in the boat, and some people fall out (or in some circumstances, jump!) This is particularly painful when it's family. They're supposed to stand by you. They're supposed to stay in the boat and help you paddle, right?

These people that fall (or jump) out of the boat, may not be able to deal with your grief. It scares them, even terrifies them. They look at their own lives, and loved ones, and they think it could happen to them. Being around you was safe but being around a 'grieving you' is just too scary.

Your old life is gone, while their life hasn't changed. The gap between them and you gets too wide. So, they abandon ship. Your ship is sinking, and they want no part of that.

Maybe they're just busy, or maybe they're just avoiding you. Whatever the case may be, the result is the same. They're not there. They fell out of the boat, or they just jumped. Unfortunately, as if loss isn't bad enough, it also alters friendships and family relationships. Grief scares those that haven't been touched by it yet.

But here's the good news, the people that fall out of the boat (or jumped) are most likely not the kind of people you need on your grief journey anyway. They're not going to be supportive. They're not going to say or do what you need. So, their absence will just free up space in the boat for those new people you'll pick up on your grief journey. People that have also lost a piece of their heart and understand.

The ocean of grief is full of people struggling to swim. You'll throw them a life ring, pluck them out of the rough ocean, and bring them aboard.

These new people will be able to understand your loss, and add buoyancy to your boat, and they will become your new support system.

JANUARY 12

An Uninvited Guest

After a loved one has died, you may feel like you can be in a crowded room and still feel lonely. Even though you may be surrounded by other people, the physical and emotional void can be accompanied by an overwhelming sense of loneliness.

This is especially true if you lost a spouse. It's normal to feel a sense of deep grief when someone dies. You miss the physical absence of the one you love, and in their place an uninvited guest moves into your life. That guest is loneliness.

These feelings of loneliness can intensify before they lessen. This can make you feel hopeless, and those around you, because everyone expects things to get better with time, and when they don't, you can feel like something is wrong with you.

A part of you will always feel your loss. But there are ways you can cope with the loneliness while moving forward and incorporating the loss into your life. Don't place expectations on your grief in how you think you 'should' or 'shouldn't' being doing it. Follow your gut and heart as to what feels right in the moment.

Give yourself things to do, it will give you something to look forward to while allowing you to have some social time around other people. But not all activities need to include interacting with others. Sometimes it helps to just be in the same physical space as other people.

Avoid isolating yourself, even though all you may want to do is stay home and be away from people. This usually happens because you feel like no one understands your grief, or you're constantly reassuring others that you're okay.

Remember, loneliness may be an uninvited guest, but it's not the same as being alone.

JANUARY 13

Grief Changes Relationships

Grief changes the nature of your relationships. It's essential to realize that your relationship with other people will be affected and change after a major loss. Some changes may lead to a positive experience, but sometimes it's not as positive.

These changes, whether positive or negative, have a lot to do with the personal stress you experience as you navigate the feelings that are common to the grieving process.

You might expect that sadness may be the most prevalent feeling that you would have, but there's a roller coaster of emotions such as guilt, anger, disbelief, denial, and more that are part of the grief experience. The impact of these feelings can challenge the previous dynamics of your relationships, sometimes exacerbating already present issues.

Even though it's upsetting and distressing to experience this shift in your relationships, recognize those closest to you are going through their own process of mourning. This may include their perception of losing what they have come to expect in your relationship with them.

You have to realize that as you try to cope with the loss, and find new ways to move on, your prior ways of thinking and being will be affected. You may also find that the role you may have previously played in your relationships is now changed.

As a result, close friends and family may feel equally challenged by adjusting to your new role and needs. This adjustment can place even more strain on the dynamics of your relationships.

Remember, any change, significant or minor, can create a sense of loss. And when your relationships change, or you change in the relationships, this can result in the other people feeling disoriented and often uncertain how to respond to you.

People you were once close with knew how to respond to you, but now they may not know how to respond to a 'grieving' you.

Don't allow yourself to be discouraged by what may appear as the unsupportive actions of other people. Try not to take their reactions personally. You'll only increase your own pain if you do. Focus on your own healing, while being as clear as you can about what you're feeling and going through.

Express what your needs are without any attachment to how they should respond.

JANUARY 14

What Is Your Greatest Challenge?

For you, this question may seem ridiculous, the answer obvious.

Your loss, period.

That's probably your greatest challenge.

But I think it's more than that.

As the loss impacts every part of your day, and everything you do, and everything you touch, you may find that your challenges in relation to the loss can change day in and day out.

Maybe for you every day presents a different challenge, like trying to raise your children, being productive at work to make a living, or just getting out of bed in the morning.

Perhaps it's the loneliness or the lack of motivation to move forward in a life that seems pointless.

The question goes deeper than you think, and in order to find the tools you need to move through each difficult day of grief, you need to know what you're truly up against.

So, as you read this, in relation to your loss, think about what's your greatest challenge?

Maybe by sharing your greatest challenge, you can find comfort and support from others walking the same road of grief.

JANUARY 15

'Normal People'

I always refer to those who haven't experienced the significant loss of a loved one as 'normal people.' If you lost someone you love, then you have been in the trenches, survived the battle with grief, and have seen and heard things that can't be unseen or unheard. The aftermath of a major loss can haunt you for a long time, if not forever, and there are just certain things only you can understand.

If you're not one of the normal people, then you're a warrior. In the past you probably turned to the normal people who knew you best for support when struggling with the trials and challenges of life. But everything changes after a significant loss, especially in the early days, and there's no change more evident in yourself that now separates you from the normal people.

Maybe this is why you seek out others who have had a loss similar to your own. At a time when there's so much uncertainty, and so few things that make sense, you feel the need to make connections with those that make you feel understood. Everything that connected you to the normal people seems to have become unraveled. Because while so much of this experience is foreign to you it may seem even stranger still to the normal people. You now have the responsibility to educate the normal people.

I just want to remind you that everything you're thinking, feeling, and doing, is very 'normal,' and very much an expected part of the grieving process. So, try to forgive the normal people in your life who don't understand. They can only know what they know. You can't blame them for what they don't know, and you have to forgive the normal people for what they can't understand.

You're in a special group now, you're perceptive, and compassionate, a person who has been through a loss and came out the other side. You've become one of the most understanding and sympathetic people you'd ever want to meet. One day when the normal people experience a loss of their own, they'll be fortunate to have you by their side.

JANUARY 16

Grief Is Everlasting

One day I woke up, and it occurred to me that 8 years is a long time. That's how long it's been since my spouse died. But I still never underestimate the power of grief, how it can make my chest tight and bring tears to my eyes.

Sometimes words are the only way for me to make sense of what I feel, to make sense of the everlasting grief that is always present in my life.

I know this might sound strange, but I consider grief a friend. You probably think that's crazy, but I really do. I consider grief my friend because it's an emotion and experience that has been with me for 8 years now. I've gotten to know it well. You see, I don't want to ever forget about my grief because then I might forget about who I've lost, and I can't let that happen.

Grief taught me to be patient with people having a bad day, whether they can express that or not, because we all have silent battles to fight. Every single one of us. Grief taught me to reach out to people, and to express myself, and to find my voice.

Grief led me to do the work I now do, and I'm grateful for that. Grief taught me to continue to use my voice and know that the impact spreads farther than I might imagine. Grief is a good teacher. I found that out when I decided to make it my friend, instead of fearing it. I'm glad I let grief in. I'm committed to my relationship with it.

I don't claim to know it all, I never do, but grief taught me that even when you do all of the right things, grief can still turn up and throw everything out of order. I know that grief is everlasting; it's been a long journey, one that I know will never end, but I'm confident that neither will my relationship with the one I still love. That's everlasting too, because death ends a life, not a relationship.

I shouldn't let grief take me by surprise after all this time, but in the same respect I'm still getting to know it; maybe grief will always just be that ever-changing dance between sadness and joy.

JANUARY 17

Love or Loved

Did you ever noticed when someone you love dies, in the context of grief, they become your 'loved' one? All the sympathy cards say it, as in, "I'm so sorry for the loss of your loved one."

This in some way insinuates a past tense situation, you no longer 'love' them, now you 'loved' them, as if you don't anymore. See what I mean?

I have an issue with this, and I'll tell you why.

When my spouse was alive, and we would both go to work, we were separated, yet our love was the same as when we were physically together. So why should that be any different now that we're separated by death?

When someone you love dies, their physical absence leaves a void, and their presence is what you ultimately miss and mourn. But there's also a new reality that their absence represents, and that's the love you have for that person is still the same, so in a sense they're still here, just not physically.

This is why you often want your grief to end, but also don't want it to end. You want to cling to their absence as long as you can and still think about all the memories you have of them, knowing they hold both the deepest joy and the deepest pain.

When they're physically gone you learn something you couldn't know while they were living. You learn just how deeply you're capable of missing them. You learn how much pain their absence has caused, and how holding onto that pain sometimes keeps them close.

Even though death has taken them physically away, you learn about a type of love that comes along with the grief they left behind. It's an even deeper and more intense love. Love is everlasting, so for that reason, someone you 'love', can never only be someone you 'loved'.

JANUARY 18

Making Room for Loss

The thing about loss is it can't be undone, but spaces for mourning the loss can be rebuilt. So how do you do that?

First, acknowledge that you'll be anxious, vulnerable, and disoriented. Don't just pretend that things are normal, share your experience, invite people to share theirs, and make that behavior normal. Even just sharing what you miss most about the person, how you're struggling to learn how to deal with it.

Second, offer the truth. What this means is, let people know what you're dealing with right now, at this very moment. It can soothe your anxiety to be heard, even if who you're telling doesn't have the answers.

It's hard to make long-term predictions, so it's better not to make any. Sharing your current concerns and fears can be more useful than giving people an idea about what you think the future will look like for you.

Grief erases your sense of importance and doing something when you feel powerless, no matter how small, can make you feel that you can still complete something. It's difficult when you have no idea what next week will be like, let alone the future.

I don't mean to say, with all this, that you need to just get on with an ill-defined 'new normal.' That would be like telling you that you'll 'get over it.' The reality is you never do.

But staying in the present, focusing on the reality of uncertainty, can keep you going and connected as you learn to live with your loss, slowly growing through it.

You need space to share and soothe your grief and making room for loss is about turning from the future to the present.

It's about regaining your footing and finding hope.

JANUARY 19

A Grieving Heart

If someone you love died, your heart is probably broken. Your heart is now a grieving heart. So how do you live with a grieving heart, a heart that's broken?

The answer isn't how you fix it, or move beyond it, it's learning to live with your grief as an ongoing way of being in the world. It's the way you honor that which you love.

Here's what I'm proposing, that with enough healing, living with a grieving heart can become natural, and very normal.

As you embark on your healing journey, you'll start crying a whole lot more. Not just to clear the pain, but for the simplest of everyday reasons, and out of nowhere. You'll cry when you see a dragonfly, a photograph, a familiar place, you'll cry even when you look at a star in the night sky.

These random things will make you cry. The heart is designed to grieve, it wants to grieve, it needs to grieve, especially when it's broken.

This is the price you pay for love. The loss of the life you thought you had, the life you once knew and held so dear. Loss of a dream you believed was true. But you can also find and feel grief in opening your heart. Opening it to love and to new possibilities. Opening it to what the future holds.

Isn't that what life is all about? Endings and beginnings, closings and openings?

The heart was designed to navigate you through this forever winding adventure called life. But you have to be willing to feel and to live with a grieving heart. You can learn to live with your broken heart, by befriending your grief.

JANUARY 20

What's It All About?

After my loss, I began to question the meaning and purpose of my life. I questioned the philosophy of life and explored the religious and spiritual values I had up to that point. I was searching for meaning for going on living.

I asked a lot of "How?" and "Why?" questions.

How could God let this happen?" "Why did this happen to me?" The death of my spouse reminded me of my lack of control. It left me feeling adrift in a sea of emotions. The person who died was a part of me. At times, overwhelming sadness and loneliness became my constant companions. I felt that when my spouse died, part of me died.

I was now faced with finding some meaning in going on with my life, even though I felt so empty and alone. The death made me confront my own feelings about dying and spirituality. I doubted my faith, and all kinds of questions were racing through my head and heart. Sound familiar?

But take comfort in the fact that all this is normal and part of your journey toward renewed living. Talking about grief and loss is not something people want to do but talking about it helps us to heal. The more you share your story and experiences, the more you're able to understand your pain and make sense of your loss.

In time, you can begin to learn how to 'move forward' while taking your loved one with you, instead of 'moving on' and leaving them behind.

You can begin to integrate your loss into your life and live in a way that you remain open to the opportunities presented to you.

This was something really bad that happened to you, but it doesn't have to define who you are going forward. There are still good things up ahead, and if you have the courage to keep walking, you'll discover the journey is worth it.

JANUARY 21

What I Believe

I believe when we die, we'll see the one we love again, not in a physical form, but more in the form of energy full of love. I think if you're looking forward to seeing the one you love again rest assured, you will.

I believe the people we love can hear us talk to them, and I know when you're grieving, you're talking to them in your mind, or maybe out loud when you're alone. They hear you and can hear you when you talk out loud or when you think thoughts their way. Thoughts are energy, and they're energy.

So, if you've got something to say, just say it. They're listening!

I believe they visit us. They're around you, sometimes trying to get your attention. Listen and you might hear them. They might even have something important to tell you, so pay attention. Look for them in your dreams, it's the middle ground where they can easily broadcast, and you can easily receive.

Are you not good at remembering your dreams? I'm not either, but I'm working on that because they can't do all the work.

If dreams aren't your thing, then look for the signs. Their photo falling to the floor mysteriously. Their favorite song popping onto the radio while you're thinking about them. The 11:11 on the clock, the dragonfly or the cardinal in the tree. They're trying to get your attention, so you have to be watching and listening.

I believe they aren't suffering, both emotionally and physically. No more pain. Well, no more body really, so that sort of solves that. I don't think they suffer at all. I think they're happy. I think they're probably in better shape than we are, because I don't think death is the end of life. Death is just life without a body. So, basically, what I believe, is that your person is just a thought away, so send them some love!

JANUARY 22

My Best Chapter

The day my spouse died; my life stopped.

The early days were hard, as I struggled to cope with all the tasks I had to do alone. I had to learn how to take care of the finances and figure out how to live on one salary, instead of two. I had to figure out what my purpose was, and what my life would be like without the confidence and courage I once had.

I tried to stay busy, but I always felt like an outsider looking in. Deep down I was scared. So, scared. Nobody ever told me that grief would cause so much fear. I was scared of all the responsibilities I now had, which I'd never done before. I was trying to be brave.

When I couldn't sleep, I'd spend hours in the middle of the night writing in the pages of my journal. If people asked, I always said "I'm doing okay", even when I wasn't. Nobody wants to hear how miserable somebody is feeling.

I still miss my spouse every day, and I even talk to him. I feel so blessed to have had the love I did, and the time we had together. It was the best chapter in the story of my life.

I now spend my life living one day at a time. This is my own personal strategy, and it works for me. I can't worry about tomorrow, because sometimes tomorrow never comes.

Nobody knows what the future holds, so I'm just grateful for what I have, and I don't want to dwell on what I lost. I consider myself lucky to have met and married such a caring and special person. Our years together were a gift that I will always treasure.

Each day is the start of a new chapter, and I hold on to the hope of it being the next best one.

JANUARY 23

Comfort Zone

I'm a survivor, and I only tell you that to give you hope if you're grieving a loss.

When I wrote my first book called *"Surviving,"* I knew from a literary standpoint my book was far from good, but I didn't care. I didn't write the book so it would win a Pulitzer Prize, I wrote it so that people suffering a loss could read it, find support, and feel less alone.

I can remember sitting down to write *"Surviving."* I was frightened. I remembered my loss and thought back over all the sorrow. I endured so much pain just to get to the point where I could even bring myself to talk about it, never mind writing about it.

I doubted my ability to write anything that could possibly make a difference. I just wanted to help other people that were going through what I had to go through. Knowing I had to do something about it, I started to write.

I didn't really think much about if the writing was 'good', I just hoped that the words on the pages would touch hearts, meet readers in their grief, and bring some comfort, hope, and healing.

Have you ever felt strongly about something, but when you think about doing something about it you get frightened? That happens to me a lot. It was especially true for me early on after my loss. I had to wait five years before I had the courage to even think about telling my story.

I've found over the years that almost every major positive step I've taken in life was hard, and scary, at the time.

Sometimes you want to be comfortable, but the reality is that your comfort zone doesn't lead to healing and growth. Over time, a comfort zone can numb your heart and keep you stuck. Grief can paralyze you. Healing and growth take great courage.

A comfort zone is a beautiful place, but nothing ever grows there.

So, try stepping out of your comfort zone, you'll be surprised at how much you can do and achieve.

It really does promote healing when you reach out to somebody or do something that honors the one you love and lost.

It's not easy, trust me I know!

It took courage to write my first book, but I'm glad I decided to step out of my comfort zone, and I'm excited that my book is helping people, because that's really why I wrote it.

JANUARY 24

Dining Alone

Grief is a thief, and when you lose a partner or spouse, it steals your self-confidence. Suddenly, you're left to explore the world all by yourself, and that's often really hard to do.

For me, even every day ordinary experiences became really daunting. Eating out alone as a widower became my biggest fear, so I just didn't do it.

My grief counselor told me I needed to do it to learn how to get myself back into the world of the living. She said I had to turn that activity from one I dreaded into something I could look forward to, or at least find some pleasure in, so I gave it a try.

I brought my iPad so I would have something to look at, and I thought it would make me look confident, even though I was dying inside.

I walked in like I owned the place and asked for a small table by the window, so I could look out and not feel like everyone was staring at me.

Almost everyone was too interested in themselves and their own meal to pay much attention to me. I realized even though I thought everyone was staring at me, thinking, "oh that poor guy", it was just my imagination, because they were all centered on themselves, not me.

The staff were super friendly, and that made me feel comfortable, and the food was good, but it just wasn't the same.

I survived that first dining adventure, but it was still sad to do alone. I really just wanted my spouse to be with me. But I proved to myself I could do it, and I could do it again if I wanted to, but I didn't. Eating out alone just isn't my thing.

It did, however, make it easier for me to do a lot of other things alone that I was afraid to do, so it wasn't a total waste of time.

JANUARY 25

At the End of My Journey

I just want to let you know I'm okay. I still feel your presence in my everyday life. I talk to you all the time and I see the signs you send me.

I smile when I think of something you would say to make me laugh. I can still hear your voice in my head and feel your love in my heart.

I don't feel like you're gone just because I can't see you. I know you're now just a part of me. A very important part, just as you've always been.

I try really hard not to feel quilt, regret or anger because those emotions only make me feel further away from you. I'm also not sad all the time. I know you would hate to see me that way.

I talk to you just as I always have, sometimes even out in public. I don't care what other people think. They don't know us, and they don't know our story.

I know as much as I tried I couldn't save you. I did the best I could with the knowledge I had at the time. I made the right decisions based on what I believed was best for you and us. I know you know that.

I'm here and you're there and I hope where you are is better because I'll see you there someday when I find my way back to you.

Thank you for being a part of my journey even though I wish it could've been longer and for teaching me about the promise of never-ending love.

Until we meet again I promise you I'll continue to honor our relationship by releasing the anger that no longer serves me, forgiving myself for what I might have done wrong and living the best life I can with no regrets.

I'll honor your memory by living my life for both of us and at the end of my journey I know you'll be waiting.

JANUARY 26

Love in Heaven

I never talk about religion. The reason for that is I was always taught not to discuss religion in a public forum. The topic just causes too much controversy.

But I'll be honest, I believe in Heaven. Maybe not necessarily the Heaven that everyone talks about with angels, harps and pearly gates. I picture Heaven as being more of a peaceful place full of love. I think when we die the pain and sorrow dies with us, and all that's left is love.

I don't think our loved ones are sad. I mean, what kind of Heaven would Heaven be if we spent all of our eternity missing the ones that we love the most once we get there? I think instead of missing us, they love us. I think the love in Heaven is unconditional and everlasting.

I think the people we love that died know without a doubt that they'll see us again when we get to Heaven someday. I don't think there's any sense of 'time' in Heaven. Even though we may spend years missing them, when we get there, I think for them it's only the blink of an eye.

They didn't want to leave, and I think they can see you cry from Heaven, and they know you cry out of love. They hear your words to them as you speak with them. They hear you think to them in moments of silence.

You're living, and they know that living isn't an easy thing to do. Life is filled with lessons of love and strength. We grow the most through our struggles. Their passing was one of the biggest lessons of love and strength that you've ever worked through in life.

I think there's nothing we take with us to Heaven except all the love we gave and received here on Earth.

So, continue to love them, cry your tears when needed, but most of all, know that they still love you.

JANUARY 27

Healing Doesn't Mean Forgetting

"How can I ever laugh again?", "What would it mean if I laughed?", "How can I do anything that's fun?", "How could I enjoy a party?", "What do I have to be happy about?", "God forbid I should fall in love again.", "Why would I even want anyone else?"

My mind screamed all these things, and so much more, over and over. But there were a few things I didn't know.

All the nights of crying myself to sleep, going home alone from a family gathering, grocery shopping solo, climbing into my empty bed, eating by myself, and trying to find my way, have taught me that pain is actually an agent of healing.

Grief drops you into the burning inferno of shattering loss, and day-by-day the fuel for the fire burns down. Each painful experience is the burning of another piece of timber, until you've lived through one more thing you thought might kill you. And it didn't.

Bit by painful bit, you blaze through the hurt, the anger, the loss, the fear, until you find that you aren't afraid of healing anymore. Because healing doesn't mean forgetting. Instead, true recovery from a loss that's so life altering creates embers that light your heart, an illumination that only grows brighter with time.

I've learned that healing doesn't mean forgetting. You still smile. You still love. You still give. You still believe. The pain won't stop you from living. Healing means you remember everything, but it doesn't hurt anymore.

JANUARY 28

The Wrong Decision

Some caregivers blame themselves for having made a 'wrong decision' in their loved ones' medical care.

I remember one man whose 85-year-old grandmother had always said she wanted to be at home when she passed away. As she grew weaker, he even moved into her home to care for her, so her wish could be fulfilled. But, when she fell and fractured her hip, he followed the doctor's recommendation to bring her to the hospital by ambulance.

The trip to the hospital was traumatic for her, and she cried out in pain and confusion. Unfortunately, just hours after entering the hospital, she passed away. He felt horribly guilty. "I should have kept her home," he said. "It's all my fault she died the way she did."

This is a difficult story. In retrospect, perhaps it would have been better for his grandmother to remain at home. With time, however, he came to realize that he made the best decision he could with the information he had at the time. He didn't know she was going to die when she did.

All he knew was that his grandmother was in pain, and the doctor recommended bringing her to the hospital. It wasn't his fault. His grandmother was very ill.

Similarly, whenever you feel you've made a wrong choice, it's important to ask yourself whether you made the best decision you could given what you knew at the time.

No one is to blame for not seeing the future, including you.

JANUARY 29

Death Keeps Knocking

I'm sure you've heard the expression, 'when it rains, it pours.' We usually use this to reflect the idea that when one tragic thing happens, other tragic things follow. This seems to be the case for me since my loss, or maybe it just feels that way. But I'm probably not the only one who feels this way. Maybe you do too.

I suppose it would be nice if every time we suffer a loss, we could have time to process that loss, and integrate it into our life, before we suffer another loss. It just seems like sometimes that's not the way it works.

It's all too common that a death is followed by another death, it's known as 'cumulative loss.' I've lost several people in the past year, including my father. I'm not telling you this for sympathy or anything, I'm just bringing it up because it made me think about how death keeps knocking.

It didn't seem to knock as much before my loss, maybe that was just because I was younger, who knows? It's not really important, but what is important is how I chose to deal with my cumulative loss. Avoiding it doesn't work, that I know. Unfortunately, there's no magic answer. Cumulative loss does put us at a higher risk for prolonged grief, and one thing I sure don't want is prolonged grief! Time isn't a factor when death keeps knocking.

Death doesn't always happen in immediate succession. My father's death has occurred many years after my spouse, yet it still managed to bring up that loss. That's just the way it works for me now. Every death is a "new death" for me, and I know I need to grieve it. Grief is as unique as each person I lose, so I know I can't rush grieving my multiple losses.

Though it can be tempting to think that grief is grief, and I can just lump my 'grief work' together, I know the reality is that I have to grieve every loss individually. I'm going to continue to pay attention to each loss in order to integrate them into my life, because death keeps knocking.

JANUARY 30

The 'Club' You Never Wanted To Join

If you've suffered a major loss, I'm sure you've heard this expression.

Whether you lost a spouse, partner, child, parent, sibling, friend, pet, or any other loss of a loved one, you joined a club, maybe not by choice, but you did.

Several days after my spouse died, I started to think about other people I knew who had lost a spouse before I did. I was somehow compelled to generate this list, and in a way, I continue to maintain it, because it's growing as time goes on.

After my loss, when all my friends that were a 'couple' began to fall away, I started to reach out to the people on my list. My loss has connected me to the people on this list instantly and intensely.

Many had lost a spouse before I did and revealed their experiences to me following my spouse's death. Their communications served as a sort of new member initiation for me into this club that I can't imagine anyone would choose to join.

If you've lost a loved one, you already know that you've experienced a life-altering event, and you probably find yourself seeking out others who 'get it,' these are usually people who've suffered a similar loss. You're now in their club, whether you wanted to be or not.

The death you've experienced has probably knocked you down with a force you could never have imagined. Now you find yourself stumbling around in the landscape of grief. If you're doing that, it helps to find these other club members that have gone before you down the road of loss and grief, because they can help you find your way.

The benefit to this new club membership is that the others in the club will say things that you can actually accept hearing. They may say, "I know what you mean" or "I know how you feel", and this will be music to your ears, because you know they do. These people can support you from a place of actual experience, not just empty platitudes.

You may have a question to ask and only another club member may have the answer. It's the people that have the most in common with your loss that can provide the assistance you need.

They're your new club members, and they share your pain and truly understand it.

You may not have wanted to be a member of the club you never wanted to join, but it may be the one membership you'll never let expire.

JANUARY 31

Opening a Closed Heart

Pain and sadness are usually indications that something's wrong, and that you should find ways to alleviate the pain, but pain, and feelings of loss, are experiences most people try to avoid. But, why?

I think it's because the role of pain and suffering is so misunderstood. Some people think you should be able to control or suppress your feelings of sadness. But nothing could be further from the truth. Your sadness is a symptom of your loss, and the only way to lessen your pain is to move toward it, not away from it.

I know moving toward your sadness isn't easy to do. Every time you admit to feeling sad, people around you may say things like, "don't be so depressed" or "just think about what you have to be thankful for." Comments like these don't help. If your heart is broken, your grief is something you have to attend to, not avoid.

You'll learn over time that the pain of your grief will keep trying to get your attention until you have the courage to face it. Suppressing the pain is actually more painful.

The pain that surrounds the closed heart of grief, is denying how the loss has changed you. Acknowledging the change is necessary, and it's important in the healing process.

I've learned that you can't go around the pain of your grief, instead you need to open your heart to the pain. You need to acknowledge the inevitability of the pain, and honor it.

Your pain is actually the key that will open your closed heart, and once you embrace it, the healing will begin.

The capacity to love, requires the necessity to mourn. To honor your grief is not self-destructive or harmful, it's necessary to survive.

FEBRUARY

FEBRUARY 1

When the Bough Breaks

Grieving a loss is hard, but grieving the loss of a child, of any age, is some of the hardest work you'll ever do. It's coming to terms with the fact that your child is dead, one who loved you back, whose needs gave shape and focus to your days. You can never have your child back, they can't be replaced, and what you want most you can't have, because your child is gone forever.

I know this sounds harsh, but if you've lost a child, you know it's all true. If you don't grieve the loss of your child, you'll stay frozen in your pain. You have to build a life in which your child doesn't live, but it's important to keep your child alive in your heart and memory. The truth is, if you've lost a child, you're left with a tremendous amount of pain, and you'll have a harder time coming to terms with your loss.

Along with grieving the loss of your child, there's guilt. The nature surrounding the death of your child influences your grief response. If the death was a suicide, you may be experiencing feelings of guilt, thinking you should have been more observant, or it was really your fault.

If you lost a child, you need to tell stories about them, reminisce, and keep pictures of them. You need to choose ways of remembering that are comfortable for you. Think of happy times and of your child's personal triumphs and special times of joy.

You know you'll never forget your child; however, you need to keep their memory alive in a positive way, which eases the grief.

The death of a child is a HUGE loss. The grief needs to be understood as being something very deep inside you for healing to take place....and it does need to come out.

There's no right or wrong way to grieve the loss of your child, it's a lifelong struggle.

FEBRUARY 2

Grieving Alone

I imagine you'd agree with me if I suggested that grieving people tend to isolate. While that is true, and isolation is a major problem for grieving people, it's not a natural tendency, it's a learned behavior.

Let me explain by writing a phrase and leaving out the last word. Most of you reading this will automatically put in the last word. "Laugh and the whole world laughs with you, cry and you cry-----."

I know that before you got to the last word your mind had jumped ahead and added the word 'alone.'

In order to explain how false that idea is, I'll ask you a question. "What's the first thing you want to do when you get good news?" Nearly everyone's answer is, "Share it with others." In particular, you want to tell your spouse, or your parents, or your children; in other words, someone important to you.

Whether you realize it or not, your natural impulse upon receiving sad or bad news is actually the same. You want to tell someone you trust. But after a lifetime of being told "Laugh and the whole world laughs with you, cry and you cry alone" and "If you're going to cry, go to your room" or, "Don't burden others with your feelings," you begin to lose the normal impulse to talk about sad or painful things with people you trust.

Isolation isn't natural, it's learned, and it's dangerous. The antidote to isolation is participation.

Start by having a little chat with a few of the important people in your life. Tell them that you'd like to change some of the guidelines and make it safe to talk openly about some of the sad or painful things you feel.

What you say should be simple statements or comments about things that have affected you. Keep it short, just to get it out and be heard. If the person you're talking to asks you what they can do, say, "Just listen."

FEBRUARY 3

Crying

Almost everyone has some questions and confusion about crying and grief. How much crying is enough? If I start crying, will I be able to stop? Do I have to cry at all? I've cried and cried but I still don't feel better, is there something wrong with me? Are men and women different when it comes to crying?

Don't be alarmed if you recognize yourself in some of the scenarios highlighted above.

Let me pose a couple of other questions here, have you ever known anyone who cries all the time, but never seems to change or grow? Have you ever known anyone who uses crying as a manipulation to get something?

There's a high probability that you'll answer yes to both questions. Both of those questions are designed to explain the fact that crying, in and of itself, does not necessarily lead to completion of the pain caused by death or any other losses. At best, crying acts as a short-term energy relieving action, and relieves, temporarily, some of the emotional energy generated by the loss.

As our society has evolved, we've seen a quantum shift in the public display of emotion. In today's world, it's not at all unlikely to see a retiring professional athlete, often the paragon of masculinity, weeping openly in a televised press conference. It's hard to imagine that same scenario occurring thirty or forty years ago.

Older parents are liable to be less willing to communicate sad, painful, or negative emotions than you. But you should try to fight the trap of applying your emotional value system to others. It may seem odd, since your parents taught you, that you have different emotional views than they do.

But most of all remember this, it's okay to cry. You lost someone you love very much, and the natural reaction is to cry. Tears heal the heart.

FEBRUARY 4

How Do You Survive All the Sadness?

Living comes with the side effect of feeling. Feelings are created from our experiences in life. A kiss from a lover, the loss of a job, the birth of a child. There exists so many emotions ranging from fear to joy, and while one could argue that the purpose of living comes from all the various things and emotions there are to experience, we have these emotions because we're alive. But when we die perhaps suffering and sadness can never lay their heinous hands on us?

There's a chance you'll live a fulfilled and happy life, and there's a chance you won't. There's a chance you'll find love and comfort, and there's a chance you won't. There's a chance you'll be entirely satisfied by all you have accomplished and possess, and there's a chance you won't.

What are the chances of getting all you want out of life? It just doesn't always work that way. With the good, comes the bad. With the love, comes the grief. With the happy, comes the sad.

The best advice I got after my loss was, "Do everything now with no expectations." When you're grieving that can be some very powerful advice.

So, what can you do to survive the sadness? Keep trying!

There's something powerful about naming this sadness as grief. It helps you feel what's inside of you. It's important you acknowledge what you go through. Take the time to feel sad. Your work is to feel your sadness and fear and anger. Fighting it doesn't help because your body is producing the feeling. If you allow the feelings to happen, they'll happen in an orderly way, and it empowers you. Then you're not a victim.

It's absurd to think you shouldn't feel sad right now. You have lost someone you love very much. You miss them. Let yourself feel the grief and keep going. It's okay to feel sad. It's important to remember that what you survive is the grief. Sadness, like happiness, is a part of life and living.

FEBRUARY 5

Grief Bursts

Someone grieving a loss once said to me, "Time is different now. I think I'm making progress, but it feels so slow."

You might think that grief is negative. It's an inconvenience in your already busy life. You view it as an item to check off your to-do list. Get it done. Efficiently. Quickly.

Grief, however, takes time. It has no timetable. Every loss and each heart are unique. Grief is not a straight road. You can't see very far ahead. You don't know what's behind the next tree. Sometimes the path itself seems to disappear. At other times, it seems to double back on itself or go in circles. The journey is full of shocks and surprises.

The truth is that you may always grieve on some level. When do you stop missing them? When does your love for them cease to exist? If you love, you will grieve. Your grief, however, changes over time. As you process your pain in healthy ways, the loss settles into your heart and mind.

Memories that brought only tears and longing begin to bring smiles and gratitude. The mental fog lifts a bit. Your mind become clearer and sharper. Your emotions hijack you less. Your body begin to recover.

Grief bursts, however, can happen at any time, anywhere. Your grief is triggered by someone or something, and suddenly you're right back in the throes of intense, powerful emotion. These grief bursts are normal and common.

The grief is inside you. These sudden bursts are simply opportunities for the grief to come out in a concentrated way. Such expressions of your love and grief are inevitable.

Loss can be powerful and deep. Your heart is complex. Give your heart time. Healing often takes longer than you anticipate.

FEBRUARY 6

Dreams

Do you dream of your loved one?

The first year after my loss I never had a dream about my loved one. I would pray it would happen, but it never did. My grief coach told me that I wasn't having dreams about my loved one because I was too sad. It didn't make sense to me at the time, but in the second year when I began to heal, I started having dreams.

In grief, sleep patterns often change. You might have dreams of your loved one. You wonder what they mean. You wonder about a lot of things.

Grief often brings sleep changes and dreams, and this is designed to be healing. It's been said that we heal while we sleep. Your body rests and rejuvenates. Your mind often grapples with what you can't consciously process during the day. All this makes sleep a more unpredictable adventure during your time of loss.

Your heart is at work, even while you sleep. Dreams can be an attempt to reconnect with your departed loved one and to somehow make more sense of what happened. Your inner pain and fears can surface. Not everyone has dreams of their loved one, and not every dream is a positive or reassuring one. Your world has been shaken, and most likely your sleep will be too. Your mind most likely won't rest well after a loss. Just as your world was shaken, your sleep is also affected.

Your dreams reflect your heart's pain, hopes, and fears, and if dreams of your loved one come, you naturally want to know what they mean. In most cases, the best place to look for an interpretation is in your own heart.

Some dreams might generate more questions. Others might reassure you and bring more peace to your heart. Still others might stir or intensify your longings for your loved one. Either way, try and use your dreams to grieve in a healthy way.

FEBRUARY 7

Creating a Life After Loss

If you have lost a partner or spouse this may be difficult to read. You just may not be ready to hear what I have to say, and that's okay. Just stop reading. I understand.

But if you're a few years out in your grief journey, you may want to keep reading.

I've been facilitating grief support groups for people that have lost a partner or spouse for over 7 years now. The most frequent comments I hear are, "I will never love anyone again." "I could never get married again." "Nobody will ever replace my spouse." I can understand these feelings because I felt the same way at the time. It was unimaginable to even think of ever loving anyone again or as much as I loved my spouse that died. I would never do it!

If you also can't imagine it, I'm here to tell you I was wrong. I'm always so filled with joy when members of my support groups contact me months and years later to tell me about their new love for someone special that has entered their life. They tell me about how they have created a life after loss.

The way I see it, we have two choices after losing a partner or spouse, we can get to work on living, or we can get to work on dying. I think our loved ones would want us to live until it is our time to join them again. They loved us, and I think they would want us to be happy.

Loving someone else doesn't mean you are forgetting the person you love and lost. If you think about the time before the person you lost was in your life, I'm sure you can remember other people that you loved. The chapters of life are full of love and loss. People come into our life and leave over the years. It's like orbs that collide. Some for a brief moment in time and others for a lifetime.

Creating a life after loss is not easy; it requires courage, strength and the willingness to keep moving forward with an open mind and heart. Although you may not believe it now, you will come to a place where you are able to open your heart again to the possibility of love and happiness.

This doesn't mean you're letting go of your loved one or that you will ever forget that chapter of your life. You will just find the courage to turn the page and enter the next chapter of your life, knowing that doing this is not a way of disrespecting your loved one.

It is my hope that you'll have the strength to find a way to hold onto the love you have for the person you lost, while moving into the future with hope.

If you're at a place where this doesn't seem possible, at least keep it in the back of your mind for when the day comes that you are ready to turn the page.

FEBRUARY 8

"I Never Got To Say Goodbye"

If you didn't get to say goodbye to the person you love before they died, you could feel greater pain about their loss. So, what can you do to ease your grief?

How about saying, goodbye.

Find yourself a private, quiet location. It could be in your house or a place that was special to the person you care about. Bring an object or photo that symbolizes their life or your memories together. Take this moment to say anything you need to say.

You can also write a goodbye.

Writing a letter, diary entry, poem, or email can provide an outlet for your emotional or physical pain. Speak directly to the person you care about when you write. Tell them everything you would have like to have said while they were alive.

Creating a ritual can also help you heal and give you an opportunity to reflect on your loved one's life. You can place flowers on their grave or scatter their ashes in a meaningful place (Please check local and state regulations if you do this.) You can conduct the ritual alone or with a group of close friends and family.

You can also make a vision board by gathering images from magazines or other sources that remind you of your loved one, and glue them to a poster board, or consider donating money to a charity they were passionate about.

Doing all these things can call up happy memories and keep your loved one's memory alive, while helping to heal the pain of not having a chance to say goodbye.

FEBRUARY 9

Tears

Let your tears fall with pride for they're not a sign of weakness or self-pity, but an authentic expression of sorrow. It takes great courage to experience your feelings, to express your feelings openly and honestly. It takes great strength to tend to your sorrow.

Crying is not for the faint of heart. Crying expresses what few words can or ever will. Your work in grief is to feel, to express, to accept, to integrate, to heal. Grief work takes guts, persistence, patience, self-compassion and courage, lots and lots of courage.

Tears are the sweat of grief work.

It is not your job to make others comfortable with your expression of grief. It's your job to grieve. To grieve is to actively feel and express sorrow. If your tears appear to make others uncomfortable, calmly speak your truth, teach them about your tears.

Tell them you cry because you're grieving. You cry because you're profoundly sad over the loss of your loved one. You cry because life will forever be bittersweet. You cry because there are no words to adequately express how you're feeling. You cry because you're brave enough to face another day, to endure, to push forward, to live with grief in your heart. You cry to express, to relieve, to release.

Witnessing the tears of friends or family reminds us of our own fragility, powerlessness, inability to fix or lessen the pain and suffering for another person. The most compassionate and supportive thing we can do is create space for those tears, to breathe, to sit with the discomfort and to understand that crying is an expression, a release, a healing, not something to be analyzed, feared or stopped.

Crying is good for your health, your mind, your body and your spirit. It's a natural cleanse stimulating the release of pain. Give yourself permission as well as the time and space to work through your grief, to feel and to express your feelings as they come.

So often we judge our healing by our tears. Find solace in knowing that tears are an expression of your unspoken words, your sadness, your pain leaving your body.

There will come a day when tears are not a part of your daily expression. Until that day comes, let the tears fall and know that they're a powerful component of healing.

Practice self-compassion, patience, and the active nurturing of your soul, and remember that every tear shed carries with it pain and stress.

FEBRUARY 10

Dorothy's Shoes

After my loss I just wanted to go back to my old life. I was wishing that nothing had changed. Maybe I was just wallowing in the complicated lush denial that my old life, the one I had with the person I love was gone. I just wanted to go home! But where was my home? Without the person I love it was gone.

So, is it that it's hard to teach an old dog new tricks? Was moving into a new and different-looking life just too tough for me? All I know is I just wanted to go back! I wanted to go home!

I was reminded of Dorothy in the Wizard of Oz, always wanting to go home. She was trapped in this new, odd world and couldn't find her way out. "Surrender, Dorothy!" screamed the witch.

I felt like Dorothy, wishing she had never left her sweet Kansas home, missing her family, her life. And look! She was now in this world that had color, flowers, unusual people, music; but also, a world that could be terribly dark, lonely, and foreboding.

The problem was Dorothy had the shoes, but she didn't have the vision.

Here she was, in a place where impossible things could become possible; horses changed color, straw men could walk and sing, and monkeys could fly. Think of all she could have done if she didn't want to go home!

It was a brave new world for me like it was for Dorothy. But much like her all I could wish for was to go home. But the fact of the matter was a click of the shoes was never going to take me back home.

But then I began to think of all the things I could do in this new place I was swept into, if I simply had the vision, and the courage to stay.

FEBRUARY 11

Fearing an Avalanche of Loss

If you lost someone you love, you're probably afraid you'll lose other people you love. Few things in life are scarier than the thought of losing a loved one. On some level, most of us realize that everything comes to an end. We usually do our best not to think about it.

But some things can bring it to the front of our minds, for example, when someone we love gets sick or dies. Or during a major crisis like a natural disaster or a global pandemic. We want to scream, "No More! Please!"

Shortly after my spouse died, my best friend died. I was already fearful others I loved would die. So, when this occurred, I even began to have the crazy notion that anyone that loved me was doomed to certain death.

What I came to realize was that these crazy thoughts were actually normal. Fear and anxiety often come from uncertainty. There are some things you can never know for sure: What will happen to my loved ones, and when? What will happen to me if I lose them? You can't see the future.

Understand that you're not alone, it's totally normal to fear losing someone. The fear of loss is something everyone has experienced at one time or another.

Focus on what you can control. One way to cope with fear is to think about whether there's anything you can reasonably do to control the situation. If there is, do it. If there isn't, try to let it go. Once you've done all you can, worrying about it more won't do any good, it will only wear you out.

I wish I could guarantee you that you won't lose any of your remaining loved ones. It's heartbreaking to say, but losing people is a part of life. I understand that now, and make every effort, every day, to let the people I love know how much they mean to me.

FEBRUARY 12

If Grief Could Speak

If grief could speak it would say, "I love you."

"You may not love me, but I love you. I love how you love the person you lost. I love how you keep taking care of the space your loved one took up even though they're gone. How you let them live a little longer in the things left behind. I love how you don't let the world forget they were here, that they mattered, that they were a part of you."

If grief could speak it would say, "You can survive."

"I know you may not want to. I know life may not be worth living without them. I know the earth collapsed beneath your feet. I know a part of you died with them. But I know you can survive, one breath at a time, one moment at a time, one day at a time."

If grief could speak it would say, "I'm proud of you."

"I'm proud of how you continue to care for those that you love and how you continue to be the compassionate and caring person you've always been. I'm proud of your courage and your strength to go on in the aftermath of your devastation."

If grief could speak it would say, "I'm sorry."

"I'm sorry it's me that arrived at your doorstep after your loved one died. But I'm made of love too. In fact, it's because I love so much that I hurt so much when you lost the one you love. It was not me that took your loved one away. I only came to sit with you in your sorrow. I will stay with you for as long as you need me until the day I'm replaced by the joy and happiness that will one day return. I'll be waiting in the wings when you need me. I'm sorry that you're suffering, I know your loved one would not want that, so together we'll find our way."

FEBRUARY 13

"Will I Ever Be Happy Again?"

Sometimes, feeling as if you'll ever be happy again can seem hopeless. Losing a loved one is a very traumatic event. When something like that happens, you feel like you can't go on or find joy again. Although you'll grieve, and most likely for a long time, there will come a day that happiness will once again become a part of daily living.

I never imagined I would find happiness after the loss of my spouse, but there did come a day when I found myself laughing and finding enjoyment in activities I was doing. I understood that while life would never be the same for me without my loved one, happiness was possible if I remained open to the opportunities that were available to me. It was a process and a journey that I had to take that included finding the courage and strength within myself to go through the pain and find my way back to a place of happiness.

It's perfectly normal to feel sad after a major loss. I've always felt that sadness is a necessary emotion, especially when you're grieving. It includes a willingness to move forward and work on getting through the pain and allowing it to run its course. Understanding that sadness lets you look inward to heal, helps you navigate the grief journey. How you deal with the grief determines whether you can truly be happy again.

It was only when I got to a place in my journey when I finally realized my loved one wasn't coming back, at least not in a physical way, that I began to move forward. This can be an exceedingly difficult transition because getting through the grieving process is one thing, but allowing yourself to feel, live, and even love again, can be extremely difficult.

There are ways to make this happen and one of them is time. Most people that have lost a loved one hate to hear the platitude, "time heals", including myself. But time is a key element in moving forward. The reality of life is that time goes on, it waits for none of us, and certainly not those of us that are grieving.

There's something you can do to help yourself get through and move forward without feeling that you're dishonoring your loved one. Holding onto fond memories is one way to keep the non-physical love alive. You spent a lot of time making the memories you have, and they'll stay with you forever to be cherished and saved in your heart. Nobody can take your memories away.

The best way to honor the ones you love is to live and remember those you love who remain.

Humanity goes on even though this terrible event has occurred. If you focus on the moment and the love that still exists, not only for your lost loved one, but also for those that remain, moving forward becomes less painful.

FEBRUARY 14

A Broken Heart on Valentine's Day

I have to admit that since I lost my spouse, Valentine's Day has always been a day I wish I could just sleep through. If you've lost someone you love, I suspect you can relate to what I'm saying.

Any holiday can be a tricky event after a loss, but Valentine's Day can be extremely difficult for the surviving partner (or partners). While people who are grieving feel their grief every day, holidays can trigger a flood of emotions and memories that can be devastating in ways that ordinary days do not. I understand that grief is different for everyone, and that what works for one person might not work for you.

If you're grieving on Valentine's Day, know that you're not alone.

Yes, Valentine's Day is typically a celebration of romantic love (whatever that means to you), but it can also be an opportunity to show other people in your life some love. If you're not up for seeing anyone you're close to, you may want to use this as a chance to show love for your community through volunteer work or even just by doing something nice for a random stranger.

Part of the reason holidays can be so tough for those grieving a loss is because holidays are usually steeped in all sorts of traditions or rituals. If you used to spend Valentine's Day with a partner who is no longer there, reminders of traditions you used to share together can be especially painful. You don't have to force yourself to follow those traditions just in the name of the holiday, you can create new traditions for yourself.

This is just another day that will most likely be just as difficult as the day before it, and the day after it. How you decide to spend it is up to you.

Valentine's Day will never be the same without your loved one, and that's okay.

Just remember, love never dies.

FEBRUARY 15

Moving On

The phrase 'moving on' is common in the grief and loss world, but it isn't very well understood or, frankly, all that helpful.

What does it mean? What does 'moving on' look like? How does one actually do it?

Unfortunately, there isn't a clear answer to those questions.

However, there are things it can be helpful to know about "moving on" after the death of a loved one, including that you're not responsible for how others feel about your grief process. It feels like what those around you mean by "moving on" is for you to stop hurting, stop talking about it, stop remembering, stop crying, and just stop grieving. They talk about wishing you would stop dwelling on the hurt and encourage you to just let go and accept what happened.

The truth is what they actually want is for you to stop making them uncomfortable about your pain. Let's face it, being with someone who's in pain and grieving isn't the easiest of experiences. It's difficult to watch someone you love hurting so deeply.

But other people's discomfort with your grief is their business, not yours. You're not responsible for making them feel more comfortable.

Moving on also doesn't mean forgetting. I suspect that the primary difficulty you have with the phrase 'moving on' is that it often feels as if you're being told to forget your loved one or the relationship you once had.

That's not what moving on means. It's not about grieving or forgetting, happy or sad, black or white. It's shades of gray. It's about learning to live a full and happy life even as you miss and long for what you've lost. It's about remembering and honoring the one you loved while also embracing the beauty and fullness of the life you still get to live.

Moving on also doesn't mean the end of grief. Grief doesn't mean a static end. It doesn't mean suddenly you're done grieving and will never hurt again. Moving on is more about moving forward than being done.

Grief and loss are complex. Loss and your experience of grief are integrated into your life, not something you get rid of, it changes and morphs over time. You get stronger as you carry it, the edges of it round and dull, and with time it begins to take up less space in your life. It doesn't simply disappear.

You move forward with life, embracing the fullness of it, even as your loss becomes part of who you are now.

FEBRUARY 16

Making Space

No one asked you here, Grief. Things were just fine without you. In fact, I had hoped that we'd never have to meet. And now you're everywhere. You're persistent and needy. Tenacious and tough. Above all you are diabolically patient, and you won't be ignored.

I know that I've tried. I kept busy. I smiled when I didn't want to. I swallowed tears and somehow got out of bed and got dressed every day. Well, almost every day.

What's so strange is sometimes I feel like I'm the only one who can see you. The people around me, my friends, family, coworkers, it's like they don't even know you're there.

Maybe that's what's so isolating and lonely about this. To be shadowed by such an invisible burden. To be feeling strangled by you, Grief, as those around me stand by and smile as if nothing has changed.

I have wished you away. I have closed my eyes, covered my ears, and held my breath in the hopes that I could shut you out. I have spent endless nights in restless sleep, hoping that I would awaken to find you were nothing more than a bad dream. But I'm learning.

I'm learning to pay attention. To appease you. To be patient and make room for you and realize that in some way or another, you'll always be around.

While I hope your presence can quiet some, and I may find a way to resume some semblance of a life without you inserting yourself into every single moment of it, I know that I need to keep space for you.

I have come to recognize that I am capable of a bittersweet life, where the happy will still be tinged with sadness. Where peace may still be edged with longing. I will make space for you Grief, and I know that once I do, contentment, peace, and perhaps even joy, will find their way back in too.

FEBRUARY 17

It's Okay To Laugh

I know laughing and grieving don't seem to go together or even sound appropriate. Clearly, when you're sad and missing a person you love, the last thing you feel like doing is laughing.

It's okay to cry, and it's also okay to laugh. Grief is hard. It's messy. Being sad and crying 24 hours a day for 7 days a week is exhausting. It's okay to take a break from that and laugh.

A good friend of mine lost her husband Jim and had him cremated. She called me after the funeral and said, "You are so good with all this grief stuff, would you come with me up to the mountains to scatter Jim's ashes in the lake? I don't want to go alone."

I said, "Sure!", and off we went.

After some long hours of driving and hiking to a good spot, we finally came upon a beautiful body of water nestled among lush green pine trees. The perfect setting. She said Jim would love it.

She scattered the ashes in the water, we cried, we talked about Jim and our memories of him, and said a prayer. It was a heartfelt time for both of us, but she was just crushed with her grief and sadness.

When it was time to leave, we were exhausted from all the emotion and finality of the moment.

After we said our goodbyes to Jim, we began to head back to the car. But just as we turned around, we saw a sign posted that had been partially obstructed by the trees. It said, "Absolutely No Dumping. Municipal Reservoir."

It was drinking water!

She turned to me and said, "Oh my gosh! I feel terrible! What will happen now?"

I replied, "I have no idea? But I guess everyone in town will be having a little drink tonight with a splash of Jim."

She began hysterically laughing, which caused me to laugh, and we couldn't stop for a very long time. But the laughter broke the tension of the moment, and our task, and we also agreed Jim would have laughed as well.

It's perfectly normal to cry when you lose someone you love, but it's also okay to laugh. The laughter releases the tension, and your loved one would like to hear the sound.

FEBRUARY 18

Out of Control

You probably already know this, but grief can make you feel 'out of control'. It sometimes (okay, most of the time) can feel like driving a car that has no brakes.

I remember feeling very out of control after my spouse died, and this feeling seemed to last for a long time. I felt as if I was "out of my body" and did not feel present in my own skin, mind and life. I began to experience emotions that I had either never experienced before or at an intensity I had never experienced before.

My experience with anger had changed in ways that felt very unfamiliar, uncomfortable and shameful. I was irritable most of the time, and I noticed that my tolerance level and patience level became non-existent.

Up until my loss, I was never quick to anger and did not experience anger too often. I had always prided myself in my ability to have a tremendous amount of patience, and a high tolerance for stress. Now I had no patience, felt very stressed, anxious, angry, frustrated and irritated all the time. I felt bad about this. I noticed that I was acting out toward the people I loved, and it made me feel horrible about myself. It was very difficult to process at times. I was just so sad and confused.

I felt very disconnected from reality. I seemed to experience my life in a fog. I found myself regularly dissociating, daydreaming and fantasizing about things that were very irrational.

I became obsessed with the idea that my spouse was still alive. I would regularly experience two distinct thoughts that seemed to co-exist at the same time: One part of my brain could rationalize his death. I knew logically he was gone. At the same time, I experienced a complete opposite thought that suggested he was very much alive and that his death never happened. I could not accept his death. It was too powerful, too intense, and carried too much pain.

Control is a tough subject, because as much as I thought I was in control of things before my loss, I really had no control over anything. I certainly didn't have any control over his death. If I did, he would still be here.

So, I don't worry anymore about being out of control. I think control is overrated.

I just get up each day and say, "Okay, show me what you got!" Then I let the flow of life, and the direction of the road ahead of me, take me where I'm going.

Maybe it's not so much where I want to go, but maybe it's more about where I'm supposed to go.

FEBRUARY 19

It's Not Fair

It's not fair that I have to wake up each morning and relive your death, because sleep has a way of giving me a break of crying and thinking about you. When I'm sleeping, I believe that everything is all right, that everything is normal. Then I wake up. But as soon as my eyes open, I'm reminded that you're gone. By the lack of sound and emptiness in the house. By the emptiness of my heart.

It's not fair that you were such a good person, full of kindness, and yet your life ended just like that. All of that kindness shining inside of you didn't earn you a few extra years. A few more minutes of life. A few more seconds with me.

It's not fair that I have to act like it's just another day when the anniversary of your death rolls around again. Or when your birthday passes, which is empty of all meaning, because death preserved your age. You're not the age you would have been now. To me you will forever be frozen in time at the age you were when you died.

It's not fair that I have a future looming in front of me when your future was taken away. That my life is continuing, that I'm getting up and going about my day and growing old without you.

It's not fair that my life is full of new experiences that you are not a part of and that I still have so much to experience, examine and explore. But you've learned all you ever will. Saw all you'll ever see, did all you'll ever do, because your life is past tense while mine is present.

It's not fair that I have so much leftover love for you, but no place to put it. I can't squeeze your hand or hug you. I can't smile at you or buy you presents unless I'm putting them on your grave.

It's not fair that I'm meeting new people that never got to meet you. That they've never seen you, aside from in photographs and their mind's eye whenever I tell another story about you, and I'm always telling stories about you. Your name is always on my lips.

It's not fair that I have a million things to say to you, but no way of knowing if you can hear any of it. Even if you can hear, even if you're settled right beside me, I won't get a reply from you. It won't be a real conversation. It'll just be me.

Alone.

It's just not fair. But nothing seems fair now that you're gone.

FEBRUARY 20

Time After Time

I always think about how time relates to grief. I'll always be waiting for that day I see my loved one again. As I turned my clock forward and backward each year, I think about how awesome it is that, for a brief moment, I'm manipulating time. It makes me think how much I wish I could turn back time all the way back to before my loss. Back to the time when things were better, easier, happier, before the grief and pain. But I was limited to only an hour.

Or, how nice would it be to turn time all the way forward to that place where we hope the pain has lessened and some healing has begun.

Time does not heal grief. While we feel it should help us heal, just as it helps following a surgery or an argument with a friend, time doesn't hold the same predictable path after a major loss.

So, if we continue to use time to measure how we 'should' be doing, we'll find we're continually let down, since most often the pain of grief can get worse as the days and months go by.

There's no denying that time is also the healer that allows for some room to adapt, and adjust, to find support, and to learn how to be where we are and who we are now that this loss has happened.

It's confusing, I know, and hard to reconcile as we try to figure out if we're on the right track. What matters is our perspective, and most importantly, our expectations.

I can tell you that you're exactly where you are supposed to be on your grief journey. Don't use time as a measure of your success in healing. Don't compare yourself to others, and don't allow anyone to dictate what this experience is like for you.

Take all the time you need. Grief isn't a race because there's no finish line.

FEBRUARY 21

Year #2

There's a theory on grieving that the first year is the hardest. The loss is so new, and you spend all your time in a fog, living in shock and disbelief. I totally agree with that. This is true regardless of if it's a sudden loss or a long-drawn-out illness. There is still the element of shock and disbelief. The reality is, there is nothing that can ever prepare us to watch someone we love die.

Grieving people that I work with are always surprised when the first year is over and they feel worse. They are always under the assumption that if they survive all the "firsts", like birthdays, holidays and anniversaries, that it will be easier in the days ahead.

But then year 2 happens.

I found year 2 more difficult and this is why, in the first year each day was a day I could look back and remember what I was doing the last year with my loved one; in year 2, I could no longer do that. That somehow made it more final for me, emptier, and sadder.

For me, year 2 was actually more of a challenge. I think it was because I expected to feel better, and then feeling even more disappointed and sad when I didn't. It also marked a whole entire year without my person. It was a year longer that I didn't see his face or hear his voice.

I'm not trying to scare you if you're in your first year, I'm just being honest. If you're in your second year now, or even further down the road, you probably understand what I'm talking about.

I know there's no timeframe for grief, and I'm pretty sure you know that by now too. So don't compare yourself with anyone else you know that has suffered a loss. Don't listen to that friend that thinks you should be dating again because your partner died a year ago, or that cousin that thinks just because you lost your son you should feel blessed to still have your daughter.

These people have no clue. They have no idea what you are going through or what your grief feels like, regardless of how much time has passed.

Grief is sneaky and crafty, so you have to be able to learn how to understand it. Try not to expect it to be predictable, because it's not! Never expect today to be hard and tomorrow to be easy. It's different for everyone.

Honor the place you are right now at this moment in time, regardless of whether it feels uncomfortable or hard, because this is probably exactly where you should and need to be.

Never give up hope; there will be a better tomorrow. I promise you one will come; you just can't set a date for when it will arrive.

FEBRUARY 22

Butterflies

Do you see butterflies since you suffered your loss?

Did you know that butterflies can symbolize the transformation of grief for some people? There has long been a parallel drawn between the transformation of going through a personal grief journey and the transformation of a butterfly. From egg to caterpillar to chrysalis and the formation of a beautiful butterfly, the journey is nothing short of amazing.

The grief from losing a special person in your life can be thought of in the same way. It's a unique process to go from the pain of loss to being able to celebrate that person and what was important for you together.

No one can tell you how long that journey takes because everyone grieves in their own way.

Like the butterfly in the cocoon, you can't rush the process of grief. With tons of work, you can navigate the process in order to reemerge as a new stronger person. If you're going to fly off to your new destiny, you have to do the grief work with help and trust.

Your loss stays with you but transforms from devastating pain to acceptance of loss then on to strength to move forward with your life. The journey through grief is a transformation to a future where you can celebrate the amazing person you lost and the impact they had on your life.

The release of a butterfly can be seen as a symbol of the release of the pain of grief. You may see symbolism in the release, not of the grief or your loved one, but the pain.

This also offers an opportunity for you to embrace a future in which your loved one is remembered and honored.

FEBRUARY 23

Lost Always Follows Found

It's the reality of life that every beginning has an ending, just as every relationship on this Earth will end.

I know this sounds really negative, but it only hurts because when you love someone you never want that relationship to end.

But I would never forgo the relationships I had to avoid the pain and grief, because by avoiding the hurt, I'd also be avoiding the love.

I wouldn't pass up the heart connection, just to avoid the heartache.

I've often speculated about which is 'better' (as if that's possible when it comes to grief and loss), to lose someone suddenly or gradually.

I'm not sure which is better, or which is worse. Loss is loss. But what I do know is grief only comes because something mattered.

So, if you have people in your life that matter to you, and I hope you do, this might be a good time to tell them so and appreciate the time you have left with them.

Lost always follows found, and I'm just glad I had the people I lost in my life for the time I did, because the way I see it, not having them would have been a greater loss.

FEBRUARY 24

What I Need...and Don't Need

I need to talk about the person who died. I often need to tell my story over and over again, and sometimes I might even need to ask you why it happened.

I'll probably tell you my story so many times, you'll get sick of hearing it. But I do it because it helps me to face the reality of what I've lost.

I don't really need your advice, especially if you haven't experienced the same loss as I have, but I do need you to care about me, and maybe even give me a hug.

I don't need you to judge me or be afraid of me, I'm still trying to be the person I've always been, but my loss has changed me. I'm grieving and trying to figure it all out.

I need you to listen to me, but I don't need you to tell me you know how I feel. I just need a lot of time to find my own way to healing my pain.

I don't really even know what I need, so please don't ask me if there's anything you can do for me, aside from bringing my loved one back to life. I don't know how to answer you.

What I need most is your support, your patience, your understanding, and your willingness to walk along beside me as I try to find my way forward.

Most of all, I need you to know I'm not going crazy, I'm just grieving.

FEBRUARY 25

Why Being Alone Feels So Lonely

If you're lucky, you were born into some sort of family. But maybe after time that family fell away as you grew up and created your own life. The separation from your birth family can sometimes seem a little like losing a limb. Even if that family still exists, it may be separate now, living its life without you, maybe feeling the same way.

It's an odd kind of loneliness moving from your starter family into whatever new family you create. Maybe you found a spouse...or you didn't find one at all, or you got really lucky with someone and made a kind of home inside your heart you'd never known before. Sometimes just the busyness of life becomes your family, friends, work, all those things that bring you joy.

Regardless of the road you've traveled in life, eventually loss steps in.

The imperfect relationships, the beautiful ones, the work, the friends, they disappear in some way. A person important to you dies, and it's a big reminder that all of this is temporary. No matter how much of a home someone makes in your heart, one of you is going to disappear someday.

It seems in some way we are always left with ourselves. Whether your heart is empty or full of love, it's still there, providing you a strange kind of companion. You're the one person you can be certain to never lose. The only one who will be there from the moment of your birth to the moment of your death.

We're all born alone, and we die alone. So why can being alone feel so lonely?

I've been wondering if it's possible to love others in a big way without losing a limb of our own when they die. I'm not suggesting that grief is avoidable, I know better than anybody that it's not. But can we find a comfort in ourselves that's at least as large as the one we seek in someone else?

I don't really know the answer for sure, but I've spent an awful lot of my adult time searching for people who could make me feel shielded from the scariest parts of life, as though having family and friends around me would protect me from my own fears.

But I realize now that this is not a job for others, and no one else can promise you that they'll never die and return you to yourself.

So, I think the best we can do is try to comfort ourselves, knowing that we're the one person we can count on, especially in times when being alone feels so lonely, but also keep loving others anyway.

FEBRUARY 26

The Price of Love

It's difficult to strike a balance between the act of grieving and your total lack of control over it.

Living with a broken heart makes it hard to have the will to continue living life and making plans.

When you're grieving, there's an array of thoughts and emotions you continue to face that are somehow invisible and unfamiliar to everyone else. The only people who can understand this are those who have lost a piece of their heart.

After someone you love dies, it feels like everything you say and do is foreign to the outside world. It's like carrying this invisible, massive boulder, cradling it between both your arms, trying hard not to drop it, praying that at any second, it won't fall and smash your feet.

How do you explain to people, who have no idea what you're experiencing, that it's been several months and you're still crying yourself to sleep? That you're always sad? How do you show them what you had to witness with your own eyes, or explain to them why you still just want the person you love to come back?

Well, you can't.

When someone you love dies, it's not just their death that you struggle with, it's also the regret of all the things said and done during the time in which they were still alive. And it's in all the things you can't say or do now that they're gone.

It's not just about the last interaction you had with someone, it's about all of it: the birthdays, the holidays, the hugs, the talks, the trips together.

It's about the lifetime of good memories.

When someone you love is taken from you suddenly, your brain has a way of doing whatever it does when you experience a traumatic event, it holds onto it tight and constantly floods you with thoughts of it.

The unfortunate truth is that you're susceptible to grief because you're able to love. The risk of love is loss, and the price of loss is grief.

Living with a broken heart means learning to accept the fact that every day is just another day without your loved one in it, and that will never change.

The problem with having a broken heart, is nobody can see it.

FEBRUARY 27

A Special Gift

I have a special gift. I can look at people who are suffering and feel immediate empathy for them. I'm not bragging, it's true. It's because I've been through my own unique brand of hell.

Eight years ago, I lost the love of my life. When I tell someone this, they always say, "I can't imagine." They're right, they can't.

Fortunately, time is indeed a great healer. My pain and emptiness have mostly receded, but they sometimes come swimming right back to the surface when I see someone else in pain.

The question then becomes, how do I respond? Do I allow these feelings to overwhelm me, and retreat into the dark sorrow I know so well, or do I try to stand silently for a moment, letting myself feel the other person's pain? I ask myself, "Is there something I can do to help?"

Often the best thing I can do for the person is simply to listen to their story. To ask questions like I'm really interested, which I am. To stay with them until my heart tells me it's okay to leave.

All this can be a special gift for someone who's having a terrible moment or a terrible day. I know from experience, and when I comfort others, simply by being present for them, it's also a special gift for me.

People tell me I'm a strong, and after my loss my first instinct was to declare war on my grief. For a time, I tried pushing through, powering on with my life despite what happened, but my life had lost its meaning.

Gradually, I realized that I might be able to find meaning and purpose again if I set out to help people make it through their own empty moments. To my amazement, I found that simple acts of kindness and compassion helped me rekindle the light that lives deep inside me.

I often wonder why comforting others seems like something I'm compelled to do. I think it's because having walked through the fire, I feel specially equipped to help others do it too.

So that's my special gift, a willingness to look at suffering full on, without flinching. Taking a chance and extending a hand to others has been for me both a lifesaver and a way to honor my loved one.

I decided instead of just struggling to carry the stone that had become my heart, it made more sense to reach out to others...and so now my special gift lies within three simple words, "Can I help?"

FEBRUARY 28

Your Spouse Died - The Relationship Didn't

You wake up every morning, and you're still shocked with the realization that they're no longer beside you. Your friends and family hope your grief will go away, but you dread the day it does. It's your grief that reminds you they existed.

While you're still shocked by their absence, you can still hold onto their presence. They're still alive to you. Their voice still rings in your ears, and you can still see their face so clearly. In your heart and mind, you're still a 'we.' You say, "If you're out there, send me a sign." You look for birds, butterflies, feathers, pennies, dragon flies, anything to know they still exist.

You're a person with a dead spouse. They're not 'lost,' and they haven't 'passed.' They're absent but not erased. Your spouse died, but your relationship outlives them.

You were dependent on them, and when they died, that dependence forced you to be independent. You're learning to carve a way forward in the new world. But this independence has always been, and still is, indelibly connected to their love, being there for you to depend on when needed.

Their love remains a secure base from which you can confidently head back out into the world. The shape of your love holds firm, and you continue to be fortified by it, turning to it for comfort and encouragement as you bear your grief and navigate life.

It's that love, and that relationship, that continues, and on which you can rely.

MARCH

MARCH 1

Sitting in Silence

If someone you love has died, you most likely have been told, "Sorry for your loss."

This phrase is so overused that it starts to have no meaning, especially if you lost someone you love. I'll admit, even though I don't like it, I say it myself. But it's become such an obligatory gesture, mostly directed at those of us grieving. It's said in kindness and caring, but it really doesn't help.

Do you agree?

The problem I have with this phrase is the fact that someone is sorry for 'your' loss, automatically makes you feel even more isolated. It's 'your' loss, not their loss. Then there's the word "loss", insinuating it was your fault. The person you love died; you didn't lose them like you lose your car keys.

I think the best thing to hear when someone you love dies is, "Damn! This sucks!" I'm sure you can relate to that much more than you can to, "Sorry for your loss."

It's perfectly okay to express how much the death of a loved one sucks.

Because it does.

It really sucks to have someone taken away from you, and all you really want is someone to acknowledge how much it sucks.

No words will ever be enough to take away your pain.

So maybe you don't need to hear anything at all. The best condolences can require no words, a hand to hold, a hug, or just being passed a box of tissues. Just knowing that someone is willing to just be there for you.

There are times when the moment calls for just pure and simple…silence.

MARCH 2

I'm Still Me

Every day I wake up, and I'm still shocked by the realization that you're not beside me. My friends and family hope my grief will go away, but I dread the day it does because it's my grief that reminds me you existed.

Even though I'm still shocked by your absence, I try to hold onto your presence. To me, you're still alive. Your voice still rings in my ears; I can still feel your arms around me, and I can still see your face so clearly.

In my heart and mind, we're still a team, still a part of each other, still a 'we".

If you're out there, send me a sign because I still look for you in all I see. I search for you during the day when I look out over the ocean, when I'm driving in the car, shopping in the store, or gazing up at the stars in the night.

I take these moments to remind myself that you still exist.

You see, I'm still me but different without you. But you're not lost, you haven't passed away. You're absent but not erased. I'm still here and you're not, but our relationship will outlive us both.

I was dependent on you, then you died, and that dependence forced me to be independent. I'm learning to carve a way forward in this new world I've been thrown into, but this independence has always been, and still is, indelibly connected to our love. It's still there for me to rely on when I need it.

Our love still remains a secure base from which I can confidently head back out into the world.

The shape of our love holds firm, and I continue to be fortified by it, turning to it for comfort and encouragement as I try to navigate life.

Yes, I'm still me, and I still love you, and it's that continuing love I can always depend on.

MARCH 3

A Grief Like No Other

Every loss is tragic. Every loss is heartbreaking. Every loss is significant.

There are so many different types of losses by death that can occur, and I always make it a point to talk about how difficult and trying most of them can be, especially the loss of a spouse.

I know the most about that one, I've "been there."

Grief following sudden death, trauma, suicide or murder can be very hard to deal with, but no matter how one loses a child, whether by prolonged illness or sudden death, the loss of a child is perhaps the most profound, the most overwhelming, and the most inconsolable of losses.

The reason for this is that it violates the natural order of things; your children are not supposed to die before you. The love you have for your child is unconditional and so pure. It's one of the most profound of attachments. The death of a child evokes rage at the injustice of it all. It's not fair for an innocent child to lose his potential and fail to see his dreams fulfilled.

Then you have to deal with all the guilt. As a parent you're responsible for the well-being of your children. No matter how random the accident was, you will probably feel like you let your child down. You may feel responsible for the death, even if that blame is not justified. Guilt is almost always present in the death of a child.

It's also very common for a parent to have a strong need to blame someone for the death of their child and to find the cause. You should be careful to avoid unfairly blaming other family members or your spouse.

Hold your tongue now so you'll have no regrets later.

Following the loss of your child, you might find that some of your friends avoid you. The death will make them very uncomfortable. It may force them to contemplate the mortality of their own kids. They start thinking that maybe it will happen to them.

Friends and acquaintances just don't know what to say or how to help you. If only they knew that all you wanted was for them to listen. Sadly, emotional and social support are often withdrawn when you need them the most.

Parents who have lost a child can feel alone and unsupported in their grief because they usually are. Support groups of other bereaved parents can be really helpful to you because those folks will understand better than anyone else the pain you feel.

MARCH 4

Memories

Those of us that have lost someone important know the death of a loved one changes life's landscape forever. The people we've lost are like missing pieces in a puzzle, without them the picture can never be whole again. We can try to recreate the scene, but there are elements of life before loss that can never be recaptured.

Things have changed, we have changed.

People always say things like, "At least you have your memories." Yes, memories are comforting, but only because they are all we really have now. As Barbra Streisand sang, "Memories, may be beautiful, and yet, what's too painful to remember, we simply choose to forget."

Not all our memories are good, especially the memories of how our loved one died. Sometimes those memories are just too hard to forget.

I find the memory of places I went to with my loved one to be sometimes painful as well. When I've been away from a special place for a long time, I'm always a little bit nervous to return. My mind tends to romanticize places, and I know I will find it much smaller, shabbier, and unimpressive than I remember it. I think this is because there is something very important that's missing, my loved one.

We are never so kind as we are to people, places, and things that are gone, which I suppose is both a blessing and a curse. On the one hand, I always have a safe haven to return to when life gets overwhelming (even though it's only a memory in my mind). Nothing else can ever seem to measure up to the one that was given to me by someone who is forever gone.

I think it's unfair measuring the past against the present. They can never be reconciled because the 'now' can never win.

I look at a picture of my loved one and me smiling on a vacation and I think, "ah yes, we were so happy, I was so happy," and then I don't recall whatever worries were bothering me on that day. These memories light the dark corners of my mind.

Were there things hiding behind our smiles? I don't remember. If there were, they are all now forever melted by the warmth of my memory. Maybe it's just easier to try and forget the bad memories.

As Barbra sang, "So it's the laughter, we will remember, whenever we remember, the way we were."

MARCH 5

The Calm After the Storm

Is it possible to ever be happy again after a devastating loss? They say that grief is the price of love. Once you've experienced loss and are wrapped up in all that pain, you might think that your life is over. But not only is grieving normal, it's also a necessary part of processing your loss. It's a heavy price to pay, but if you think about it, you know it was worth it.

But the question still remains, do you ever 'get over' the suffocating feeling of losing someone or something precious in your world?

I can tell you that the good news is that although it never disappears, you can develop coping skills and a new reality. Eventually, you will feel empowered by your pain.

Whoever said that time heals all wounds was very wrong.

True, the emotional loss may diminish over time, but the scars are long-lasting. If you've suffered a devastating loss, you can find healing in your own time. When you're grieving, give yourself the same compassion you would give to a friend or loved one.

Happiness is fleeting and circumstantial, while joy is a decision. While you walk through the shadows of grief's trials, don't feel guilty when you bask in the light you will eventually see. No matter what your loss is, you will discover peace in your own time. Your forever scars are proof of your strength and humanity. Allow yourself to feel the pain to its fullest so that you can properly heal.

Finding joy after a crushing period of grief does not mean you've forgotten your loved one or the situation. Many people postpone their healing because they feel guilty or believe they're being selfish. Again, extend the same kindness and empathy to yourself that you would give to others.

The only way to truly find peace after the storm is to walk right through it.

MARCH 6

Grief Is Like a Shipwreck

You've probably heard the expression, "grief comes in waves".

When someone you love dies, it's like when a ship first gets wrecked, you're drowning with wreckage all around you.

Everything floating around you reminds you of the beauty and the magnificence of the ship that was and is no more, and all you can do is float. You find some piece of the wreckage and you hang on for a while. It can be a physical thing, a memory or a photograph.

Maybe it's another person who's also floating, going through the same pain that you're going through, and for a while, all you can do is float and try to stay alive.

In the beginning, the waves are really high and crash over you without mercy. They come seconds apart and don't even give you time to catch your breath. All you can do is hang on and float. After a while, maybe weeks, maybe months, you'll find the waves are still really high, but they come further apart.

When they come, they still crash over you and wipe you out. But in between, you can breathe, and you can function. You never know what's going to trigger the grief. It might be a song, a picture, a face in the crowd or even the smell of a summer day. It can be just about anything, and the wave comes crashing.

But in between the waves, there's still life.

Somewhere down the line, and it's different for everybody, you find that the waves are smaller, and while they still come, they come further apart. You can see them coming. An anniversary, a birthday, a wedding, or maybe just shopping at the store.

You can see it coming, for the most part, and prepare yourself. When it washes over you, you know that somehow you'll come out the other side. Soaking wet, still hanging on to some tiny piece of the wreckage, but you'll come out.

The waves never stop coming, and somehow you don't really want them to, but you learn that you'll survive them. Other waves will come, and you'll survive them too.

If you're lucky, you'll have lots of scars from lots of loves and lots of shipwrecks.

MARCH 7

"At Least"

These are two words you probably never want to hear if you lost someone you love.

If somebody sends you an email, card, or starts off a conversation with these two words stop listening.

I'll give you some examples: "At least they didn't suffer." "At least you still have other children." "At least they're in a better place."

The problem with these statements is that they imply that you should actually be grateful for what happened. They belittle your pain. People that say these things to you want to point out to you how your situation could be worse.

Seriously, when you lose someone you love could your situation be worse. I think not. All these statements do is make it worse.

I heard many "at least he's not suffering anymore" comments after my spouse died. For me, there were no "at leasts." There was only one thing that overshadowed everything else, including every reason to be grateful and every reminder of how my situation could have been worse, that was the loss of the person I love.

His presence was once my whole world, and his absence (despite knowing it was coming) was extremely painful. It brought an end to all that could have been and now would never be…and there were no 'at leasts' in that. I didn't even think there should be any.

There's nothing bad about loss and pain. We shouldn't be made to feel guilt for being sad someone we love died. In my opinion, it's just not okay to tell someone grieving how they should or shouldn't feel.

You aren't weak just because you're mourning someone you love. At least, that's what I think!

MARCH 8

No Guarantee for Tomorrow

I have learned that those who have not experienced great loss may not understand the grieving process, at least not until it happens to them. Grieving for a lost loved one doesn't end in this lifetime. You may accept the loss and move on, but the realization of lost tomorrows doesn't ever go away.

At first, the loss is felt in every breath you breathe. Then minutes will go by before you feel the stab of loss. Eventually hours and days go by without crying and feeling pain. Sometimes even weeks. But don't be fooled; the reality is that at times it will grip you all over again with the same intensity as it did the day it happened.

Then there are the times when you'll be reminded that they won't be there to see your accomplishments, for special moments and milestones you would have shared, and they won't be there to hold you when you're sad.

It doesn't help when people tell you that other people have had it worse. It doesn't help when they tell you that time heals all wounds. The time will come for complete healing, it just won't be in this lifetime.

I know for a fact when you're young and lose a spouse, it doesn't help when someone tells you you'll move on and be okay. The thought is just too devastating. Losing my spouse at a young age made me aware of just how temporary we really are, how we aren't invincible like we thought when we were young.

It's hard to go on knowing you'll never see them again for a lifetime. You have a heightened awareness of how precious your time with one another is.

Even today, when others who married around the time we did, celebrate milestone anniversaries, I'm sad that we were robbed of that opportunity. I know this all sounds a bit depressing, but I just want you to remember how important it is to enjoy today because there's no guarantee for tomorrow.

MARCH 9

The 'Inside Out' Theory

Have you ever asked yourself, "If I feel happy, then I can't be sad, right?" Wrong!

This way of thinking goes back to the false belief that you can only feel one way at a time. The reality is that you can feel many things at a time. One emotion doesn't replace or cancel the other out. So, in the example above, happiness doesn't replace sadness, it exists alongside it.

After someone you love dies, people always ask, "How are you doing?" It's a simple question. You know your options for an answer, but I would bet that you usually just say, "I'm doing okay."

The problem with grief is that sometimes you feel like somebody turned you inside out. Am I right? I call this the "inside out" theory. (This isn't a real thing, at least I don't think it is, I totally made it up.)

When you're grieving, you don't always feel just one thing at a time. Even though you answer, "I'm doing okay" you're usually feeling a million other things. It's just taking too much effort, that you don't have to talk about all of them. The real answer is so much more complex.

The reason grief makes you feel so turned inside out is because when you lose someone you love, you can actually feel both happy and sad at the same time. If you feel this way, I can tell you that it's something you eventually learn to live with because this bittersweet reality is just unavoidable.

The first time you find yourself laughing or experiencing happiness again, you'll feel guilty.

That's when you'll say, "If I feel happy, then I can't be sad, right?"

Wrong!

95

This is where my "inside out" theory comes into play. Grief is hard work for so many different reasons. Grief forces you to stretch your heart and mind to create enough space for all your thoughts and emotions to exist alongside one another.

You have to learn to be flexible enough in your thinking to accept that it's okay to feel two totally opposite things at the exact same time. Grief is like a sun shower, sunny and raining at the same time. Different emotions that exist in the same moment. This reality can make you feel like you've been turned inside out.

In time, you discover that the pain of loss can exist right alongside things like, happiness and hope. But this is actually a good thing, because it means that you never have to leave your loved one behind as you move forward.

MARCH 10

L-O-V-E

Sometimes I think I talk way too much about grief and not enough about love. It's almost impossible to find a grieving person that hasn't heard the phrase "Grief is Love". So, what is grief in relation to love? Honestly, I think they're the same thing.

The problem with love is that we often think of it as hearts, hugs, kisses, and all kinds of romance, but I think love is much more complicated. I know that love can be wonderful and amazing, but I've also learned it can cause the worst kind of pain and sadness.

I believe the most painful kind of love is called grief. I learned all about grief when the person I loved was taken away with no hope of returning. Grief was confusing to me because I didn't know how to love someone who was gone. How do you love someone that isn't even here anymore?

Along with my grief came this incredible amount of frustration, anger, and bitterness about the whole concept of love and resentment at death's destruction. I loved someone, and they were unfairly taken away. But in time, I realized that for love to survive and truly thrive, I had to find new ways to connect. I had to believe that 'grief is love.' It wasn't just some saying that people post on social media. It was actually true.

I learned that grief is love's unwillingness to give up. It was about stretching my bond with my loved one and creating a space where I could still love him even in his eternal absence. I know we can't ever be physically together again, but my love has never changed.

I know you might not believe me right now because your grief is so intense, but there will come a day you feel just as connected to your loved one as you always did. It will just be in a different way.

I just want to remind you that underneath all the emotions of the grief you're feeling right now, there's still LOVE.

MARCH 11

Grief Lasts Longer Than Sympathy

"How long does grief last, after a death?" This question is like asking, "How long is infinity?" Everyone grieves differently, so there's no answer that would be true for everyone. There's also no right or wrong way to feel after losing someone you love.

Grief is painful. You probably already know that. It can be overwhelming, so it's natural to wonder if there's an end to it, a time when you'll start to feel better.

I wish more than anything that I could tell you when that will be, but I can't. What I can tell you is that you're grieving because you have a special bond with the person who died. You will never stop missing them. But don't worry, that doesn't mean you're always going to feel as terrible as you probably do right now or that you'll never be happy again.

Over time, grief tends to soften. The initial shock and pain become something more manageable. Eventually, you'll find that you'll spend less and less time hurting, and more and more time feeling okay.

Just because the sympathy cards stop coming in the mail, doesn't mean the grief stops too. In the early days after a loss, it's normal to feel shocked and numb. But once everyone else has moved on, that's when your feelings can surface. After the shock has worn off, the most common symptom of grief is a deep sadness or depression. But it's not uncommon to find yourself cycling through a variety of emotions. Anger, guilt, denial, shock, and fear of being without them, these are all normal.

Eventually, you'll feel okay most of the time, but there will likely still be 'triggers' that set you off, like birthdays, anniversaries or certain activities you used to do together. These may also get easier with time.

Notice how I said these 'may' get easier, that's because grief last longer than sympathy.

MARCH 12

Problems

After my loss I came to see that every life has its share of problems. I never met anyone that didn't have problems of one sort or another. If we find ourselves without any problems, it's just a matter of time until something pops up. That's life!

Don't worry if you think you're the only one facing challenges. If people around you don't seem to have problems, that just means you don't know them well enough to see their troubles or they're very good at hiding them. Problems are inescapable for all living beings. No one can avoid problems.

Living a joyful life, I've found, is not about trying to avoid the unavoidable. Joy comes from summoning a strong life force to overcome problems, from the smallest irritation to the biggest disaster.

You may have been born with a natural enthusiasm for facing your problems.

I sure wasn't!

Though I didn't run away from my problems, I also didn't really see the point of facing them.

Whatever difficulties came my way, my motto was always, "I'll go on." Somehow, I found the will to keep going. Even after my loss. But I didn't face what was holding me back.

It wasn't until I experienced the worst possible event, the loss of my soulmate, that I turned my attention inward, and I discovered the concept of solving my problems instead of letting them destroy me. The reward is not so great without the struggle.

The way I see it, there are two rules in life. Rule number one is to never give up, and rule number two is to never forget rule number one. What really matters is not whether you have problems, but how you go through them.

MARCH 13

Making It

"I don't want to live in a world where my loved one no longer lives." Have you ever said this? Have you at least thought about it?

Maybe you don't want to admit it because it sounds suicidal. Maybe if you say it, your family and friends will want to check on you constantly and think you're going to do something drastic.

But I bet sometimes that's exactly how you feel. If you sometimes feel like you don't see yourself making it, you should know that you're not alone. There's this whole alliance of us who are fighting the same fight. We're all scarred and bruised, and just trying to find our way.

The thing about writing is it's both a vast and open world of possibility, and a small and confined space of honesty. So let me be totally honest, sometimes I just don't see myself making it.

So, there it is, out there in the open. I'm not afraid to say it or feel it because I know it will pass. It always does, and then I keep moving forward.

My life is a wonderful life, but sometimes it's also hard. That's just the way it is, if there weren't bad things in life, how would we know what was happy?

Life is hard, but there's always hope. I think 'making it' is all about never letting go of the hope that things will get better.

Yes, I wish I didn't have to live in a world where my loved one no longer lives, but I still have hope that each day brings a new chance for making it. A chance to keep my heart open enough to accept that sometimes life is hard, but it's also full of possibilities for happiness.

We're still here, right?

Sometimes that's enough for me; I'm still here, and I'm making it.

MARCH 14

No Attachment to Outcome

"How do I deal with the fact that I had to make the decision to end my loved one's life?"

By feeling guilty, you get a sense of having control over the situation. If you can assume guilt for the death, then you can impose some order on chaos. You create cause and effect, saying to yourself, "Because I did this, then this happened." But these self-inflicted emotional wounds plunge you even further into despair. Regardless of what happened, you really had no attachment to the outcome. You did the best you could with the knowledge you had at the time.

So, what can you do to relieve yourself from the torment of these self-accusations?

Start by apologizing to your loved one. One of the ways to release guilt is to talk it over with the person to whom it is linked, even though your loved one isn't here. Visualize your loved one sitting with you or speak to their photograph.

Talk openly from your heart. Be specific about the action or omission or other reason for your guilt. Talk about why you did (or didn't do) the thing that now causes your pain. Explain how it makes you feel now and how you would change it if you got a chance.

Then ask for forgiveness. Discuss the forgiveness you need and the reason it's so important to you, and then focus on the aspects of your relationship that were purely positive.

I'm sure there were many more of those moments than the one you're feeling guilty about. Realize that by living within the cell block of your own guilt, you're creating a jail for yourself. Give yourself permission to free yourself of all those negative emotions, and instead embrace the love and positive memories you shared.

MARCH 15

Hiding From Grief

Since your loved one died, I bet it's been difficult to face the reality of never seeing that person again. It's really painful to pick up the pieces and move forward.

Am I right?

Don't you wish you could just find a safe place where you could be free of grief and all the emotions that go along with it? Wouldn't it be nice to simply decide that you just won't deal with those situations that make you feel uncomfortable, afraid, or emotional? Wouldn't it be great if you could pick and choose exactly what you want to happen in your life, how it happens, and when it occurs?

It sure would be great, but the bottom line is you can't run away from fears all of your life; you don't have the option to write that perfect story of your life. More importantly, you can't hide from death, it's a part of life. The only other option is to be in the moment today, live life, and face every single experience that comes your way, no matter what.

So, let me ask you these questions, are you hiding from your emotions and your grief from the loss of your loved one? Do you find yourself burying your guilt, anger, resentment, and other emotions because it's much easier to do this than it is to face each feeling? Are you afraid of what you'll go through as you face each emotion?

If you're like me, you've answered 'yes' to at least one of these questions. I get it! I totally understand.

If you don't face your emotions, your grief, or your fears, you're only hurting yourself in the long run. You're setting yourself up for even greater pain, guilt, or anger, or whatever the emotion may be. You may not realize it, but burying your feelings, or hiding from fear, or running away from your grief, closes off a part of you that deserves to live.

It's really important to your health and well-being to face your fears, emotions, and grief head-on. If you don't face and accept it when the situation occurs, you'll be reminded time and time again throughout your life until you do work through it.

I know it's not easy but try facing your feelings. Be honest with yourself regarding your emotions. Accept the fact that you're in this situation. When you face your feelings about the death of your loved one, and you move through the grieving process, you then have the strength and courage to continue forward with your life in a healthy way.

You can't escape grief. It follows you wherever you go. So instead of trying to avoid it, try to accept it, and instead of running from it, learn to live around it.

MARCH 16

Do What You're Afraid of Doing

Have you been wondering what you're going to do now that your loved one is gone?

It's hard to think about when the passion to live has been taken out of your life. Nothing seems to matter as much as the life that you lost when the person you love died, right? Everything pales in comparison.

So, how do you find that passion again?

Have you ever thought that maybe the grief is covering up the things you care about? Is it a way of staying safe while you heal? Don't forget the fear. You're moving into a strange new life, and you're probably wondering who you are without your loved one. That's scary!

You may be also wondering why you haven't moved ahead on some things that were meaningful to you before. Maybe it's the fear of becoming that new person. The person without your loved one. It's the 'new normal' everyone talks about, and all grievers hate to even think about.

Or maybe you're just downright afraid you won't find your way back to living again. You have to do the thing you're afraid of doing. That's how you learn, grow, and heal.

Maybe you haven't lost your passion so much as you're just afraid to live without the person you love and lost. Maybe you just think you can't actually be happy again.

Eleanor Roosevelt said: "You gain strength, courage, and confidence by every experience in which you really stop to look fear in the face. You must do the thing which you think you cannot do."

Make a commitment to do the things you've been putting off and take a chance. Do what you're afraid of doing.

MARCH 17

Waiting

At some point after a loss, you stop waiting. You stop waiting for people to react to your loss. You stop waiting for the person you lost to come knocking on your door. You stop waiting for the grief to stop breaking your heart.

But most of all, you stop waiting to become you again.

It takes a long, long time for the waiting to turn into acceptance. No matter how many people walk away or enter your world, nothing is more apparent that the old version of yourself died too.

One day you wake up, look in the mirror, and don't recognize yourself. You get really frustrated and even angry at the idea that you have been on this road of grief for so long already and still seem to have no direction. You feel so alone.

You aren't alone. There are so many people that are going on their own unique grief journey and trying to find a new identity.

They have stopped waiting.

Sometimes it takes reconnecting with previous identities to find your way to healing. Grief has a way of cleaning out your closet, and that's not always a bad thing.

Feeling a little lost is part of being found and finding yourself again.

Once you stop waiting, you can start moving.

MARCH 18

Living Like I Was Dying

It always seemed like I had so much time, until someone I loved died. I wish I knew then that time was slipping away. It wasn't until the death of my spouse that I realized how much time had gone by, time I spent 'being busy' instead of 'being with' the person I love. We got so busy with our day-to-day lives, often just trying to make ends meet, that we forgot that the time we spent interacting with each other could end so soon.

The problem is my mind was always so distracted. I spent so much time worrying about work, paying the rent, getting done all the things that now seem so unimportant. When I was doing all that, it was really hard to enjoy the moment we were currently in. I was always dwelling on the past, dreaming of the future, and ignoring the present.

Instead of spending so much time worrying about what I had to do, maybe I should have put as much effort into making the most of the time we had together. That's the problem with losing someone you love; you don't learn that lesson until it's too late. If I had to do it all over again, I'd spend a lot less time working and worrying, and a lot more time being with the person I love.

So many times I said life was too short to do something. Usually that 'something' was forced on me by circumstances, like working too much because I really needed my job to make ends meet. But looking back on my life, most of the things that I wasted my precious time on were necessary and inevitable. The problem was I didn't make enough time to do the things I really wanted to do with the person I loved. Now it's too late.

I'll always regret that I didn't always live in the moment and learning that lesson cost me a price I was not willing to pay, the loss of the person I love.

I often think about what I would do if today were my last day to live. I imagine how different my life would be if I lived like I was dying.

MARCH 19

What Matters

It recently occurred to me that we spend so much time talking about things that don't matter, and little about things that really do.

The reason grief is so isolating is because talking about death in our society is off-limits. People don't want to talk about people that died. Even the people who care about us don't want to talk about death and dying. It's the forbidden topic.

I lost my spouse many years ago, and my dad more recently, and nothing makes me happier than someone asking me about them. This is because the last thing I want to do is lose memories of them too. I think the last thing they would want is for their deaths to define their whole life.

The way we keep our loved ones alive is in conversations, memories, and the way we live, because the end of life in no way translates to the end of the relationship.

If you're anything like me, you probably spend a lot of time trying to find answers that don't exist. Why me? Why them and not me? Thinking of these questions is inevitable, and the answers just don't exist. It was only when I tried to stop making sense of the 'loss' and started making sense of the 'life' that I began to get out of the mess I had created in my head.

If I can celebrate every moment just the way they would want, I think they would be very proud of me. I know that nothing in this world can bring them back, nothing can ever replace their presence, and nothing can ever explain my loss. But acknowledging their presence in my life, and living a happy and purposeful life, is the best way I can honor their memory.

If you're yearning for your loved one, you should know that there's no end to grief, but I hope you can also see the beauty in grief. If you grieve, it's because you love, and how lucky you are to have experienced that love.

MARCH 20

When the Tears Won't Come

You might wonder if your grief is normal. If you're not crying, you may feel you're not grieving as you should, and it can make you feel uncomfortable. Yet, grief can be surprising and unpredictable; you may well feel emotions you hadn't expected. It's good to remember that your relationship with the person who died was unique, so the way you grieve this person will be unique as well.

If someone dies after a long illness, it's possible that you already experienced something called anticipatory grief. This is an emotional response to loss before it actually happens. There's already been some acceptance of the death for some time. If this has happened to you, that is, you've felt some grief before the actual death, then it may ease your sense of loss at the time of death and affect the way you grieve.

You may feel numb when someone dies and feel intense grief much later. These intense moments can be triggered by celebrations, anniversaries, surroundings, or even people who remind you of the one who died. There may be no triggers at all, and it's hard to predict whether grief will come later.

Grief can be very private, and you may wonder how your feelings compare to the grief of other people.

We all find our own way of coping with the feelings that surround death. It's important to remember that if you feel overwhelmed, there are people who can help you try to understand what you're going through.

The benefit of joining a grief support group is that you may find it helps to know you're not the only one grieving, and to see how others are grieving, and to hear how they're managing grief.

Grief is not a pathological condition, it's a normal reaction to losing someone you love very dearly.

MARCH 21

Weekends

"I hate weekends" isn't something you hear too often. Most people look forward to, and live for, the weekends. But it's not always the case for those that are grieving.

If you're grieving, you may feel this has become the story of your life. Every weekend. There are aspects of grief that make loneliness seem inevitable and unsolvable. Primarily, the fact that what you desire is your loved one, and what you have is an emptiness molded so precisely to your loved one's likeness that no one else could ever fill it.

Add to this an 'empty' weekend. Sometimes the fun things you did were on the weekend, or maybe the weekends were when you spent the most time together.

I was working all week, so my mind was at least semi-focused on something else for 8 hours a day. The weekends felt like a giant black hole I would tumble into on Friday night.

I've come to understand that loneliness after the death of a loved one is many things. Above all else, it's the ache of having loved someone so much that pieces of you became them, and pieces of them became you. Weekends are for fun. Without them, weekends are just extra time to cry.

When the person you love left, they took pieces of your shared life with them, and now you have to live a life that feels incomplete. You lost one of the few people in this world who really truly 'got' you.

Once your brain starts thinking in an "I'm on my own, so I have to look out for myself" kind of way, it may start to guard against others by pushing them away. This includes doing things with them on the weekend. So as much as you may not want to do it, try to do something on the weekend, even if it's something small, like a walk or going shopping.

You can't easily solve loneliness caused by grief. It takes time and effort. You will never fill your loved one's void, that simply won't happen. Instead, you have to find other ways to connect and fill in the empty spaces, like the weekends.

How do you do this? I sadly can't answer that for you. I guess I would say that when you're ready, open yourself up to the love of other people in your life.

You can hold on to your loved one while at the same time accepting the company and support of others. And maybe, if necessary, seeking out new people in the process.

It won't be easy, and it won't be perfect, but perhaps in time, you can partially fill the hole left by your loved one with the love of many. Then, maybe your weekends will be something you look forward to again.

MARCH 22

Running

I had an appointment to do some grief coaching with a woman who recently lost her husband. We met for an hour and a half, and I thought the session went well. She asked me if I would meet with her again this week. I agreed.

When it came time for our session she said, "I don't want to do this anymore."

I asked why, and she replied, "It hurts too much to talk about it. I would prefer not to ever talk about it again."

We will all face great loss in our life at some point. It's one of the few things of which we can be certain. Every one of us will be forced to make choices about how we deal with it. Some of us will face our loss and grief head on. Others, like her, will try to run.

I explained to her that she can run away from it; she can run away from her own grief, and she can run away from others' grief. She could ignore her grief and push it down; she could live, and even function, but she would live a very narrow emotional life. I told her that running away from it just means she would never recover from it.

We started to talk about grief instead of her loss. We discussed how embracing it, moving through its agony, and allowing ourselves to just 'be' while it washes over us, is the only way to survive it. We have to feel the worst of it in order to let it change us, and then we can start to find out who we are going to be in the wake of it.

I shared with her what I have learned about how at the beginning, and this is especially true of a traumatic loss, the grief is all-consuming, but over time you find you are starting to live again. The mistake some make, though, is believing they can go back to being the way they were.

e say, "This isn't going to change me." But that's not how it is. recognize that loss is a life-shattering experience and that you must grieve and rebuild, you can move on positively into a new phase of life.

I told her that she didn't have to forget the person who's gone; she could never do that, and she should not worry that she would. Instead, she could fold her husband and her loss into the new person she would become, and maybe that, in the end, is the greatest tribute she could make for him.

We talked for almost two hours, and she cried, and sometimes laughed, as she talked about her husband, but she realized running away from her grief was not going to take her to a place of healing.

MARCH 23

Being Broken

When my spouse died, I kept going back and forth between missing him and hating him for leaving. At times the mixed emotions felt like I was literally sinking into insanity. One moment I would cry and the next I would yell. I was no longer myself.

Nobody told me that grief does that to people, and because I didn't know what I was feeling was normal, I felt broken.

I had never heard of the five stages of grief until my loss. That's when I learned that a person goes through denial, anger, bargaining, depression, and acceptance after the loss of a loved one.
But what I also learned is that there is no specific order to these feelings. It felt more like being on an emotional rollercoaster. One that was going too fast for me to jump off. But it's important to know that this emotional ride is normal, and you will get off of it alive and stronger.

The problem is when you do finally get off the rollercoaster, you're not the same, you're broken.

I know what it feels like to not want to get out of bed. I know what it feels like to not want to take a shower or brush my teeth or even eat. I know what it feels like to lose twenty pounds in six weeks, and to lose friends and family.

I know what it feels like to be broken. I know the feeling that the world has ended, and I'm left behind alone and miserable.

I've been there, so believe me when I say that there is hope.
There is, in fact, a light at the end of this dark grief tunnel. But the only way to get to that light is to walk through it. There is no way of getting around the process, and the earlier you begin the journey of mourning and recovery, the sooner you'll reach a place of healing and peace.

The grief journey is long, but it's not a race or a competition. It's a journey with yourself. There will be days when you'll feel stronger than ever, and some days will bring you back to your knees.

Being broken is a casualty of grief. The process is the journey. So even when you are down, feeling as if you've made no progress, remember that progress is being made every day you choose to be alive. Every time you take another breath.

I may be broken, but I'm alive.

You may be broken, but you're alive.

Together we'll survive.

MARCH 24

Changing Perspective

Nothing can change the circumstances of loss, but sometimes a shift in your perspective can make a difference in helping us to move forward.

Viktor Frankl was a therapist and Holocaust survivor known to help those through the darkest and lowest of times.

When an elderly widower spoke to Frankl about the suffering he faced following the loss of his wife, Frankl asked "What would have happened if you had died first, and your wife would have had to survive you?"

"Oh," replied the man, "for her this would have been terrible; how she would have suffered!"

Frankl replied, "You see, such a suffering has been spared her, and it is you who have spared her this suffering."

The man said no word but shook Frankl's hand and calmly left his office.

It would be great if we never had to know what it feels like to have people we love die and then suffer their loss. But that's just not the way life works.

Death is a part of life.

So, what if we could view our loss as having saved our loved one suffering, and we could find strength and pride in loving them enough to shoulder the burden?

There's no right or wrong answer, but sometimes we need something to turn to, and I hope this thought can help you today.

MARCH 25

Living in the Moment

We are always told that peace and happiness come from embracing and living fully in the moment, but I often wonder what should we do when the moment sucks?

How do we embrace the pain of loss without suffering sorrow?

I don't know that we can entirely. What the years without my spouse have taught me is that to live in the moment, I really have to do just that, whether the moment sucks or not.

During the first weeks after my loss, I allowed myself to wallow in my misery, yet at the same time I didn't just feel the pain; I did something about it. I responded to it, I listened to its needs, and gave it attention. Even though the pain didn't totally retreat, in time, it lost its hold on me. The more I allowed myself to feel the pain, the more I cried, and in time the tears healed my pain.

You can't run from the pain when you lose someone you love. You can't drown out the feelings by numbing yourself to them. Don't refuse to talk about it by burying your feelings. If you do, they'll only grow stronger and eventually catch up with you.

It's been many years now for me, but I don't miss my spouse any less. There will always be a hole in my heart. But by learning to embrace the awful moments, the sad moments, the inevitable times when I remember he's no longer at my side or in the next room, I have learned that they, like everything, are not permanent.

So, how do you live in the moment even if the moment sucks?

Talk about the person you love and lost; by doing this it keeps them alive. Share the memories, the laughs, the good times, and even the bad times. Giving a voice to who your person was allows other people to do the same.

When the sad moments come, when the ache of missing them washes over you, embrace them. By acknowledging your loss and sadness, and giving it the space it requires, you'll feel better and can move on to other parts of your life.

Living in the moment is easier than looking too far ahead, even if the moment sucks. I find it comforting to think about my spouse and cherish that moment, and embrace it, even if it's not all I would like it to be.

So, my advice is to embrace the moment for what is, and then make the best of it. In doing this, you'll limit pain's hold on you, and you may even turn that moment of sadness into a moment of joy.

MARCH 26

Stopping In to Say Hello

I went to the cemetery the other day. I stopped in just to say hello. The tears flowed from my eyes the moment I knelt down on the grass. They came so fast and so quick I didn't even realize they were there. I was there alone trying to catch my breath.

The grief comes in ebbs and flows these days. There are so many moments in the day I think of you, and my heart aches a little for what might have been. It's hard to understand the grief that comes with losing someone so long ago. Some days it's fresh in my mind. Some days it's so distant. I'll always grieve for the loss of what could have been. I'll always wonder what it would be like if you were still here.

As I sat there on the grass, my eyes filled with tears, my heart ached. I was reminded life isn't always easy, and you never know what life will throw your way. There are moments I think I should be over it, but I'm not. I will never be over it, but with each passing day, I know tomorrow the grief will feel different. Even though tomorrow will be different, I'll still always wonder.

I wonder what it would feel like if you walked in the door. Would you think I looked different? Act different? Would you even recognize this person I have become or this new life I have created for myself...by myself?

I will always wonder, but even though sometimes these thoughts fill my mind, I know I still feel your love. The love is different, yes, but it's not any less. I know that even though you aren't here, you're watching and waiting.

As I sat there alone, I realized it won't always be this way. I know every time I stop in to say hello, the sadness will be different. Sometimes it will overwhelm me. Sometimes it will be a distant memory.

I know I will always wonder what might have been, and what it would be like if you were still here, but I also know you are with me, always.

MARCH 27

Talking About Death

I knew grief was going to be painful. What I didn't know was how lonely it would make me feel.

Our society doesn't cope with the idea of death. We fear it, and because we fear it, we ignore it. We refuse to consider death and illness as a part of life. We irrationally believe that it won't happen to us or our loved ones. This makes us totally ill-equipped to deal with it when it does happen to us.

But the pain shouldn't be compounded by society's inability to deal with our grief. Most of us will acknowledge that grief is a process that takes time. But sometimes, some of us aren't ready to accept the responsibility that comes with it.

We who are grieving know we won't just 'get over it' with time, the experience of loss has changed us deeply and forever.

As a society we have a responsibility to acknowledge the pain and help other people. We need to accept that it won't always be this hard, yet it will never be the same. Dark, awkward, depressing, sad, painful, and uncomfortable: grief is all this.

It's not something we want to think about. It's not something we wish on anyone, but it's something that will happen to all of us.

We need to be here for each other when it does. And for this, we need to be prepared to deal with the bad and the ugly.

We need to talk about death.

MARCH 28

Keep Trying

I was coaching a man who told me he lost his wife a few months ago. He said to me, "I've read both your books, I read all your blogs, and I talk to you every two weeks."

I said, "Yes, that's true. Are you finding any of that helpful?"

He replied, "Yes, but…"

"But what?" I asked.

He asked, "What would you tell someone like me who's done all this and is still feeling overwhelmed with grief?"

I replied, "Keep trying."

There's something powerful about talking about our loss and acknowledging our grief. It helps us feel what's inside of us.

It's important to acknowledge what you're going through. One unfortunate byproduct of our society is we're the first generation to have feelings about our feelings. We tell ourselves things like, "I feel sad, but I shouldn't feel that; other people have it worse."

The 'grief work' is hard. It doesn't happen overnight. If you loved your person for a long time, why would you think it's not going to take a long time to grieve them? It's just not possible. It takes work and time.

If you allow the feelings to happen, they'll happen in the order they are intended to happen, and this will help you to go forward towards healing. It's not easy, and sometimes you're going to want to just give up. But don't!

If you feel like all the work you're doing hasn't changed a thing, then my advice to you is keep trying!

MARCH 29

There's No Letting Go

Being told to "let go" sounds the same as being told to "get over it." If you lost a piece of your heart, you know there's no letting go. You need to sit with your grief for a long time!

Some people wait months or years before they're ready to sort through their loved one's belongings, and some cling to anger at God or doctors who they blame for the death.

You can't be hurried or pushed. It's when you allow yourself to fully express, explore, and process your grief that you become open to healing and growth.

A year after my spouse's death, I realized that I'd stopped crying every day. At two years, I'd stopped needing to talk about the death all the time. At three years, I still carried a great burden of guilt about what more I could've done.

I'll always be a survivor of my loss, but I've loosened my grasp on that identity today, compared to the early stages. I'll never fully let go of my grief because it's bound up with love, and it's formed me over many years. Some feelings of grief still surface, and that's okay.

So, I ask you, what comes to mind when you think of 'letting go' as you move through your own grief? Do you think it's possible?

If you answered "No," I agree with you. There's no letting go; there's only noticing that healing is possible. It can be helpful to step back and take stock of what has shifted over time with or without your efforts.

Do you cry as much as you did weeks or months ago? Have some physical symptoms of your grief subsided? Do you notice even the slightest lifting of the pain you carry every day?

Instead of focusing on 'letting go,' maybe it's better to just take note of the ways you're moving toward healing in your own time.

MARCH 30

Life Happens

I'm one of those people that always tried to control everything in my life, and then my spouse died. Just when I thought I had it all under control, everything came to an end. Life is so inconvenient sometimes.

But you name it, I've tried to control it. I wanted ultimate control of everything. I never thought it was a bad thing to do, but it was stressful. I just figured I might as well try to control what I could since life was going to be random anyway. Besides, it also gave me satisfaction that I was shaping my own destiny. Boy was I wrong!

I think I adopted this way of thinking because I wanted to control things to protect myself and feel safe. But then my spouse died, and I had zero control over that.

I don't try to control anything now, and that's something that's still hard for me to do, I still struggle with it daily. But somewhere, deep down, I know that life happens FOR me, not TO me.

I figure nobody can predict the future. I was stupid to do that when I believed my spouse and I would have way more time together than we got. If I could predict the future, then I should've been playing the lottery.

But the reality is I can't foresee what's coming down the road. I can only choose my attitude when I hit roadblocks along the journey, and that's what ultimately shapes my choices. Now when life doesn't go as planned, I embrace the change.

Life is like the chapters of a book, when one ends, another begins.

I've learned to accept that life happens and goes on. I have no control over that, but it also gives me a chance to look forward to the next chapter and maybe create something bigger and better.

MARCH 31

Learning To Be Alone

My spouse and I were best friends. We didn't really need to socialize; we were just happy being together.

But that all changed when he died.

I thought I'd die of loneliness. It was so hard watching him slowly dying as the cancer ate away at his once strong body. I felt so helpless watching him disintegrate that way, when there was nothing I could do about it.

But even worse was being alone after he died.

One of my biggest regrets was that I didn't try to make and cultivate friendships over the years. Then maybe I would have had a support network. I couldn't expect people I saw only casually to fold me into their lives when I needed them.

I didn't realize at the time how important it was to invest in other friendships. I never imagined how much I would need them after my loss.

I had some friends I'd collected over the years, but when I needed someone to hold on to me really tight, there was nobody there. I was alone.

It didn't take long to figure out that some friends didn't contact me because they were uncomfortable talking about death. Not knowing what to say, they stayed away.

I needed to feel connected, but I didn't know how to do that. In the months after my spouse died, sometimes my only daily contact with people was in the bank or the post office. I would go whole days without talking to another person.

Eventually, I learned to work on my loneliness. I started to reach out more, be willing to be vulnerable, and to tell people I was a widower trying to make friends.

I also needed to learn to be alone, to enjoy my own company.

If you're feeling the heavy weight of loneliness after losing someone you love, I can tell you that alleviating that loneliness requires a real connection, a feeling of being understood.

Go easy on yourself. It can take a long time to learn how to cope with loneliness, to reach out, to want to live, but when you're ready, it will happen.

APRIL

APRIL 1

The One Left Behind

I hope this finds you well. I'm not holding up good at all. I don't know how to cope with losing you or how to heal the wounds that I can't see.

I don't know how to be me without you and didn't realize how empty the world would feel without you here. Now that you're gone, I feel so alone, so isolated, and so sad.

I'm finding it hard to do anything other than think about you. Everyone tells me I need to let you go, but that will never happen. I can't and won't do it.

I can't stop thinking about the fact that I won't see you again, ever, at least not here on Earth. Honestly, I don't know how to fill the void that you've left. The place you had in my life is empty, and all I have left is a giant hole in my heart. I know that nobody else will understand how we loved to be together, just doing the things we loved to do.

Nobody else can fill the hole in my heart because no one else deserves that spot because no one else is you. I'll never stop loving you, missing you, and wanting you back.

But I'll be strong because I know you would want me to be, and I'll move forward as best as I can, being as brave as I can. I'll be looking for you in everything I do and every place I go.

I know that you're watching over me and still loving me, and for each breath I take, I'll take one for you. You'll always be a part of me, and I'll always treasure our time together. I will never forget.

I know that you're at peace now, and I pray that you're happy, and when the day comes that my journey here is over, I know you'll be saving a seat for me.

I love you, still.

APRIL 2

Shattered: A Life in Pieces

If you've lost someone who was dear to you, then you know what it feels like to live without them. You probably feel like you're falling apart and have no idea how you're going to put yourself back together.

It sometimes even feels like someone is reaching inside your heart and squeezing it tight, and the squeezing never stops. Every time that person pops into your head or you're reminded of what you've lost, the squeezing starts again, and if it gets too tight, your heart is going to disappear altogether.

When you voice your grief, some people find it awkward. They don't know what to say and are afraid of saying the wrong thing. Well, the truth is sometimes you just want someone there as a sounding board, someone who can listen and accept that you're broken. There's really nothing they can say that's wrong.

Okay, maybe there's one thing, 'it will get easier' because at the moment it feels like it will never get easier, and saying that it will, suggests there'll be a time when the person you lost will become less important, and that thought can terrify you.

I know when you're grieving, people want to hide under a rock when you get upset or start talking about the person you lost. Maybe you don't want them around, but maybe sometimes you do. If anything, they can be a distraction from your shattered life. Death and loss are tough topics for anyone. It probably scares people, and you remind them of that.

One important thing you need to know is that you're not just going to snap out of it in a year or so. You don't just 'move on' when a certain amount of time passes. Instead of ceasing to exist, grief tends to evolve and change.

If you feel like you're falling apart, you could attempt to put all the pieces of your life back into the same overall shape, but it will never, ever, be as good as new again, It will just be different.

APRIL 3

I Wish

I wish my loved one hadn't died….and I wish I had him back.

I wish you wouldn't avoid saying his name and asking me about him. He was really important to me, and I'd like to know that he was important to you as well. When I cry because you do talk about him, I wish you knew it wasn't because you hurt my feelings.

I cry because his death makes me sad, but if you allow me to share my grief, I'll be forever thankful.

If it seems like I'm grieving too long, I wish you wouldn't think I'm not dealing with it well because for me there's no end to the grief I feel. I'll suffer my loss for the rest of my life, and I'm trying my best to live with that reality.

I wish you could understand that I can't help thinking about him. My life was shattered when he died, and I'm doing my best to put the pieces back together. That may take a very long time, so please be patient with me.

I wish you knew that I have to hurt to heal.

When I say, "I'm doing okay," I wish you could understand that I don't really feel okay, and that I'm just saying that to make you feel better because inside I'm sometimes slowly dying.

I wish you could realize that I do all I can to just make it through each day, and that grief changes people because when my loved one died, part of me went with him. I'm not the same person I was before he died, and I'll never be that person again.

I wish that you could understand my loss, my grief, my pain, my silence, and my tears, but to be honest, I wish that you'll never have to understand.

APRIL 4

The 'Dark Cry'

After the loss of my father, I was left feeling sad, but it really knocked the wind out of my mother. They were together for over 66 years, and his absence has left her so lost and devastated.

I asked her how she was holding up in the aftermath of my father's death, and she replied, "I have my good days and bad days. The worst part is the lonely hours at night when I miss his presence, that's when I really have the dark cry. You know that cry that comes from someplace so deep in your soul you don't think you'll ever survive?"

Unfortunately, I'm familiar with the dark cry.

If you're grieving over someone you lost, you know how overwhelming and consuming it can be, it can really take over your life at times.

But don't be alarmed, the way you grieve is unique to you, and that's okay.

Acceptance is a process, not only learning to accept what's happened, but also accepting how grief is affecting you day to day, focusing on how you feel in that particular moment.

Don't fight or try to avoid your emotions. Cry if you need to cry, even if it's the dark cry.

Grief is an emotional roller coaster. Sadness is a big part of it.

Give yourself permission to feel sad and try your best to keep to your normal daily routine (e.g., eating, sleeping, and regular social contact).

The natural grief process needs to be at your own pace and in your own time. Embrace the pain, it's a reflection of how much that person meant to you.

Have a good cry, it's important, even the dark cry will help you heal.

APRIL 5

Stinking Thinking

You're grieving, this means your thoughts aren't the same as before your loss. So, what's going through your heart and mind right now? I don't know what your future plans are, but I suspect you want to be happy. We all want to be happy, don't we?

The good news is that happiness is achievable, even if you're grieving a loss.

This might seem like a 'way-too-simple-solution' but if you dwell on thoughts and feelings that make you feel good, you won't feel so bad. If you find yourself sinking into grief and loneliness, try choosing to think about happier times.

You probably have so many negative thoughts in your head right now, like "How can I go on without them?", "What's left for me now?", "I'll never survive this!"

I call this 'stinking thinking'.

It's when all you do is think about all the negative things that you're feeling. If you constantly think about all the bad feelings you have, you're going to feel bad, but if you try and stop the stinking thinking and focus on the good in your life, you'll feel good.

Nobody is happy all the time, but you also shouldn't be sad all the time. You're not your thoughts, you're simply holding onto them.

An example would be you may be thinking, "Life has no meaning now because someone I love has died." This stinking thinking can be changed to, "How blessed I was to be loved." I could give you a thousand examples, but you get the point.

Your thoughts are merely the passenger, not the driver, no matter how difficult they feel, they're temporary.

APRIL 6

Grief Is Ugly

Nobody does grief well. It can make you really angry.

Grief can be really ugly, and nobody likes ugly.

No one can really cope or is cut out for angry grief. But never underestimate the need and power that anger has in the face of loss. That resentment, blame, and judgement is a level up from feeling hopeless and numb.

It might be ugly, but it's something; it's a feeling, a lifeline.

When you're angry, you're fighting for something. It gives you a sense of control. You're fighting for yourself and sometimes even for your life.

A lot of the people I work with that have lost someone they love, feel such overwhelming despair and hopelessness that they just want to die. The pain and grief are just too much.

Grief may be ugly, but rage and anger help you to fight and survive.

Your anger can help you get out of bed, shower, eat, and face a day you don't want to participate in. The ugliness of grief, and the anger that goes along with it, can help you move through your sadness and despair.

It can help you to act.

I think the best thing to do is to accept that anger is normal and DON'T try to avoid it. It's just another way you're fighting your way through the ugliness of grief. Remember that anger is a reasonable and appropriate stage of grief.

So, look your grief in the eye, stare at the ugliness, and then love yourself anyway.

APRIL 7

Maybe NEVER

When does grief end? When do you stop feeling the pain and missing the person you love that's gone? When do you feel "normal" again, and stop crying, maybe, NEVER?

The problem with grief is it doesn't affect just one person. It affects a group of people. For me, after losing my spouse, it seemed as though everyone just went back to living their lives as usual. But recently losing my dad has meant that my family is still going through their own grieving process. They didn't really know what it felt like to lose someone close to them, but I did.

When my spouse died, I did my best to deal with my grief in my own way without involving them in it. That may or may not have been a mistake, but what that means is they didn't realize that I was grieving until more recently, as I've shared information about what I went through in a way they can now understand.

What they didn't understand is that loss continues to grow as time passes, and because I was the first member of the family to suffer a major loss, they ask me when it gets better, easier, but I hate to be the one to tell them, maybe NEVER.

You never go back to who you used to be, and I kept waiting to be the person I had been before, and I think other people expected that's what would happen, too. They imagined that I would be sad for a while, and then be back to my old self. The person I had been that day my spouse died, also died and I couldn't make myself be him again, no matter how much I tried.

Grief becomes part of who you are, and I used to wish that it wasn't true. I guess that's a part of denial, but I did think that if I'd accepted grief then I wouldn't feel so much pain.

When I'm asked when the pain will go away, my answer is always the same, maybe NEVER.

APRIL 8

Smile!

Just because you're grieving the loss of someone you love doesn't mean you can't have periods of grief sprinkled with smiles, laughter, and happiness.

Grief doesn't have a time limit, and while it's important to dedicate time to processing a loss rather than skipping through it, it's not helpful to judge others or yourself for moving forward 'too quickly'.

You feel guilty when you're grieving anyway, so piling it on with judgement just makes it worse. When you're grieving you can feel pressured to live up to what grief is 'supposed' to look like.

You can feel you have to cry, you can't live a normal life, and moments of fun come tinged with guilt, as if you're not even allowed to have fun. But realistically, even in the deepest grief you can experience happiness, and that doesn't take anything away from the very real loss you've experienced.

Instead of questioning or judging those moments of happiness, as proof that grief isn't real, you should be enjoying them while they last, understanding that sadness and anger will most likely return anyway.

Your feelings change, sometimes good and sometimes bad, but the reality is, you'll always have feelings about the person who died. Enjoy the moments of happiness, grief is like the weather, sunshine and rain.

Be kind to yourself and let whatever emotions you feel come and go as they will without pressure to meet a certain set of feelings. It's not disrespectful to the person who died if your grief doesn't manifest in the way you think it 'should'. Stop worrying about how you 'should' be feeling. If you feel happy, be happy about that. If you're sad or angry, that's okay too.

I'm sure you would never wish eternal misery on someone, and your loved one's death shouldn't change that, so think of them and smile!

APRIL 9

Spencer's Mom

I have a dear friend; her name is Kym. She lost her son; his name is Spencer.

I knew the love and light Spencer gave to this world, but I don't know the pain that Kym now feels.

Here's what I do know: everyone has times in life that are, let's just say, less than good, but nothing compares to a parent that has experienced the death of a child. That's just plain devastating.

These parents, like Spencer's mom, aren't strong or even brave; they survive because they have no other choice. They have other family members that need them. They have jobs, homes and other commitments. They do these things when all they really want to do is quit living.

They go on, they breathe, they live, but not because they're tough, they're not that at all. What they really are is weak, tired, and broken.

Their reality is different than what they show their friends, families and the world in general.

They don't show others the true depth of their pain. It's too personal and too raw to show anyone that hasn't experienced it themselves; they know that people can't understand the sorrow of losing a child unless they've lost one.

These parents can't be completely open about what they're going through because they're trying so hard to just survive. They may not cry because they know if the tears start, they won't stop. This is their reality.

They'll go on living, but they will never be quite the same as before they lost their child. The pain of losing their child will always be a part of them, yet with time they do find their way forward, but how they do that will remain a mystery to me.

APRIL 10

Living With a Ghost

After my spouse died, I didn't want to change anything in our home. In my heart, it was still "our" home. I left everything the way it was: his bathrobe hanging on the hook, toothbrush in the cup on the bathroom sink, clothes in the closet, glasses on the side table; you get the picture.

In my heart I believed he was still there, well, his spirit maybe; I was living with a ghost. It was the first time in my life I really wanted to believe in ghosts. I know about the living, and I know about the dead, but I think there's also a place between them both, an in-between, where the bonds of love can still dwell. I believe some things exist in the in-between. Someplace between the dead and alive, and the present and the absent, I believe my loved one exists. Gone, yet still here.

Living with a ghost means remembering his actions, character, and yes, I think I can use the word, 'spirit'. It literally helped form my own pathway forward so that the way he thought, and his little idiosyncrasies are dwelling in me.

I know living with a ghost is not a good way to move forward, but I think there are pieces of him that move forward with me, and the love still exists to play out in joy, confidence, and bravery. I often wonder when people we love die, do we just naturally look for signs of them to deal with our grief? Are we making meaning from nothing?

When I get up in the middle of the night, I still feel that anxiety about the shadows; I won't lie. I still worry about seeing a creepy old man ghost hovering in the hallway looking for his missing head, but there's also still a part of me that wishes I'd see my spouse too.

So, yes, sometimes I feel like I'm living with a ghost, but I believe love, unlike everything else, finds a way to live. The only problem with living with a ghost is it was keeping me from living with the living.

APRIL 11

The Truth About Time

People always say, "time heals", but you won't hear me say that very often. It's just one of those platitudes that doesn't really seem to help, especially in the early days and months after a major loss.

Sometimes time only seems to make it harder. If you lost someone you love, then you know that it's really just more time without them.

It's more time without seeing their face, hearing their voice, feeling their hug, having them to talk to, all those things you never seem to stop missing.

Sure, time heals the intensity of the pain, but I'm not convinced it changes anything when it comes to how much you continue to miss their presence in the world.

You can never really be prepared for how much their absence can hurt.

Time doesn't make the grief go away; the grief just teaches you how really amazing what you had was, and why losing it hurts so much.

But maybe the person you love wouldn't want you to spend too much time missing them and would prefer you made the most out of every day you have left. To take every opportunity and try your best in all that you do.

The only truth about time is that it marches on, and maybe the best way to honor the one you love and lost is to be kind to yourself and continue to live.

APRIL 12

My Letter to Heaven

I want you to know I still think of you.

Just because I don't talk about you as much, doesn't mean I've forgotten you. You see, it's just that other people don't want to hear it. They don't understand. It makes them uncomfortable.

I still experience flashbacks of that day I held you in my arms, and you took your last breath. You whispered, "I love you", and then you were gone.

What other people don't understand is there's really no way to forget something like that. I still dream of you now and then. I still drive past that beach where we first met, and sometimes the tears start falling out of my eyes. I still wear the shirt you bought me, and I still carry your picture in my wallet. I still see your smile and hear your laugh.

When it gets very hard, when the memories jumble and force themselves to splash out of my head, I sit silent. I think about how much I miss you. I think about how much I want to see you. I think about how much I want to feel your presence beside me.

The other thing people don't understand is that thinking about you is what reminds me that I'm going to be okay. Your memory is what reminds me that life goes on. That even when you died, it's still your memory that makes me feel alive.

Just because I don't talk about you as much, doesn't imply that you're forgotten because I still love you. No matter what happens, you're still a part of my life, a very important part.

So don't you worry because I'm okay. I'm happy. I've let the pain go. I've finally learned how to embrace loss and happiness all at the same time.

So, thank you for stopping by my life; I'll see you again when it's time.

APRIL 13

Filling the Emptiness

Grief can leave you feeling empty. Death comes so suddenly, even when you know it's coming. Then after it happens, it's so final. There's no "wait a minute, I have something else I want to say and do" and there's no "not now, I'm not ready to say goodbye!"

When it ends, it's over!

This leaves you with an empty feeling. The feeling of nothing left to do, no one to care for anymore, a life you have experienced for so long, is gone. Even in the midst of feeling good about something, the grief that comes with loss can still leave you with a sense of emptiness.

It seems like everyone is grieving something these days. We're living in a world where so many people are getting sick or dying. We're all experiencing losses we haven't before, and therefore, we're all grieving.

I think you need to understand that your loss is real, and that your grieving is real as well. Grief will continue for a long time to come. You can't rush grief. It has to play out in your life in its own time. To rush it or cut it short, keeps you from feeling the pain in your life.

We all want hope, but to get there, sometimes it begins with suffering. It's the pain that will eventually strengthen you and help you to move forward to achieving a new sense of joy and peace. It really is the stuff in life that knocks you down that gives you the courage to get back up.

If grief has left you feeling empty, then now is the time to fill that emptiness with whatever it is that brings you joy and feeds your soul. You'll always miss the person you love, but you can take the love they gave you and spread it around.

Another way to stop feeling empty is through gratitude. Instead of only focusing on what you lost, think about what you have, and be thankful.

APRIL 14

The Invisible Anchor

Grief, I have learned the hard way, is like being tied to an invisible anchor. You won't see it for hours or days until you start feeling like it's no longer holding you back and it's gone, and then all of a sudden when you least expect it, it will tug at your heart.

This will happen when you see or hear anything that reminds you of your lost loved one. It can be driving by the hospital, or looking at a cereal box in the supermarket, or even just looking out the window at nothing at all.

There's no warning when that invisible anchor will start pulling and dragging you down. There's nothing you can do to prevent it or stop it. It will often happen in a public place, and it's never a matter of seeking attention, because if anything, you just want to be as invisible as that anchor of grief.

The invisible anchor of grief can drag you down into a dark well of depression. It can make you struggle with everyday things, you lose your ability to concentrate, to decide, to respond. The pull of the anchor can be heavy if you don't have many friends with whom you have daily conversations or you're someone who doesn't socialize much.

The invisible anchor of grief can make it difficult to move forward as it continues to pull you back, unseen by others around you.

Because nobody else can see your invisible anchor of grief they will give you unwanted advice. Things like, "look at the positives in life," "be practical," "you have so much to live for," "they're in a better place." But you still feel the pull of the anchor.

What's worse is that the anchor doesn't show; there's nothing that can testify that there's something there holding you back and that the torture is real.

Then comes the worst low; you think there's no way you will ever be able to cut the line and let the anchor go. Just because the anchor is invisible, doesn't mean it isn't heavy.

The invisible anchor of grief always stays with you, it just becomes less heavy. The line that has been holding you back starts to lengthen, you start to be able to move forward, further each time, before you feel the tug of the anchor. You'll get stronger, and you'll be able to drag the invisible anchor of grief with you.

In time the anchor will be so light you'll sometimes forget it's even there, until you see or hear anything that reminds you of your loved one; that's when you once again feel the gentle tug.
Just because the anchor of grief is invisible, doesn't mean it isn't there, you just get stronger and better at dragging it around.

APRIL 15

Coming to Life Again

The loss of a spouse is an extraordinarily difficult experience, I know this firsthand. You may wonder if there's life out there after your loss. It's important to reaffirm that you can find life after your loss, a changed life, but life, nevertheless.

Coming to life again beyond that loss won't be easy, but it's possible.

First ask yourself, "What do I want to take from my old life into my new life?"

Maybe there are memories you want to retain, or even objects that remind you of the person who died. You may want to recapture the joy and confidence you once had. There might be relationships that you want to preserve and carry forward.

Then ask yourself, "What do I want to leave behind?"

As you adapt to a changed life, there may be pieces you don't want to bring with you. These may be feelings such as anger or guilt that you still struggle with in your journey. There may also be memories or images that you haven't explored and need to release. There may be relationships that no longer seem significant, constructive, or meaningful.

Lastly, ask yourself, "What do I need to add?"

As you move into a new life, you may need to develop different skills that you now need to survive alone. You may need to develop new relationships, interests, or support.

Even in loss, there are choices. But ultimately, the choice is whether you'll choose to survive. Even as difficult as it seems now, you can thrive in this changed life.

APRIL 16

A Vacation From Grief

Stepping back from grief recharges your inner light; it allows you to appreciate where you've been, refocus, and provides clues as to what you want to learn as you continue your grief journey.

Take a vacation from your grief today and look at all the beautiful things and people, you have in your life.

Taking time away from your grief to make progress may seem counterintuitive. You may feel like you can't do it, and if you do, you'll be judged. The question you have to ask yourself is this, "are you willing to risk the judgment of others in order to discover breakthroughs about yourself and your purpose in life?"

One way to do this is to look at alone time as an opportunity instead of a punishment. Isn't it time you took a break from any guilt you may be suffering, and take some time to focus on you?

In today's on-the-go society, taking time for yourself is often looked upon as being selfish or unproductive. You have a job to do, kids to take care of, meals to cook, bills to pay, and the list goes on.

How can you possibly justify taking time out for self-care without feeling guilty? If you feel like you need to take time for yourself, there are many ways to do it.

Even if you have a chaotic life where there seems to be only seconds to spare on any given day, it's possible to carve out time for yourself by simply planning ahead. Make this a monthly occurrence to begin a healthy self-care habit. Do something nice for 'you'.

You deserve a vacation from grief, and don't feel bad about it because grief will be waiting.

APRIL 17

Not Knowing

I sometimes get obsessed with wanting to know what the future holds. Even when I start reading a book or watching a movie, I always want to know right away how they end. I've always been kind of envious of fortune tellers; I wish I had the power to get a glimpse at the future.

Then I think about how horrible my life would have been if I actually knew well in advance my spouse would die so young, six months was more than I could handle.

I guess my anguish about knowing what the future holds stems from my discomfort with uncertainty. So, I've decided to embrace uncertainty and celebrate not knowing what comes next, how the book or movie is going to end, or who will die next.

Maybe peace and happiness are only possible if we simply let go of the need to know?

In order to let go of my need to know what the future holds, I found myself living more in the moment, instead of always making plans for a future that may never come.

So now I don't sneak a peek at the last chapter of a book I'm reading or fast forward through a movie to the end. I also say goodbye to the people I love as if I'll never see them again just in case that turns out to be what happens.

I consider every day a gift, and I don't take any of them for granted.

I'm actually enjoying not knowing what the future holds; I keep reminding myself that if I have no expectations for tomorrow, I'll never be disappointed.

I realize I don't know anything for certain, like when I'm going to die, so I'm just going to make sure I remain grateful for every day until then.

APRIL 18

Relapse

You probably know that grief is like a roller coaster of emotions. One moment you feel terrible and the next you feel okay.

I used to think the word "relapse" only applied to a setback in someone's recovery from addiction, like smoking or drinking or the deterioration of someone's health after a period of improvement, but you can also experience a relapse in your grief.

After making significant progress on your grief journey, it can be extremely discouraging and infuriating when you feel like you've gone all the way back to 'Start'.

Everyone stumbles from time to time on the road of grief. It doesn't matter how far you think you've gone; grief has a way of pulling you back. We all relapse sometimes, but a relapse is temporary, it's not forever.

There's one commitment you can make, and even help others to keep, and that's the commitment to keep trying.

You still have the power to choose what your life will be like from this moment forward. New beginnings start with each breath and step you take.

When deciding on your new path in life, instead of focusing on how far you've slipped back, focus on how far you moved forward.

APRIL 19

Existing in the In-Between

Has this ever happened to you…?

You're having an 'okay' day, then you suddenly run into someone that doesn't know your loved one died. They ask how they're doing, and the day quickly goes from 'okay' to 'not okay.'

There's this awkward moment, where for a brief second, your heart actually stops. You realize you now have to relive the worst thing that's ever happened to you all over again. There's actually a tense that isn't past or present. In many ways, this is how you feel when you're grieving, that you're existing in the in-between.

Living in the in-between is when your head is in the current day, but your heart is back in a time when the one you love was still here with you. You know you can't go back, but you also feel incapable of moving forward.

This can be extremely difficult when you're faced with situations that occurred during times spent with your loved one. So, here's my advice on how to play it…

The question, "What are you and your loved one doing this weekend?"

Your answer, "We're going to spend it like every other one…together in love."

Now, think about it, all of this is technically true and it's pretty neutral timewise. This is slightly more advanced than using body language or completely falling apart. You can use this response when you're asked a question about your dead loved one, that stings your heart, from someone that doesn't know they died.

It's not easy living in the in-between, but this technique, when employed correctly, can dodge a lot of bullets.

APRIL 20

Ordinary Moments

Shortly after my loss, a hospice chaplain told me that there could be joy and gifts that come from grief. At the time I thought she was really in the wrong profession. Joy and gifts from grief? No way!

Then one day, many months later, I found myself laughing. I considered that a gift. I never imagined I would ever do that again. Then I found myself actually looking forward to doing something that alone brought me joy, since I had no hope of ever doing that again either, so I felt normal doing these things.

Grief is so complex; it's a combination of joy and pain.

Everything after a loss becomes bittersweet. I laughed and looked forward to something, but I was still always looking back at the loss that was causing my pain. This made it hard to recognize the joy and the gifts. But now I understand better what that hospice chaplain was talking about. I see more clearly.

Sometimes I'll walk on the beach and look out at the ocean, and I find joy in that ordinary moment. To me that's a gift.

I've learned that I have to find the joy and gifts of grief wherever I can. It can be in the eyes of my dog when she looks at me with unconditional love, or in the voice of a friend who calls just to see how I'm doing, or a sunset over the ocean.

I know I'm not here forever, but I'm here right now. So, I can choose to live always in my grief, or I can experience these ordinary moments and consider them a gift.

Try looking for the ordinary moments in your own life, if nothing else, they can be a distraction from the suffering you're feeling most of the time and be the joy and gift that push you through the pain.

APRIL 21

If It Brings You Comfort

What to keep and what not to keep. That always seems to be a common dilemma after a loved one dies. I think it comes down to asking yourself what brings you comfort and what brings you pain.

A tangible item, like an article of clothing, a favorite book, or, in my case, a pair of sneakers, can build a strong connection.

Yes, you heard me right, in the back of my closet is a pair of my spouse's sneakers. I still can't bring myself to let them go. In some strange way I guess I've always thought that if he came back, he would need them. I know that's silly, but I think the real reason is that to maintain the advantage of holding onto my loved one's sneakers, to me, makes him still seem relevant.

Maybe I've channeled my longing for the person I lost onto the sneakers. By keeping my spouse's sneakers, I'm not seeking independence from him. Instead, I'm relying on them to deal with the anxiety and feelings of grief around our final separation. The sneakers are my transitional object, they help provide security and a symbolic link for me. The sneakers being in my closet somehow bring me comfort.

When you're faced with a home full of your loved one's belongings, knowing what to keep as one of your transitional objects can be daunting or straightforward. So ask yourself this question, "Will keeping this bring me comfort?" Then think about how the person you love and lost would feel about it.

You don't have to get rid of everything. Keeping anything that holds meaning or brings you a sense of peace can be what keeps you connected to your loved one.

Knowing that he wore those sneakers every day keeps us connected, and I imagine they'll always be the item that brings me comfort.

APRIL 22

"I'm Just Sad"

I was talking to a little boy who just lost his dad. I told him I also just lost my dad.

My heart hurt for him since he was so young. At least I had my dad in my life for a long time.

When I asked him how he was feeling about it, he replied, "I'm just sad."

If you're old enough to love, you're old enough to grieve.

I think if I asked anyone that lost a person they loved, they would respond the same way as this little boy.

So simple and to the point, "I'm just sad."

It doesn't seem to be saying much, yet in so many ways it says it all.

When you're grieving, you can experience so many different emotions in a day. At the end of it all, the energy it takes to experience so much pain can wear you down. Nothing is left but a weary sadness, and there's absolutely nothing you feel you can do about it.

Loss is defeating, and even the strongest of souls can be defeated by the sadness that great loss brings.

In the end, loss is sad, and sometimes life is sad, and being sad along with it may be the only thing you can be.

APRIL 23

Life Is Fragile

If you're like me, you probably don't spend a whole lot of time thinking about your mortality.

But I'll admit I do it much more frequently now that I suffered a major loss than I ever did it before.

It's uncomfortable to think about dying, yet it's the one thing that is certain in this life along with our choice of how we show up and navigate each day.

As I reflect on the years since my spouse died, I think of all the missed milestones that have marked my life both big and small. From the fun everyday moments to the can't miss celebrations.

This year in particular is bittersweet. It marks the year we would have been married 20 years. Another important milestone that I'll celebrate without him, and it makes me sad.

But he's been with me all along the way in spirit. Sometimes I hear his voice. Sometimes I sense him around my house. I can still feel his warm hugs and see the twinkle in his eye when he really saw me for me.

I continue to tell my story. To remember who he was as a husband and friend. I share his jokes and his love for peanut butter and fried clams.

It's the little things that we remember about people. How they make us feel.

I consciously choose to live with no regrets. I try to acknowledge the people I encounter with care and kindness. To be aware of the energy I'm putting out there.

I'm not perfect. I make mistakes. I sometimes unintentionally hurt other people. But I continue to try to do my best to be thoughtful in my interactions and make amends when I screw up.

APRIL 24

Don't Compare

When you lose a person you love, the worst grief is your grief, so don't compare it to anyone else; it's never going to be the same.

Try not to compare yourself to your expectations. The best thing to do is to let go of your expectations about grief entirely. Throw things like grief stages, tasks, and timelines out the window because individual grief is unique and unpredictable.

Your relationship with the person who died is unique, so comparing it to anyone else will only make your journey through grief more difficult.

I realize how scary it can be to look at grief as a complete unknown, but in doing that you'll allow for a more flexible and accepting understanding of your experiences. Try to learn what you can from the grief experiences of others, but don't compare your experience with grief to theirs because this won't help you. Don't compare your methods of coping because everyone copes with grief differently.

And finally, don't compare your overall healing to your perception of how others are healing. Grief is a story without a true end, and your ups and downs will happen at different times and in different places. Most importantly, don't compare yourself to yourself.

When you try to think about or assess how you're doing in grief, you make the mistake of comparing yourself to the person you were before your loss (who, by the way, you'll never be again, and that's okay) or some idealized idea of who you will be "when you feel better."

Making that comparison isn't fair because you discount all the progress you've made in your grief.

If you still insist on comparing yourself to yourself in grief, I recommend comparing yourself to how you felt on day 1 of your grief and how you feel now.

APRIL 25

Love in the Midst of Loss

Have you ever wondered how you can ever possibly be happy again after the loss of someone you love? I have a feeling if you're reading this the answer is, YES.

When someone you love dies, the pain of the physical loss is so intense that you lose sight of the love that still exists. You can't see love like you can see a human body. When someone you love dies, their physical body is gone, but the love remains.

Let me explain it like this, when my spouse was alive, we loved each other when we were together, but we also loved each other when we were both at work, in different places. We couldn't see each other, but nothing about our love for each other changed.

So how is that any different now that he is not physically here? He may be gone, but the love remains and continues to grow in the ashes of my grief. I knew in life he was loving me, even if I couldn't physically see him or touch him, so I know he is still loving me now.

I know this doesn't change the fact that you still wish you could hug them, and kiss them, and tell them to their face how much you love them, it's just to remind you not to forget the love remains. Doesn't that alone begin to open your heart? It does mine. It's about remembering this truth so that you act from that knowledge instead of from your own grief and pain.

So, what's it all about? Why are we here? Why do we love someone only to feel the pain of losing them? I think the answer is LOVE.

Here's what I think: I know we can't take any of our materials things to Heaven with us, but I do believe we take all the love we have collected here with us.

So, I want to make sure I collect all the love I can…so my soul is full when I get there.

151

APRIL 26

Always Go to the Funeral

It's always an interesting experience as a Grief Specialist when I go to a funeral. People seem to think I have all the answers on how to avoid the pain and sorrow of a loss. SPOILER ALERT: I don't!

When I was sixteen, my friend's grandmother died. I didn't want to go to the funeral, it just seemed like such an inconvenience. But my mother said, "Always go to the funeral." She said it was disrespectful not to go.

Sounds simple, when someone dies, get in your car and go to calling hours or the funeral. That, I can do. But I think a personal philosophy of going to funerals means more than that.

'Always go to the funeral' means that I have to do the right thing when I really, really don't feel like it. I have to remind myself of what my mother told me. I have to sometimes do things that are hard, like going to funerals. I'm talking about those things that represent only inconvenience to me, but the world to the person who is grieving the loss.

Being a Grief Specialist doesn't make going any easier. I feel the same sadness and sorrow. The thing is life (and death) sometime get in the way of what I really want to do. Most days, my real battle is doing good versus doing nothing.

In going to funerals, I've come to believe that while I wait to make a grand heroic gesture, I should just stick to the small inconveniences that let me share in life's inevitable, occasional calamity.

So, sometimes I have to do things I don't want to do, and maybe that is an inconvenience, but I was taught to, 'always go to the funeral.'

The most human, powerful, and humbling thing I've ever seen is a church full of inconvenienced people who believe in going to the funeral.

APRIL 27

Eternity

After my loss, someone said to me, "Don't you worry, someday you'll be together again for eternity." I think this was said with the intention to make me feel better, but I'm really not so sure.

I remember when I was about seven years old a teacher explained to me the concept of eternity. She explained it as something that never ends. She said it just goes on and on, forever and ever.

The idea of something that never ends was somehow scary to me. Going to Disney World for eternity would be awesome, but what about going to the dentist? I was terrified of the dentist. I didn't want to go there for eternity!

Even if I made it to Heaven, I didn't want to be there forever. I was excited about seeing the angels and flying around (I was absolutely sure this was part of the deal), but beyond that, I would miss all the people I loved here on Earth. It seemed like a great place to visit; I just wasn't sure I wanted to stay there for eternity.

The problem is, as a child, I was mostly worried about my own fate. I assumed everyone I cared about was going to live forever, or at least as long as I did. Of course, as I got older, and my understanding of the world became more complex, I found out people do die, and sometimes before me.

"Don't you worry, someday you'll be together again for eternity."

That statement still doesn't seem to bring me the comfort people feel it should when they say it. Maybe it's because my focus is no longer on my own fate, but on the person I lost.

So maybe the answer I'm looking for is to the question, "Why can't we just be together again for eternity right here and now?" Maybe sometimes just being sad and missing someone are all we need; maybe we don't need promises with no guarantee...like eternity.

APRIL 28

A Broken Heart Is an Open Heart

There's no pain quite like that of a broken heart. The experience of loss in love wounds you like no other. In the midst of your pain, you cry out wishing there was something to take the hurt away. But there's nothing. There's no cure for a broken heart except for the universal healer, time.

If there is no cure for a broken heart, nether is there a guaranteed way to avoid having one. The more you risk, the more people you grow to love, the more it's possible that you will experience a separation. Yet, whenever your heart is broken, you receive a blessing, your broken heart becomes an open heart.

When you experience sadness and grief, something unexpected emerges. When you allow yourself to be broken, a gentle transformation takes place. In the midst of the pain, you feel a softness and vulnerability that are truly beautiful.

You become more accepting and open. Judgement and criticism are replaced by a compassion for others and an acceptance of life the way it is.

Think back to another time when your heart was broken, remember what it was like to feel sadness and grief. Remember how your heart was opened. If you didn't experience this opening, then see if you can allow it to happen now.

You were born to grow in love and understanding. By keeping your heart open and allowing it to experience both joy and pain, you will fulfill your highest destiny as a human being.

APRIL 29

Living in the Here and Now

A part of the grieving process is looking back at what you now understand to be 'the whole story.' You know that your time with this person has ended, so now you can look at the whole picture.

You can revisit the painful and beautiful moments. You can think about your decisions. You can let yourself experience the feelings that come with remembering regret, joy, gratitude, guilt, all of it.

You can spend a long time doing that. I'm not here to tell you not to. You take as long as you want to take; grief in my experience is limitless. How can anyone set a time frame for dealing with infinite sorrow? I can't. No one can.

When you're ready to release the past, you will. You'll be done spending your time and energy looking back. You'll pick up whatever remains of yourself and your life. You'll start moving forward. This act of acknowledging the weight of what is gone and learning to live in the present leads to acknowledging the weight of what can never be; here's where the other aspect of grief waits for you.

This part of grief will feel like a punch in the throat. This grief will come on you like a sudden storm. This grief is for a lost future, an imagined future, one that can never exist. The one who would have created it is gone. You can't recover them.

When you're not ready, a picture of that future will fly up, deliver a blow. It's always a sucker punch. How can you prepare to face something that doesn't exist? How can you predict when something imaginary will appear? You can't. So, you don't. Don't try it. It's a waste of time. Instead, know it for what it is. Another step in this journey of grief. A necessary step, important, not one to skip over or ignore.

So how can you grieve and still continue to live?

I don't know what happens next. I can tell you to release the past, but I'm not sure it's that simple. The past has a definite timeline, a beginning and an end. An imagined future has no such limit. It can extend with us indefinitely like a train track. Every now and then, the train jumps the track. I don't know that you can stop it from happening. I don't know that you would want to.

I know that an imagined future can eat up the beautiful present. I don't think you would want that. Learning to live in the here and now, fully aware, feeling it all, as grateful as you can be, is the best thing to do because if you only focus on a distant past or an imagined future, you might miss something in the present.

APRIL 30

A Source of Strength

Have you ever wondered, "How have others been able to live through this"?

You most likely know of somebody that had a major loss before you had your loss. Maybe you even admired their courage. If you could only be like them! But you are 'not' them. So don't compare yourself to other people. You are a distinct individual.

No two people are exactly alike, and relationships are all different in their own way, so not everyone brings to their grief journey the same resources for coping. This doesn't mean that there's something wrong with you. You should never feel ashamed of your emotions.

As a distinct person, you bring to your grief your own unique experience in living and your own resources in trying to understand and cope with your loss. Family, friends, neighbors, and maybe even your faith, will be some of the resources that may help you to face your grief.

But you may be overlooking yourself as a source of strength.

I remember when my aunt, who had two children, lost her husband, and shortly after that, both of her sons. I was always so surprised by how she could endure such great loss, yet miraculously she somehow still had the ability to cope with all that tragedy. I was truly amazed at how well she was able to deal with what was happening to her.

How was she able to do it? In addition to other resources, she found within herself a source of strength that I'm sure she didn't even know she had, and she was able to draw from it. That source of strength helped her, and she survived. If she could survive the loss of her entire family, surely, I could survive my loss.

Don't underestimate yourself as a possible source of strength. You're not new at living life.

157

You've made it this far in living because you have successfully learned how to deal with other difficult times. Overcoming those hurdles made you stronger and gave you added strength.

I know the loss you are experiencing now is very different from other dark times you've encountered in life, nevertheless, with perseverance, determination, faith, and hope, you can find the strength to survive this experience. You may surprise yourself.

You may find yourself drawing from a source of strength that you didn't even know you had.

MAY

MAY 1

Suicide – Remembering a Life

While the prevalence of suicide in our culture is in itself tragic, the grief of losing a loved one to suicide is often overwhelmingly isolating and literally unspeakable.

After the death of a loved one to suicide, you may feel disconnected from your understanding of the world, encased in shock that weighs on you like a block of ice only to reach out for support that you may not receive.

I lost a close family member to suicide, and I've been speaking with people that have lost a loved one to suicide for many years now. Eventually, all of my work on suicide became helpful to me in piecing together the components of my own loss and eventually, making a measure of peace and moving forward with it.

However, for a number of years following the death, I sleepwalked through my life trying to re-work all the details that I knew of that had led to the death. It has been years since this event occurred, and I still don't have a clear memory of what anyone said about it in the aftermath. I think because nobody ever talked about it.

If you're a survivor of suicide loss, please know that you're not alone.

Suicide loss survivors often tell me how wary they are to share their stories of loss because of their past experiences in hearing myths about suicide, receiving judgment from friends, family, or religious communities, or feeling overwhelmed with the burden of having to simultaneously share their story while teaching someone about the reality of suicide and suicide bereavement.

These concerns are understandable; navigating the months and years following a suicide loss is challenging enough without risking further harm from others.

I know that there are potentially tremendous benefits to telling your story or testifying your grief and having others bear witness to them. In finding trusted friends, family, or helping professionals, you may be able to acknowledge the pain that your loved one experienced as well as your own pain at the loss.

You may find comfort in undertaking your continued grieving process without bearing the burden of doing so alone, and in doing so, you may also find a community of survivors.

Moving forward with your life after a suicide loss is one of the most difficult processes you'll undertake as a survivor but identifying and building a community that can support you reinforces that you're not alone.

MAY 2

Drowning

I've never drowned, but I can imagine the panic. The fear. The fight as your body merely wants to do what is natural, just breathe. The burn in the chest. The enveloping darkness. The pound of every pulse reminding you that you're surrounded on all sides by what you can't escape.

I've never drowned, but I do know that's exactly how grief feels.

Every single reality check is your heart trying to comprehend what your brain is telling you is true. The finality of loss and the love of a life you can no longer grasp. Just gravity, pulling you down and stealing your breath.

Grief is being numb to everything but the pain. The fog of indifference envelopes you. The bills weren't paid. The plants didn't get watered. Who cares? Not you. You're just trying to breathe, and the pain in your soul drowns out all other cares.

I've never drowned, but if I did, it would be dealing with a 'first," and grief is dealing with firsts. Not just the big ones like anniversaries and birthdays but the little ones. The first piece of mail addressed to the person who died. The first trip to the grocery store where your shopping list doesn't include their things.

I've never drowned, but I know a lot about 'never,' and grief is the word 'never.' It taunts you with what will never be again. They'll never walk in the door again. They'll never hug me again. They'll never tell me they love me again.

I've never drowned, but I can tread water, and grief is like treading water. In time, the waves lessen, and you start drifting to the top again. Though the water surrounds you, it's no longer pulling you down. Your head can now stay above water with the push and pull of grief's influence.

Your breath, instead of coming in gasps, becomes deeper and steadier.

MAY 3

Worst Case Scenario

When it comes to grief, most people can pinpoint at least one thing that, since their loss, makes them feel anxious in ways it never did before. The death of a loved can create such new and distressing emotions that they test or change your existing relationship with emotion. You become so fearful because grief creates fear and anxiety.

I was never afraid to die until my spouse died. Prior to that event, I assumed that the world was a good and safe place, where things happened for a reason. I also subconsciously believed that bad things wouldn't happen to me. I became fearful and anxious. If I became sick, who would take care of me? Would I die alone?

My loved one's death led to my belief that bad things can happen to anyone at any time, and now something bad was going to happen to me.

Then one day it all changed for me. I was a participant in a grief support group, and I said to the facilitator, "I'm so worried about all the bad things that might happen to me now."

She asked, "What would you say is the very worst thing that has EVER happened to you in your life?"

I looked at her confused by her question that I believed had such an obvious answer, and replied, "Of course the loss of my spouse."

She said, "If you survived that, it's safe to assume you will survive anything else."

I agreed with her 100%. On that day I stopped being anxious about everything. I came to the realization that my 'worst case scenario' had already happened. I had no control over anything, and nothing else was ever going to seem as bad. It came down to learning to live in an unpredictable world that I can't control.

MAY 4

The Puzzle of My Life

My life was so perfect before my loss. (Well, at least that's the way I remember it.)

Then when my spouse died, it all fell apart. It was like this perfectly put together puzzle that fell off the table and all the pieces scattered on the floor. The problem was, when I picked up all the pieces, one of the pieces was missing. The most important piece.

When somebody you love dies, the life you had is broken into a million pieces that just don't fit together anymore. There's that one missing piece that connected all the others. It takes a long time to try all the pieces and try to make them fit into the same picture of the life you had and lost. But every time you do that you just keep coming up with that missing piece. Without that piece, it just won't be the same.

Eventually, you find a couple of pieces that go together. They don't look the same as they did before, but they fit. You start to look for pieces that are the same color and pattern. Pieces that you know are edges, and pieces you know are not. In time, the puzzle of your life comes together. It just looks very different.

Grief is like the pieces of a puzzle. You have to take the scattered pieces and find a way to put them back together. You have to fall apart before you can rebuild your life. It's not easy to do, and you may have to make many attempts at it, but in the end, you will piece together a new life.

It may not be the same picture, but it can be just as beautiful. My new puzzle is different and all of it has made me who I am. All of it is my life. Even the painful parts are precious to me, like that missing piece, because it represents the one I love.

Although the puzzle of my life may not be as perfect as it once was, the piece I cherish the most is the one that's missing.

MAY 5

Just One More Day

Would you trade a whole year of your life for just one more day with your loved one?

One year for one day, that's a bargain don't you think?

I can see it now; the day is a perfect, warm weather and a gentle breeze is blowing off the ocean. We're sitting in our beach chairs holding hands and just enjoying the moment; and each other.

Calm, peaceful, happy, and in love. We're both drinking an ice-cold lemonade and watching the sailboats floating by, and the sun is warm on our faces.

We talk all day long about so many things. He tells me all the secrets about where he has been. He shares with me all his wisdom about the afterlife, and the wonderful things he has seen on the other side. I tell him the things I've always wished I'd said before he died. I tell him how much I love him, and miss him, and how life has changed so much. He tells me he's proud of me. He knows how sad I have been but has also witnessed my strength and compassion.

I tell him I am who I am because of him.

I hear his voice. I feel his touch. He sees that I'm okay. We sit in silence during that beautiful time of day right before the sun goes down and neither of us feels sad or alone. As the sun starts to slowly set, I look at him and suddenly think, oh no, I only have a few hours left!

I realize that once again time is taking him away from me, and I have no ability to stop it. I need to try really hard to look at his face. Listen really close to his voice. See his smile and feel the way he touches me. The way he loves me. It's really important I remember all these things about him! My time is almost up! How can I possibly let him go again?

I begin to wonder if the heartache of him slipping away from me all over again is worth one more day. One more hug? One more time to say, "I love you." One more time to feel normal again.

I don't know if I have the courage or the strength to say goodbye again? But, then I think how some days I wish with all my heart for him to come back. How I'm tired of only seeing one chair on the sand.

So, would I still trade one year for one day? Of course, I would. I wouldn't hesitate to trade a year for just one chance to do it all again, even for only 24 hours.

I would make the trade, no doubt in my mind, even knowing it would have to end.

MAY 6

Feeling Better

When you're grieving, your main focus may be on feeling better. When will that happen? How long does it take? But what does 'feeling better' mean in the context of grief? That seems like the goal, right?

It feels like if you can just get over the pain and the sadness then everything will just go back to normal. But that's not really true, because after someone you love dies, nothing will ever really go back to normal...at least not the normal you once knew.

It also seems like everyone around you is just waiting for you to 'go back to normal,' so this puts even more added pressure onto you and your grieving heart. People just assume that in a certain amount of time, usually much less time than you could ever imagine, you will go back to being the person you were before your loss. Nope!

If you've suffered a major loss, you know it's not as easy as that. Getting better is about finding even just one small part of yourself that you recognize.

It's about finding patience with all those people that don't understand. It's about finding joy again in life or interest in something, anything, again. It's about having the energy to get out of bed in the morning, and the courage to leave the house.

Feeling better is when you're able to recognize that you're not meant to spend the rest of your life sentenced to days, weeks, months and years of suffering. It's not being disloyal to the person you love and lost to want to find your way to a place of healing, or dare I say, a place of feeling better.

I think the only way to feel better is to do it bit by bit, day by day, until you no longer feel stuck. You won't be the same person you were before your loss, but you'll know that you've moved forward, and that feeling better is really just a state of mind not a destination.

MAY 7

Being Okay With Your 'New Self'

Loss is one of the most universal experiences. You carry the remnants of loss with you every day. So let yourself grieve and feel your pain, even if other people might tell you to 'move on' or 'get over it.'

What those people don't understand is that grief never quite goes away. It's normal to feel what you're feeling. While your grief will change over time, its impact endures, and accepting this fact will allow you to begin to integrate the loss into your life.

I believe love is eternal, so on a certain level you're still in a relationship with the person you love and lost. This love is an integral part of who you are, so continue to talk about them and stay connected to the person who made such an enduring impact on you.

Remember that they will always be a part of your life.

You've changed, so don't expect to return to your 'old self.' You're learning to live your life as your 'new self' and that's a really hard thing to do.

This 'new self' has a new attitude towards a lot of things about life, death and your own purpose. Other people may have trouble with your changes but let them know that change is a natural part of living.

Letting yourself be okay about these changes gives you the strength to grow. Being open to all the new aspects of yourself, both good and bad, will give you the courage and confidence that will make it possible to survive.

Being more open about the changes in yourself caused by your loss and grief will actually enable you to live with it more peacefully.

After a death, love and loss go hand-in-hand.

Closure on one would mean closure on the other.

MAY 8

Mrs. Patrick Swayze and Me

After my loss I was searching for someone who could relate to what I was going through, someone who would understand. My spouse died of pancreatic cancer, and shortly before that, Patrick Swayze had died from the same illness.

I wondered what it must be like for his wife Lisa. Not only had she experienced the same type of loss, but she was also in the public eye. She had the disadvantage of grieving on a public stage. Then I realized being in the public eye was also an asset, especially if you are trying to get a message out to the world.

Lisa was doing great things to make the world aware of pancreatic cancer and the effect it has, not only on the people that have it, but also on those that love them. She was taking the bad thing that happened to her and making something good come out of it. I wanted to do the same thing.

I thought since the best way to learn about something you can't understand is to find a mentor, somebody like Lisa who had already suffered her loss and was on the road to finding herself.

So, I started to follow her blog page. She was posting about her experience with grief after the loss of Patrick. Each blog she wrote inspired me to keep moving forward, even on days when it seemed impossible. I believed if she were doing it, so could I!

One day I decided to reach out to her and tell her my story, how it was like her own. I never imagined that she would respond to me, but she did.

This opportunity allowed me to ask her questions I was struggling with and learn more about the healing of grief. Because of her mentorship, I was able to move forward. I read her books and decided to write my own. I listened to her at speaking engagements and created my own workshops and used what I learned about grief and loss to help others.

To be able to do something positive out of your loss can be a very healing and rewarding experience. Seeking out a mentor can be the first step to achieving that goal.

Look for someone who is doing what you desire to have for yourself. It would be ideal if you could talk to this person, but if you can't for some reason, carefully study what they have done to be at the level you strive to obtain. Follow their examples and create a plan.

The mentor you select doesn't have to be someone who did something that changed the world. It can simply be someone who has an interest that they share with you. Having someone who has already achieved it can be a good way to find your way to the same goal.

Lisa taught me that the best way to honor your loved one is to do something that makes their death, and their life, matter.

MAY 9

Life Without Dad

Today is my dad's birthday. I lost him to congestive heart failure. This loss has taught me that the passage of time is constant, it's tricky, and it sneaks up on you.

I've known for a long time what it feels like to lose a spouse, and now I know what it feels like to lose a parent.

I've moved forward since my spouse died, it's been eight years, but lately I've found myself wishing for two opposing realities, one in which I have moved forward and away from the heartache of losing my dad, and another that turns the clock back to a time when he was still here.

The last few months of my dad's life were hard to witness. Most heartbreaking was watching his body get weak, even though his will to live was strong. He wasn't just my dad; he was also a big piece of my life and a very special person to me.

My dad, true to his nature, taught me that death was just a part of life, that we all have an expiration date. He didn't want to leave, not because he was afraid of death, but because he loved life.

I know he would want me to honor him by doing the same and live on as usual after he was gone. That I wouldn't allow his death to keep me from living my life to the fullest. That despite life's challenges, I would follow his lead and continue to live the best life I can, for what time I have left.

My dad is another missing piece in my life, and another date on the calendar to dread, but that's not going to stop me from having the courage to say, "Yes, Dad. I'll be okay, and I'll continue to live, not only for myself, but also for you."

Because of the losses in my life, I've learned that we'll never control how and when the people we love leave us, but we can grow through it.

MAY 10

You're Still Here

Do you no longer enjoy activities you once did?

My advice to you is not to try and return to them right away. It's like trying to recreate something you once did that can't be redone. There will be many things about your 'old life' that just won't work anymore. Even though it may be sad to see certain things stay in the past, there can be a unique excitement in trying something new.

The problem with grief is that no matter how much time is left, and no matter how hard it may be to live a life without the person you love, you're still here.

But is a life without joy or happiness the only way to prove your love? Is living an unfeeling existence the best way to pay tribute to the person you lost? Maybe it's more about having a balance and finding a way to invite both joy and sadness into your life.

I know you're probably thinking, "What's the point? Since the person I love died, nothing really matters." I get it. I really do. I've said that very same thing myself.

When someone you love dies, your priorities shift. Before your loss you probably had a lot of plans for the future. Things you cared about. Some good. Some important. Some not so important. But when the person you love died, those plans changed. They changed because they included the person you love. Maybe they don't even seem that important now, maybe just having them back is all you really want.

The loss of the person you love changes what you once thought was so important. But the good news is, despite the terrible thing that happened, you now have the potential to gain a perspective that you probably never would have otherwise. Don't squander this insight and go to the extreme of thinking that nothing matters. Instead, use it to your advantage.

So how do you do that?

Don't sweat the small stuff anymore. Don't worry about what other people think because they're too worried about their own lives anyway. Make time for joy and recognize what can wait for tomorrow and realize that a good life is what you make of it. You're still here, so live the best life you can.

It's not easy dealing with change. When you suffered your loss, there was already so much that changed. But, you have the power to make new plans that include happiness for yourself, and by doing that you also honor the one you love and lost.

MAY 11

When the Grief Is Too Much

Grief...it's a place no one wants to find themselves, and it's often lonelier and darker than you ever would've imagined.

If you're coping with the loss of someone you love, I'm sorry to tell you that it's a hard road ahead, but you're not as alone in your emotions as you might feel right now. Your grief can feel all-encompassing or overwhelming, and it's extremely hard to see through it to the other side.

While there's no one universal secret to getting through this time in your life, know that you'll find a way through this winding path of emotional obstacles, and there are many others walking the same journey.

You may have some expectations about how and what you're supposed to feel in your grief. Part of the challenge is coming to accept that your emotions never quite manifest how you think they should.

There's no way to prepare for the thoughts and feelings that are going to come up in your grieving process but making space for them can help. Try to remember in those moments that the person you're grieving for loved you as you were when they were still with you.

They would want you to keep being that person and living a version of that life, one where you honor their memory with joy. Imagine your future life through the eyes of the person you're grieving.

Chances are they'll be proud.

MAY 12

It's the 'Nevers' That Hurt the Most

When I think about the person I love and lost, it's usually what I call the 'nevers' that hurt the most.

Never another phone call. The call to work to ask me what's for dinner or if I'd rather go out to eat. The call to share some exciting news or just to see how I'm doing and how my day is going.

Never another "I love you." What wouldn't I give to hear that even one more time? Hearing it when I was leaving for work or coming home. When I was worried about something, scared, or just sad. When I was happy and made some kind of achievement or even just for no reason at all.

Never another hug. This is the one I think I miss the most. That feeling of being engulfed in the arms of someone who hugged me so tight, and then I would hug back even tighter and feel so safe.

Never another smile. Looking across a crowded room to see that familiar face. The one that would seek me out and flash me a smile that let me know I wasn't alone, even in a crowded room.

Never seeing that face again. Only in a photo can I see what I once saw for real and in the flesh. Running my hand down a familiar cheek.

For me, it truly is the 'nevers' that hurt the most.

MAY 13

When I See You in Heaven

I could feel the slow rhythm of your heartbeat when I laid my head against your chest. Tears were rolling down my face as I held back the scream that was coming from my own heart.

Please, not yet!

I closed my eyes and thought about all the special moments of the life we shared together. Such sweet memories. Yet my heart was breaking.

I wasn't ready to say goodbye. I still had so much to say. I wanted you to know how much I loved you and how very much I would miss you.

I knew you were in pain. I could hear your shallow breathing. Your struggle to stay with me. I gently took your hand in mine and prayed for your suffering to end. I was suffering too. I wanted you to go gently, but not without me.

Please, not yet!

The clock was ticking; the sun was rising. A new day was beginning. A day that would never be forgotten but for all the wrong reasons.

The moments passed; the memories flashed through my heart and mind.

And then it was time.

Not a day goes by that I don't think about you. Even now. I can close my eyes and imagine your face and hear your voice. The tender things I've kept hidden in my heart will stay there until I see you again.

There will be no more death. No crying. No sorrow. No pain.

There will be no separation. No longer will it hurt when I see you in Heaven.

MAY 14

Taking a Break

Somebody told me everything I write is too sad. I guess most of what I write is sad because I'm always talking about grief, and grief is, well, sad.

So maybe today should be a day to take a break from grief. It's absolutely okay to do that. Just give yourself permission to mentally walk away from grief.

Trust me, it isn't going anywhere.

It will come back and demand to be heard soon enough. But for now, put it aside and take a deep breath.

Sometimes you get really tired of the pain and sadness. Grief wears you down. It's exhausting. So, it's okay to take a break once in a while.

Putting your grief aside doesn't mean you're abandoning the one you love. It doesn't mean you're forgetting them.

I'm telling you today that it's okay to take a break. Give your brain and your heart something other than sadness to focus on. Find one thing that brings you peace or joy and focus on that.

You don't always have to stay in the dark place. You're allowed to sometimes walk out into the light. Every day doesn't just have to be about your loss, or your grief. Today concentrate on you.

I'm asking you today to take a break from your grief; you owe it to yourself.

177

MAY 15

Please Don't Go

Grief is funny, you know. You desperately want it to go away, except for sometimes when you don't want it to go away. The problem is, sometimes when you're grieving, love gets all mixed up with pain and grief.

You realize your pain has become the expression of the love you lost. It becomes the way you honor your loved one, the one consistent link between life with them and life without them. You feel like the more you grieve for them, the more it proves that you love them. It sounds like kind of a silly thing to do when you think about it in that way, doesn't it?

It's like while you're wishing the pain of grief away, it turned into something else entirely. It's like grief has even come to define you in the context of your life after loss. Who are you if you're not someone grieving the loss of someone very special? And who are they if you're not here, in life, holding vigil for them?

If you're struggling with these thoughts, you're not the only one.

Sometimes you might feel like if you're doing okay, you're forgetting them, or if you're not suffering enough, you're not missing them enough. Maybe you feel like if you stop feeling the deep pain of grief, it's a sign life can move on without the one you love, and you for sure don't want that to be true!

Surely the only thing that is keeping you connected to the one you love and keeps their memory alive is your pain. Any little piece of that grief that goes away means another little piece of your loved one is going away. Again, sounds like kind of a silly thing to do when you think about it in that way, doesn't it? These feelings are completely normal. I promise!

It's very common to feel extremely conflicted about feeling better, although it may not seem rational, it's also common to gravitate towards the pain.

When it feels like the alternative to feeling pain is losing connection to your loved one, what other choice do you have?

But, what I want you to try to understand is that your loved one's memory doesn't live in your pain or grief; your loved one's memory lives in YOU.

It lives in the stories that you tell people about them. It lives in the memories you shared together. It lives in the things you do that your loved one taught you. It lives in the things you do in their honor and memory.

Your loved one is not disappearing as your pain and grief diminishes, you're just learning to live with the memory of your loved one in a different way.

MAY 16

The Ouija Board

I remember when I was about 10 years old my aunt bought me a Ouija Board for my birthday.

She said, "You can use this to contact people you love in Heaven." I was so excited! That sounded so awesome! I couldn't wait to try it out!

I only had one older brother who didn't really have any interest in doing things with me, but he would sometimes play Monopoly with me, so it was worth asking specially to talk to dead people! Who wouldn't want to do that? I really needed him because it took two people to use the Ouija Board, so I begged him to play with me. He finally agreed, so we set the board up.

One condition of him agreeing to play was he got to ask the first question, so I of coursed agreed because I was just so happy he agreed to play with me. We very gently put our fingertips on the planchette, and I was concentrating so hard because that's what the directions said to do, and he asked his first question, "Is Gary a little jerk?"

The planchette moved really fast and pointed to 'YES.' "Wow!" he said, "This is a great game and really works!" and off he went. I was so confused. I knew that the board was supposed to be a way to ask questions and answers, and it did seem kind of exciting and spooky, but I didn't expect that.

I told my mother what happened and how I wanted to contact dead people, and how my brother was no help in achieving that goal. I asked her if maybe she would help me do that.

My mom sat me down and explained that the people we love that died talk to us through our soul and not through some piece of cardboard with writing on it. Being so young I didn't realize what a soul was or how people talked through it. The Ouija Board made a lot more sense. But she said if I really love someone that died, I should instead concentrate on how much I love them, talk to them, and they'll hear me and answer.

The Ouija Board stayed in the back of my closet collecting dust for many years. When I went off to college, I took it with me. There was one time my friends and I used it, but it was mostly turned into a 'drinking game,' and then I graduated and just left it behind.

I think Ouija Boards are probably a really cool concept at the age of 10, but as an adult, I don't think you need to use a Ouija Board to connect with the people you love and lost. I believe you have a direct connection called your "intuition" that helps you connect with your loved one through thoughts, feelings, and emotions whenever and wherever you want.

So, forget about the Ouija Board, and trust that connection It will only grow stronger over time, and it's a beautiful way to stay in touch with those you love.

MAY 17

Grief Sucks!

I apologize if you find this title offensive. But if you're like me, and have lost someone you love, then I have a feeling you probably agree with it, more than you are offended by it. I'm also sure you probably have those days where you wake up in the morning and say, "I miss my person and my life sucks."

Maybe you're even having one of those days today. Sometimes when you're grieving, the day can feel like it's nothing more than a backdrop to your pain.

You might also have days where you say, "How long will this last?" "How long do I have to live before I die?"

Okay, I know I sound pretty depressing, but I think if you're reading this you probably agree with me that grief sucks, it really does.

If you do agree with me, then I'm thinking that you should let everyone know so you're not carrying the whole load alone. I'm sure you're still so mad that the person you love was taken away from you. I know it hurts.

Getting mad is okay! I do it all the time. I don't get mad at anyone or anything in particular; I usually just direct it towards my grief. I say, "No. You're not going to crush me today." I'm not a violent person by any means, but sometimes I can feel so small and helpless under the oppressive weight of grief. It sucks!

Sometimes it sucks more than other times. So, if today you're having one of those days that grief is really pushing you down with its heaviness, I hope you will do your best to not let it crush you. If that means getting mad, then I encourage you to get mad.

Maybe tomorrow you'll feel much better, but it's not tomorrow today, so do what you need to do to survive it because grief sucks!

MAY 18

What I Choose

Why do some people die young, and some people live to a very old age? Why do good people die, and bad people live? I really don't know why, and I don't have the answers.

I guess there is no answer to these questions. I think there will always be a lot of unanswered questions, and I'll just have to be okay with that. Maybe it's just part of the great mystery of life.
I've decided that life is too short and precious, and I'm not going to waste it sitting around being miserable, mean, and sad. So, I choose to have a positive upbeat attitude.

I remember shortly after my loss I was shopping for a new cell phone. I was still wearing my wedding ring at the time, and the salesman asked me if my spouse was also going to get a new cell phone. I told him that I was a widower and my spouse had died three weeks ago. At first, he was speechless. Then he said "I just can't believe that you're a widower, and you've only been a widower now for three weeks. You seem to have such a great, upbeat attitude." I told him that it wasn't easy, but I decided to maintain a positive attitude as much as I could most of the time.

I don't believe that I should waste my time on earth feeling miserable and feeling sorry for myself. I choose to move forward. I choose to be optimistic. I choose to heal, honor the past, but embrace the present. I look forward to the future. This is what I choose.

Everyone is different, but after my loss, I was falling into a darkness that scared me because I knew if I let my loss destroy me, I would never again see the light. Then one day I decided that I had two choices: I could get to work on living, or I could get to work on dying.

I decided that what I choose is living. I believe I was loved by someone that would only wish I was happy not sad. What I choose is to honor that love by living the best life I can, and I also choose to never give up.

MAY 19

Am I Healing?

This is a very common question. You may have asked yourself, "Are there ways to measure my healing?"

There are some signs that your grief work is helping. You just need to recognize these signs and realize that you're working through your grief even if it doesn't always feel that way.

You may notice that you're experiencing a lessening of the frequency, intensity, and duration of your pain. Maybe you're finally realizing you had no attachment to the outcome, and you recognize that all that could have been done was done.

Sometimes you might find yourself saying that your loved one is 'dead,' not that 'he left me' or 'she's gone.' This is a sign that you're facing the reality of the situation. Healing is all about a change in focus. Learning to live with the never-to-be-answered questions and living in the present. Knowing that things will never be the same.

When the fog begins to lift, and the dust begins to settle, you realize that life goes on and still consists of happy and enjoyable moments. You actually start to feel good about feeling good.

You make time for fun and laughter while celebrating your good memories that will always stay with you. You can't recognize you're healing if you don't step back from your grief long enough to see it.

I'm not suggesting it's easy but reinvesting your energies in new projects and new choices will give you a renewed sense of life. A purpose. A reason to go on. Healing isn't forcing the sun to shine but letting go of that which blocks the light.

It's my hope that signs of healing continue to shine in your life, on the good days and the not so good days.

MAY 20

Signs From Heaven

Have you ever wondered if you're getting signs from Heaven?

I think our loved ones send us signs all the time. I get them when I least except it, and it always brings me comfort and joy.

I'll be driving in my car and our favorite song will come on and it always seems to be right when I'm missing him the most. It's like he's telling me he's still here.

Even if you don't believe any of this, isn't it your greatest hope that you could somehow, some way, reconnect with the person you lost?

There are a lot of Mediums that claim you can do just that, but what about us regular people? Is it possible for us to do it? We're all born with intuition and the ability to feel, sense, or know something without really understanding how we know.

I believe that our loved one's energy remains after they're gone, and that we can recognize it and feel it even though they're not physically here. They can be pretty creative finding ways to grab our attention!

I think they're always trying to connect with us, and there really is no death, just a changing of worlds. They're in one, and we're in another. They want us to know that they're still a part of our life. If they know something is wrong, they want to help us. They want to get our attention and let us know they're still around. After all, they love us!

So, listen to your intuition and pay attention to the signs. Talk to them as if they were alive and try to hear their thoughts. Imagine how sad it must make them to see you in pain, and how happy they must feel to know you know they haven't really gone away, that they are still a part of your life. So, remember, the next time you think you sense the person you love has come to say hi, you're probably right!

MAY 21

Anniversaries of the Heart

After someone you love dies, you most likely will experience an "anniversary reaction." It's the grief response that's triggered by a date or an event that reminds you of the death. This anniversary of the heart will be felt in your mind, body, heart, and soul. All your memories will come to the forefront and will be heightened. All your feelings will be intensified.

It's important to remember that this is all perfectly normal.

If it's the first anniversary of your loved one's death, for example, it may seem as if you're re-experiencing in vivid detail all you went through on those same days twelve months before. Your grief may be temporarily, but strikingly, reawakened.

In my opinion sometimes these days just suck as much as all the others. You might respond only mildly or moderately to such an anniversary, or you might have a much stronger response.

My advice is to allow your feelings to flow through you, rather than expend all that extra energy holding off your feelings, that will only add to your stress. Talk or write about what's happening to you during these days. Plan a ritual or a commemoration, even if it's small or informal, as a way to honor your loved one.

Take time to reflect on the changes that have occurred, on how you've grown, and on how you might still grow.

These anniversaries of the heart, which sometimes include birthdays, wedding anniversaries, and specific holidays create opportunities for you to include others in your act of remembering.

These times can help you gain personal perspective about your courage and your resourcefulness, not to mention your love.

MAY 22

Standing in the Shadow of Grief

When my father recently died, I grieved his absence in the world and in my life. But what I found even more difficult was standing in the shadow of my mother's grief.

I feel totally inadequate with the awkwardness of seeing her pain. I always feel a little like an uninvited guest when it comes to her sharing with me her deepest part of her soul.

It's really hard to stand at the edge of someone else's grief.

What can I say when I share the pain of my own loss for the same person? I know I can't take away her pain; I'm not even sure what to do with my own.

Grief has a way of unsettling everyone that loved the person that died. I know what it feels like now to lose a parent, but it also stirs up my own unhealed parts of what it also feels like to lose a spouse. I have this instinct to smooth over her emotions, to make everything go back to normal for her....and maybe also for myself.

She needs me; we're both grieving, and we need each other. I've had so many moments of not knowing how to help. That's why I share with her my insights about what healed, and what hurt, when I lost my spouse. I want to help.

Even though it's hard sharing this journey, I'm trying. I know it's awkward and emotional and brings up feelings it would be easier not to feel. But this journey is actually as much for her as it is for me. Those broken pieces inside me, the ones that are triggered when I witness her pain, can also be healed as I share her journey.

It's not easy.

But as I sit with the pain, hers and mine, I learn that hope matters in a way deeper than words. That love prevails.

And as I feel the depth of those hardest emotions, I start to believe in a way that life is beautiful. Even in our grief we connect, love, and support each other.

Maybe that's the gift my father left both of us.

I know I'll survive the loss of my father, just as I survived the loss of my spouse, and I know that my mother will also survive.

I choose to stand with her in the shadow of grief in this place I didn't choose to stand.

MAY 23

In the Fog

Grief causes a fog to roll into your life. This fog of grief can affect your ability to think and concentrate. The fog starts right after the person you love dies. Even after the shock wears off, sometimes the fog can linger. Drifting in and out of your days and nights.

Your grief can get so heavy that it surrounds you and clouds your mind. It interferes with your ability to think clearly. You walk into a room and wonder why you're there. You put your car keys in the refrigerator. You read the same page of a book over and over, and you can't remember what it was about.

If you feel stuck in the fog of your grief, be patient with yourself. It's totally normal and will eventually lift. Just try not to do anything that's really difficult or requires a lot of concentration. If you do have to do something, ask for help.

After my loss I had to put those little yellow 'post-it' notes all around my house to remind me what I had to do. They helped, but I still found myself doing some really goofy things. One day I went food shopping and pushed the cart to my car, drove home, and realized when I got there, I left all my groceries in the cart.

If you still feel like you're living in the fog of grief, try not to make any irreversible decisions until you reach a point where you can clearly think through all the long-term implications.

I promise you the fog is only temporary, it may linger at times or come and go for a while, but sooner or later it will lift.

MAY 24

Finding Hope

I've often had people ask me how I found 'Hope' after my loss. I'm usually honest in my answer that it wasn't easy to find. Here I am eight years later, and I'm still finding myself clinging to my life preserver when grief surfaces.

I guess if I really think about it, I didn't really find hope, it found me. It happened after facilitating my first grief support group, and a member approached me after the last meeting and said, "Thank you for what you do, it saved my life."

I knew that day what I needed to do, help other people. Helping them to heal, helped me to heal. That gave me hope. But the reality is I still search for it every single day.

Finding hope for me was the first time I laughed. In that moment, I knew I might survive. I still wasn't sure exactly how, but I knew I might. I knew, I had a forever road of healing ahead of me. I knew I had no other choice.

Finding hope means there will still be dark days for the remainder of my life, but I'll also laugh every day, and that's okay.

Hope showed me that even though my heart was broken, it could still beat. It beats for the love I still have for my loved one, and I can share that with others by helping them to find hope.

Losing someone you love is like getting a crash course in learning that life doesn't always turn out the way you plan it, but if you work really hard, you can find a way to live again, just differently.

I realized that in order to survive I was going to have to find a new purpose. I needed to figure out who I was in this life without my other half.

Finding hope is knowing that no matter what you do, no matter where you go, you'll always bring your loved one with you.

MAY 25

When Soldiers Cry

It's been less than a year since my father died. I thought a lot about writing about my grief, and how it's very different from the grief I experienced when my spouse died. I write a lot about grief but it's not easy to write about it when you're deep in the belly of its awfulness.

But I know that when you keep your grief holed up inside, it twists you out of shape and makes you someone nobody wants to be around. So, I write.

Grief steamrolled its way into my life eight years ago when my spouse died. Now it has returned after the loss of my father. My father was 89, so I guess I figured his journey was getting close to the end. But still, much like a naïve child, I thought my hero would live forever.

Yes, this time my grief is different. Maybe the loss of my spouse has always felt out of sequence to me. I mean, I guess I just always assumed my father would die before my spouse who was much younger.

I learned eight years ago that life doesn't always happen the way we want it to, it throws curveballs. It's really difficult when you're a Grief Specialist and someone you love dies because everyone thinks you have all the answers, all the secrets. Not true! I'm just like everyone else, I hurt.

Sometimes the hardest thing for me to do is to allow myself to break because for me (and maybe for you too) it's just not cool when we think others think we're not coping.

Our culture celebrates the tearless soldiers, leaving the rest of us, the criers, feeling ashamed of our emotions. Men don't cry, right?

At my father's funeral, I watched all his veteran friends stifle their sadness except for his best friend. I watched tears silently roll down his face, and I knew at that moment, it was safe to allow myself to break.

MAY 26

Acceptance

Do you feel like you'll never be happy again? Do you feel like since your loved one died it's hopeless to even think about being happy again?

If you answered "yes" to these questions, you're not alone. Losing a loved one can be a very traumatic event. When life-altering moments happen, they can make you feel like life can't go on. Maybe you don't even want it to go on. What's the point, right?

This kind of thinking is actually normal and a natural reaction to a major loss. But I also want you to know that while it's very true that a grieving process should be expected, there can be a light at the end of the tunnel. It is possible to feel happy again.

Your life will never be the same again but healing and learning to live again are possible. The loss will be felt, but the sting doesn't have to be so great.

Feeling sad after a big loss is considered perfectly normal. It's what comes after the grief process has been worked through that seems to truly determine whether a person can be happy again or not. A lot of it has to do with a willingness to accept the loss.

Denial is usually the first stage of the grieving process. It's an inability to accept the death, and this is a very normal part of grieving.

Acceptance is usually the final stage of the grieving process. This is when you get to the point on your grief journey when you realize there's nothing you can do to fix the situation. Your heart doesn't want to believe what your head is telling it your deceased loved one can't be brought back.

You may not want to hear this right now, but it is possible to feel happy again without dishonoring your loved one. Getting to the acceptance stage, however, can be really hard. When a heart has suffered a big loss, it can be very difficult to even have the desire to live or seek out ways to be happy again. When the time is right, you'll try it. Trust me on this! It won't be easy, and somedays will be better than others.

You'll do it in small steps. It's very important to let the grief process run its course before even expecting to be truly happy again. Guilt, pain, and sadness all need to be worked through before living again can be a true reality.

So, how do you reach acceptance? In a nutshell, it's all about focusing on the important things and redefining happiness.

While things will never be the same, 'different' can bring its own sense of happiness.

MAY 27

Please Come Back

How often do you say this?

After the loss of my spouse, I would walk the beach every day. Regardless of the weather (rain, shine, snow or wind), I was walking. I would cry and look out over the ocean and say, "Please come back!"

Sometimes it was a scream, and sometimes just a whisper.

If you find yourself doing this, you're not alone. Yearning for a lost love is normal. It's the heart's way of refusing to say goodbye.

People will tell you all kinds of things like, "At least you have your memories," and "You'll be together again someday." Let's be honest, they sound good, but they don't really change the fact that all you really want is to have them back. Am I right?

No matter what people tell you, there will always be those times when you think about the person you love and lost and say, "Please come back."

I still walk the beach. I still yearn for what my heart wants. That will never change. I've accepted that. I know he's not coming back. I've accepted that too.

The heart wants what the head can't understand. That's what it means when grief becomes a constant companion. Your head knows they can't come back, but your heart may never understand, and that's okay!

MAY 28

The Grief Lens

When you lose someone you love, it's very easy to start looking at the world through a grief lens. You just suffered the most terrible trauma and devastation you could ever imagine, so of course everything looks foggy. It's totally reasonable and expected for you to be miserable for a while. The trouble is these negative feelings can cause you to reach conclusions and hold onto beliefs that are really pessimistic and not true.

You may not realize how, over time, negativity can impact your overall worldview. You start thinking things like, "My loved one died, and now life and everything in my life just sucks," or "I'm all alone, nobody cares, I have no friends, and nobody loves me."

When you look at life through the grief lens with a negative attitude, you may be more likely to find depressing, cynical, and suspicious explanations for everything. You start to feel like your life is awful, but everyone else's is happy. You believe this will never change; you'll always be sad.

When you're looking through the grief lens, you can get very defensive if someone tries to make you feel better, tries to love you, help you, or just be your friend.

So, when you're ready, I simply ask you to pay attention to the ways in which you see things through the grief lens, and how they can deceive you, and magnify your unhappiness.

Awareness, in my opinion, is the most important step because it allows you to understand the ways that your interpretations of life may be distorted due to your grief and pain.

I realize you may not be ready or able to take this step right now, but it's always good to know that no matter how helpless grief makes you feel, you aren't completely powerless or alone.

MAY 29

A Loss Worth Grieving

There's so much that people forget about pet loss. When we're young and we lose a pet, we hear, "Oh, don't feel bad. You can get another one!" or "That's okay, it was just a pet. It's not like you lost (insert any human name)."

I don't know about anyone else, but my dog is my best friend. I have lost pets in the past, and I still grieve the loss.

Losing a pet can be a devastating, grief-inducing, and all-around heartbreaking loss. Pets are a part of our everyday routine. They're with us every single day. They're a part of our routines and regular activities. Feeding them, taking them out, playing with them, and sleeping with them is what every day normal looks like for us. It's really jarring when that routine and normalcy are upset.

Pets give us a reason to get up in the morning. They're dependent and need us in order to live. Their dependency on us gives us something outside of ourselves to care for, so when they die, not only do those tasks stop, but that feeling of 'doing for' something outside of ourselves stops too. And that's really hard.

Pets have seen us at our best and our worst and are with us through our milestones. They sit with us and stay with us through our personal griefs and losses. Pets don't question our joy, our celebration, or our grief. They continue to love us through it. Our pets are a strong constant in a life that's always changing.

Pets are a source of unconditional love. This is it, the bottom line. Losing unconditional love is the biggest reason we grieve when our pets die.

There are so many reasons why our pets are members of our lives, and for those reasons, their death matters. Their loss is worth grieving.

MAY 30

Betrayed

What happens if your loved one's death feels like a betrayal?

After all, they promised to be by your side and to love you forever; dying wasn't part of the deal.

Feeling betrayed after the loss of a spouse is just another emotion attached to grief; you were left alone and that's not fair. You feel a variety of feelings and emotions, but the one that really hurts the most is the broken promise of a future spent together.

When someone you love dies, it's normal to keep going back and forth between missing them and feeling betrayed by them for leaving. At times the mixed emotions can feel like you're literally sinking into insanity. One moment you cry, and the next you scream.

Probably nobody told you that grief does that to people, and because you didn't know what you're feeling is normal, you feel even more alone.

I know what it feels like to not want to get out of bed. I know what it feels like to not want to take a shower or brush your teeth or even eat. I know what it's like to lose twenty pounds in six weeks, to lose friends, and to lose your sense of safety, and I know the feeling that the world has ended, and you were left behind alone and miserable. It's only natural after all that to feel betrayed to be the one left behind.

I've been there, so believe me when I say, there is hope.

There is, in fact, a light at the end of the tunnel. But the only way to get to that light is to walk through it. There's no way of getting around the process, and the earlier you begin the journey of healing, the sooner you'll reach peace.

The journey is long, but there's no race and no competition. It's a journey with yourself. There will be days when you'll feel stronger than ever, and some days will bring you back to your knees.

Feeling betrayed is just one of so many emotions on this rollercoaster journey. So, even when you're down, feeling as if you've made no progress, remember that progress is being made every day you choose to be alive.

Progress is being made every day you choose to take another breath.

Remember, you weren't betrayed, you're alive for a reason, and you're going to survive.

MAY 31

Missing Mom

Your mom gave you your life. Her face was the first one you set eyes on. She was your first friend. She's the one who rocked you as a baby, kissed your cuts, and eased your pain. In a sense, your mom is the biggest part of your life. So how do you deal with the death of this most important person?

The pain is crippling, and it hits you at random moments. One minute you might be fine, and the next minute you're curled up in a ball on the floor in inconceivable pain. If you've lost your mom, then you're probably sitting there nodding your head right now.

The first few days after your mom dies feels like a nightmare. You'll function only in that you will make funeral arrangements, contact relatives, console family members, and go forward taking care of necessary tasks. Numbness is the perfect word for this time. The funeral will come and go, and so will the relatives and well-wishers. Back to business as usual.

After the service, it's time for life to go back to normal, right? Wrong! Life will never be normal again. It will be different, but it will never be as it was. How could it be? Your mom died.

For the first few weeks, your friends and family will be wonderful. They'll offer you lots of smiles and hugs. They'll offer to help you, and they'll listen as you talk about how bad the pain is. You'll hear a lot of "I'm here for you", and "If there's anything I can do" comments during this time.

After a couple months, it will seem like people have forgotten that you lost this important part of your life. They'll stop asking how you are, and they might even look worried when you want to talk about your mom. You see, people who haven't gone through this pain think there's a period of grieving and that's it. After a certain time, you should be ready to move on with your life and 'get over it.'

But you'll never get over it. The pain will lessen, and the moments of intense grief will be farther apart, but how can you ever get over losing your mom? It's just not possible.

I think your mom would most likely want you to smile and live your life. She may have been your biggest cheerleader in life, so continue to make her proud. Make her legacy be yours to carry forward.

At some point after your mom's death, you'll find reasons to smile again. I think this is one of the greatest things you can do to honor your mom and the love you have for her in your heart.

Your mom deserves to be remembered; she deserves to be missed.

JUNE

JUNE 1

Being Human

My brain has been wired for survival for eight years now. I often wonder what the effects must be of that.

In the beginning, I was afraid that the rawness of my pain had a time limit to it, and if I didn't act and respond to grief the way society expected me to, then I would be rejected. It's that fear of rejection that continues to pull me away from sitting with my pain.

I've become hypersensitive to other people's reactions, and I can sense when my pain is too raw and uncomfortable for them, so I avoid the loudest and most consuming part of me to enter the conversation in order to make them more comfortable.

I believe that the key to healing is to embrace the sorrow of loss throughout life. Loss happens continuously, but we often forget to experience it because we glorify the illusion of always being strong and resilient.

Fear is a block to healing. It activates our survival brain and keeps us there. Never feeling safe enough to process our emotions, we continue to suffer instead. But, once you have had your authentic pain validated and witnessed, this frees up space for you to become an enlightened witness to another.

That's why I think there are so many people needlessly suffering right now. We're all afraid to confront the human condition of pain because we're afraid to lose our attachments to others. So, we mask it and avoid it and deny it at any cost.

I don't want to lose my attachments to other people, and I don't want you to do that either. I think if you do, you'll end up terrified of being alone, and terrified of never being loved again.

That would be terrible, wouldn't it?

JUNE 2

'Forever Sadness'

There's a place that's very dark and very lonely. It's called 'Forever Sadness'. You probably never heard of it because I made it up. I make stuff up sometimes just to get my point across. I'll tell you a little about this place called 'Forever Sadness.'

There are a lot of people that live there. They cry all the time and refuse to find any joy in life. They believe if they remain always sad, it will keep them connected to someone they love that died.

These people are very quick to accept that everything is bad, and they're just a little too weary or angry to be positive and constructive. They're afraid to acknowledge their pain or to let it go. The people that live in 'Forever Sadness' may not have seen the sign at the entrance that reads: A Nice Place to Visit - Just Don't Live Here.

Okay, so I know you are probably thinking I'm being really silly, but I believe feeling sad is perfectly fine, and acknowledging and feeling the full range of emotions after a loss is a necessary part of being human. Especially the pain. The trouble is, for some reason or another, people might discourage you from spending any time in your pain. Sometimes your pain comes from a place so scary that you don't want to say it out loud or talk about it. You go to 'Forever Sadness' and move in.

I don't know what you've been through, and I don't know who you have to turn to, but if you've been holding your pain inside, I would encourage you to take the first step and say it out loud. Your pain matters. Acknowledging your pain is an important first step in fumbling your way out of 'Forever Sadness.'

I know sometimes things feel so bad it seems like they'll never change. I want you to acknowledge your pain, because that's important, I just don't want you to live in 'Forever Sadness' for the rest of your life.

JUNE 3

I Want To Feel Ready

I recently told a friend that I didn't want my old life anymore. My old life is the life I had to live after my spouse died, and that's a life that was full of grief and pain. My previous life didn't exist anyway. When I look at pictures from that life, they're just reminders of what I used to have but don't anymore.

It's funny, in the beginning after I lost my spouse, I was afraid the pain would leave. It was almost like I'd lose him if it went away. Now, I'm still carrying the pain, but it takes a backseat to my happiness. But like I've always suspected, grief has a life of its own. I don't control it and it's doesn't listen to me. There came a time when all of a sudden there was a definite shift forward. A sense of 'getting on' with things.

I can tell you from my own experience that this wasn't always easy. I could decide that I was going to move forward in a positive way in my life, and still, it could feel like I was pushing a giant elephant up a stairway.

And then, the thought would pop into my head just like it did after my spouse died, "How do I get through the day, let alone the rest of my life?" Then the answer came to me; get twice as strong, and then, get stronger than that. Sometimes that thought makes me feel very tired, and sometimes I feel ready. I want to feel ready.

It's strange how much grief takes out of you in just trying to function every day, and for me, I think the reserves that were depleted during my spouse's illness, and then further smashed into smithereens after he died, have now been fully replenished.

For a long time, I felt that it'd be much easier to sit around waiting to die and never doing a darn thing. It seemed like an option.

But then I realized I still wanted my life to mean something, and that was a positive sign to me.

JUNE 4

Lost at Sea

Have you ever heard the expression, "No one gets out alive"? I think it refers, not only to death, but also grief. I would like to think that missing someone you've lost is some kind of 'romantic' pining away for that person. But the fact of the matter is, it sucks, and there's only one way to get through it, you just have to get through it.

Today is the anniversary of the day we met. I keep thinking that I'll pass these anniversaries with positive feelings and flying colors, but it just hasn't worked out that way. I still sometimes feel lost at sea.

I woke up yesterday with a sharp spear of pain going through me, out of nowhere. Ah, it's the anniversary coming! And from this pain, feeling such anger, I realized, even after all this time, I'm still so mad he died. All the ugly feelings that I would like to keep buried, the anger that is so inappropriate especially after burying someone I love. Why would I go to such awful thoughts?

And then, I woke up this morning, and before I opened my eyes, the thought came, calmly and clearly, "We've GOT to stop cancer. It's taking the ones we love. We have to keep fighting until we eradicate this disease."

My spouse was taken too soon and taken in an unfair way. And it's happening to others, and it needs to stop. And that's another thing I remembered this past week that made me angry. It's not exactly a pleasant memory. But it's real. Too real.

This morning I don't feel angry, like yesterday, and I'm glad of that. I'm glad I'm not too sad and depressed. I do still feel lost at sea on these days, but I also see hope on the horizon. I looked at a picture of our first date, and I couldn't help but smile. Yeah, we sure had some fun times.

And my hope today is that I feel your spirit with me, soaring out on the open sea.

JUNE 5

"It Will Be Okay"

After my spouse died, everyone told me, "It will be okay." I often wondered how these people that never lost a spouse were so sure about that. Sometimes when people haven't lost someone or experienced what you're going through, they can say some really unhelpful things. For me, this was one of them.

Maybe it would be okay, but when you first lose a person you love, the pain is too heavy to imagine that it's ever going to be okay. When you're grieving, there are just some things that you don't want or need to hear.

I remember I went to the cable company to take my spouse's name off the account. I waited in a long line and then when it was my turn the lady at the counter said to me, "Why are you taking his name off the account?"

At first, I thought it was really none of her business, but then I started to cry and replied, "Because he died."

She said, "It will be okay, but you're in the wrong line."

At that point it wasn't okay. Nothing was okay. Nothing was going to be okay. I didn't need or want people to keep telling me that. But tell me they did.

What I've learned is that it never really is okay. You just learn to live around it and find ways to incorporate your loss into your life.

Looking back, I'm pretty sure that lady at the cable company never lost a spouse because if she did, she would have just helped me instead of making me cry and sending me away to wait in another long line.

When people tell me they lost someone they love, I never tell them it will be okay. I just tell them it sucks!

JUNE 6

Suzanne

Did you ever feel so lonely that you didn't know how you would survive? Like a really terrible loneliness? If you lost someone you love, I'm sure your answer is, "Yes."

I remember shortly after my loss, I was sitting with someone I just met on a porch that overlooked the ocean, and I sobbed uncontrollably. For the previous two months, I had become so desperate, depressed and in pain. I remember the whole world felt like it was tipping to one side, and I had to hang on bracing myself against it to keep from falling off.

Hanging on and hanging on. Never to be happy again. That's what the fresh pain of loss felt like to me. I remember thinking at the time, particularly, this was what my life was going to be like going forward, and that I was always going to be alone. No love, no hope, no nothing.

But then life sucked me back in. That someone I was sitting beside on the porch would challenge me to feel again, connect, and dare to risk opening my heart. That someone would help me find the strength to raise myself up again and meet a new day. That someone was named Suzanne.

Suzanne knew I was so incredibly vulnerable. She wasn't afraid of my grief. Instead, she looked it in the eye and taught me how to see that I was not the only one needing help, compassion, empathy, and most of all love. She offered me a job working with developmentally disabled adults, and that job opened my heart wider than it had ever been stretched.

It's strange how this grief can weave through your life. There were times I couldn't see the forest for the trees. It's an understatement to say there were times I just wanted to give up, and times when I was so truly weak. But then, Suzanne showed me how to stop closing down my heart, and open it to those who needed it, and those that eventually filled it up again.

There will always be a hole in my heart that belongs to who I love and lost, but there is so much more room there to be filled with love. I feel so very sorry for that guy who was me that day on the porch, and how there was nothing I could do to help him.

But I tell him now that I understand. I remind him that he needs to forgive himself. For not being perfect, for not finding his way. I'd like to whisper in his ear that it's not over.

I'd like to tell him to believe Suzanne when she says that "very, very good things are going to happen, and you'll receive unexpected gifts in the future." I'd mostly like to thank Suzanne, but you see, I can't because she died.

I miss her very much, but I'm so thankful and feel so blessed Suzanne sat on that porch with me that day and taught me how to love again.

JUNE 7

Angels

Do you ever feel the presence of your loved one? Does it seem like they're trying to communicate with you? I think it's very possible they are doing just that!

I think our lost loved ones are constantly drawing our attention towards signs, and they will leave you with clues that will guide you in the right direction. Sometimes, these signs may seem small at first but can increase in frequency when they're focused on, acknowledged, and appreciated.

They also connect through sights, sounds, and smells. Have you ever noticed a particular smell, shape, or sound, and you were unable to identify the source? This may show up in the form a scent or a ringing in your ear.

There were times I saw shapes in the clouds, sparks of lights and flickering lamps. I also see rainbows and know it's a sign that my loved one is bringing me encouragement and validation from heaven.

Have you ever received a message in your mind or heard a voice whisper in your ear? This is your loved one in angel form reaching out to you. They may even be that bright star in the sky that catches your attention. They may be numbers you see that have some significance to you or a song on the radio.

Maybe you don't believe any of this or maybe you do, but I think that there are angels around us all the time. I believe that my loved one loves me enough to let me know he's still with me. I get signs all the time!

Once you begin to tune into the signs from your angel and practice present moment awareness, you'll become more conscious of your angel and the guidance and assistance they have for you.

If you notice any of these signs, be open to the message they may be trying to send you!

JUNE 8

Soul to Soul

I want you to take a moment and think about how much your loved one contributed to your happiness. Just by being who they were, they created so much happiness for you, and by recognizing this, it will remind you about the love they had for you and the place they held in your life. Nothing they added to you can ever be taken away just because they died.

I think the transition from this life to the next doesn't need to be perceived as something final. Beyond merely having faith in the afterlife is the experience of surrendering to your loved one's continued presence in your life, in spirit form.

The wind rustling the leaves of a tree, a dragonfly flying above your head, or even a dream that brings you comfort are all signs of the continued connection that exists between your souls.

When the person you love died, your life changed forever, but keeping their spirit and love alive can create a greater definition of yourself and open a new meaningful chapter in your life.

If you know me at all, you know I never use the term 'letting go', I prefer to say, 'moving forward.' Even if you aren't a fan of that term either, the fact stands that we can't go back to the past. The only direction available to us is forward. But I think there's a time when we begin to 'let go' but with love. Getting over a painful experience is like crossing monkey bars. Sometimes you have to let go at some point….in order to move forward to the next bar.

Moving forward doesn't mean you forget or go on with your life as if their life and death weren't important.

It just means that you have found the soul connection that always existed and have embraced it enough to live your life knowing you aren't letting go but taking them with you as you move forward.

JUNE 9

"Why Is Everybody Afraid of Me"

One thing about grief that's hard to understand is that nobody wants to talk about it. I talk about it all the time, every day. I try to pull it out of the closet and bring it out in the open. It exists, and it affects a lot of people. So why pretend it doesn't exist?

Before the person you love died, I bet you felt like you had a really supportive group of family and friends. Then I bet after the person you love died; you thought it would be those same people who would be there to support you. If that's what happened, consider yourself truly blessed.

But for many of you, that may not have been what happened. Maybe that network of people you thought you could turn to shrunk. How could that be? Don't they know that their support is needed now more than ever? So, what happened that those people you thought you could count on retreated when you needed them most?

I'll tell you why because they're scared.

They think because if it can happen to you, it can happen to anybody. It can even happen to them. They're scared of how this loss has changed you. You might not be the same fun, warm, and happy person they know and love. But most of all, they are scared of saying or doing the wrong thing.

Your loss and your grief have made them feel helpless. They want to help, they want to take your pain away, but they don't know how. They're afraid of saying something that will make you cry. They think if they mention their name, you'll get upset. They don't realize all you do all day and night is think about your loss.

I find most people would rather hear something, rather than nothing. I also think they would prefer someone just give them a hug or hold their hand. Basically, instead of being afraid of your grief, acknowledge it.

The problem with grief is you may not know what you need or how to vocalize it, and that's okay. Try to find the people you want to be a part of your grief journey and let them know what this experience has been like for you. Tell them how lost, isolated, and confused you feel. Educate them on the process.

It's frustrating to be the person that is suffering, and then you also have to be the one to reach out. I get it. But, when you're ready you can find empathy for those in your life who want to help and don't know how. These people really are desperate to help, they're just afraid of your grief.

They knew how to deal with 'you,' they just don't know how to deal with a 'grieving' you.

JUNE 10

Happy More Than Sad

There are times when I feel like I'm completely over the pain of my loss. Like I'm dancing on clouds. So, I'm going along like that, and then out of nowhere, I'll crash and burn. Suddenly, it's like nothing has changed at all in these past years, and it's like my spouse died just yesterday.

Do you ever feel like that?

There was a period of time where I almost felt guilty when I was feeling good. There was this unexplainable fear that if I felt good, I'd be letting my spouse go, that I'd be forgetting about him. You know, my pain was somehow keeping him close to me.

So in the months after he died, I thought bravery was daring to be happy again. But then I found that some kind of feeling good was a necessity.

About a year and a half into my grief journey, I thought I would surely die if things didn't improve. My body was so trashed by being overwhelmed with so much constant pain for so many, many months. I needed some kind of relief. Needed it or I wouldn't survive. Luckily, things did start to lighten a bit. Often, I would still crash and burn, terribly, but I was finally getting some relief!

As time has gone on, I've been happy more than sad, and I'm amazed at how long I can feel good now. It's gone from minutes to hours to days to weeks. Sometimes I forget that I can hurt so much, and it makes it even more surprising when I plummet and crash yet again.

The wound is still there. I've just learned to toughen up, building up a scar around it so that it doesn't hurt every time I touch it.

And still, sometimes the hurt rises from within.

In a strange way, I've started to adjust to these "up and down" roller coaster cycles. I've come to accept that it isn't something I can control, I just know that it's coming my way. It's coming one way or another. To some degree, I've stopped wondering, judging, and anticipating, and I just roll with it.

And when I wake up in the morning, I do my best to be grateful for whatever may come my way. No doubt about it, I'm grateful for whatever happiness I feel. The better I feel, the closer I feel to my spouse.

I think all that pain was getting in the way of feeling what's really there because what's really there has been, and still is, really good.

JUNE 11

Goodbye to the 'Old Me'

One of the most difficult things about surviving grief is saying goodbye to yourself. It's not easy saying goodbye to the person you love that died, but it's even worse saying goodbye to your whole life: your past, present, and your hope for the future.

That's exactly what happened to me. I had to say goodbye to the 'old me'. It was hard, because the 'old me' was the strong, confident and smart guy that was a happy husband, and part of a team. One half of a whole. But that person died when the love of my life died.

So, who was this 'new me'? This vulnerable guy that was crying and sad all the time. He wasn't acting in any way that was ever familiar to me. He was afraid to be home alone and sleep with the lights off. He was avoiding people for fear they might ask too many questions.

Questions the 'new me" couldn't answer. It was like some stranger was hanging out in my familiar body. The problem was that I was comfortable with the 'old me'. I never wanted to say goodbye. The 'new me' made me nervous. He seemed so out of control. He was just like a baby trying to learn how to walk.

The 'new me' had to figure out who I was, and what I wanted to do, where I wanted to go, and how the hell I was going to get there. It sure wasn't easy. I fell more times than I can count. But I always got up. I think if my loved one came back, he wouldn't even recognize the 'new me,' but I think he would be proud of what I've done to honor him and our life together.

Saying goodbye is never easy. When you lose the person you love, your heart shatters and your world falls apart. Saying goodbye to the person you were in relation to the person who died, now that's the really hard part. Saying goodbye to the 'old me' was the hardest thing I ever did in my life, but the 'new me' will never say goodbye to the memories.

JUNE 12

The Child You Lost Matters

Loss is something that's never easy, but especially excruciating when it was the life you created, carried, birthed, and held. It's so important to remember your child but also important to remember you.

Grief is one of the most uncomfortable topics in the world. When you're grieving the loss of a child, you struggle to capture the wide range of emotions you feel and to grasp what kind of support you need. But for others watching you grieve, it's awkward and sometimes silent.

If you lost a child, it's okay to take as long as you need because you'll need forever.

It's okay to feel the range of emotions, to talk about it, to cry, to not be all right sometimes.
I unconditionally accept your loss.

While grief may take a lifetime, healing allows your pain to feel like that boulder on your chest each and every day is a little lighter. It's anger, acceptance, pain, and comfort.

Your journey matters. You matter. The child you lost matters. The idea that things are different, and you might not always be able to put your finger on what's best for you at each moment, it's important to surround yourself with others who allow you to grieve in your own time and your own way.

In my opinion, losing a child is the worst. But in your grief and your process to heal, you only benefit you and your family when you begin to assess what you can and will need from yourself and from others. If you don't know right now or tomorrow, it's okay. It takes time. If it feels selfish at first, that's okay too. It's not selfish, but it can be uncomfortable to put your needs first when you're feeling the weight of such a heavy loss.

However, when you allow yourself to prioritize what you need, that will benefit your life and health. Reach out to the people who help you accomplish that; it WILL lead to healing.

Through self-care you recognize that when your mental health improves, others around you benefit and want to improve too. You remember that your journey matters and that you matter.

And the child you lost matters.

You're not alone. Many others have endured the tragedy of losing a child. However, your journey through this difficult loss is different and as important as anyone else's loss.

You deserve unlimited time to grieve and unlimited time to heal. Your grief and healing matter, so take your time because you matter, too.

JUNE 13

Embracing Your Loss

Although it has been over eight years now since I lost my spouse, some days it feels like a lifetime ago and other days it feels like only yesterday.

The one thing grief and life have in common is they're both so fluid and ever changing. My life now is so different, just as my grief has changed over the years. Sometimes I feel like if I went back in time to when it happened, I wouldn't even recognize myself. I've changed.

My loss changed me forever. The sadness and sorrow are no longer as intense as they once were, but the grief remains. It's just changed form and taken a back seat to everything else in my life. I no longer let it dominate my life, instead I live around it. It's a part of me now.

My grief is a reminder of my loss, which is something I'll never forget, nor do I want to forget. The love I had for my spouse is a part of my story.

A good part of my story.

Since my loss I've had some incredibly happy times in my life and some incredibly sad times. I believe we're all just walking each other home, and if we can do that with compassion and empathy then the world would be a better place.

I think it's important that we remember the person who died. Can you still have a relationship with someone who died? Of course! You have your memories which become your ongoing relationship to the person you love.

I still talk to my spouse every day. and I encourage you to pursue this kind of non-physical relationship. Remembering the past makes hoping for the future possible.

The future will only become open to new experiences if you continue to embrace the past.

JUNE 14

Green Acres

I'm feeling so much stronger after my loss, and you will too one day. I promise!

In all honesty, it comes down to accepting that nothing will ever be the same in your life and then learning to view your life differently. I guess it comes down to a matter of perception. Our lives are just like a mirror reflecting back what's going on with us. In time, you'll crawl out of the ashes of your loss and find the strength to actually affect some change in your life.

I can tell you this because I'm seven years into my 'widowerhood' (yes, I do hate that word 'widower', but I'm used to it now, and I'm starting to give in). After a couple of years I suddenly looked around and saw that my life had been falling apart. It's like I came out of a fog, one that I didn't even know I was in.

I thought I had it pretty together during those first few years (considering a nuclear bomb had been placed under my life and exploded), but as I started coming out of that fog, I saw that, not only was I a widower, but I was a stereotypical widower. My yard looked a mess, the inside of my house was full of expired food, everything was collecting dust, things were broken or not working. My life looked like that derelict house that Lisa and Oliver Douglas lived in on that show "Green Acres"!

Also, during my two-year haze, I made some bad choices, like cutting down trees just so I wouldn't have to rake leaves. Letting things go on the outside just because I didn't care how my house or yard looked. Beware the widower!

I tried so hard not to make stupid widower mistakes, and still I made stupid widower mistakes (much more important ones than what I've list here). They say you shouldn't make any important decisions during the first year of widowhood. And I'd say, be careful even up to two years! Even now, at eight years in, I'm still a bit shaky about the quality of my judgment on some things.

In the past, I would look around quite frequently to see what life was reflecting back at me. Is it a mess? Does everything look perfect? And at a certain point, I stopped. Why? Because it wasn't going to change anything. I mean, I didn't need to look at the condition of my house to know that I was in pain. Trust me, I already knew that. At that point, Green Acres was the place I'd rather be because nothing else mattered.

I'm so much stronger now. I'm still working on trying to bring my life back together. It's a long process. I think it might even take the rest of my life, and that's okay. It's not easy rebuilding your life from the ground up. I'm still doing it. I've made some pretty good progress.

My house doesn't look like Green Acres anymore, and that alone seems promising!

JUNE 15

A Thief Called Grief

After my loss I started to cling to everything and everyone. I no longer trusted anything if it was out of my sight. You see, grief robs you of joy, time, and sanity. You might even lose a few months of memory. Consider that a blessing!

Grief hurts. It physically hurts. Headaches, panic attacks, chest pain, aches, and fatigue. They can all be unwelcome visitors during the healing process.

But it's also a strange comfort. Grief is isolating, but it never leaves you alone. In the moments you wake up crying, the car rides with tears streaming, grief is your companion. When everyone moves on, forgetting your loss, grief remembers.

I was surprised by how much I fell in love with my grief. I nurtured it, gave it room to grow. I rarely fought it. To excuse my grief, to send it on its way, felt like a betrayal. It was all I had left.

You might not believe it right now, but the physical responses to grief do lessen over time. The tears become more manageable. The regrets are replaced with memories. But just like with anything, this doesn't happen overnight.

For a few years, my grief made me bitter, fearful, and lonely. I found myself always waiting for the other shoe to drop. Seven years later, my grief has made me more compassionate, empathetic, and loving. My joy and faith have returned.

I'm now a proud member of the club I never wanted to join. I know what it means to be there for someone, unconditionally, bringing light during their darkest times.

Grief is a thief, but I've learned that although my grief will always live with me, the bitterness didn't have to.

JUNE 16

When You Died, I Died

My world fell apart when you died. It was like the whole Earth shifted on its axis, causing me to fall and keep falling. Nothing seemed real, yet all around me people were going about their day, living their life, yet mine had ended. I had no past, and I could see no future. Just darkness. The light was gone.

When you died, I died. The only difference was I was still here, and you were gone.

I was lucky to have you. You were loving, caring, giving, and kind. The Earth was a better place when you lived on it. I learned to give to others and be generous by watching you. Losing you crushed me but also made me strong. I love that I became strong, but I hate that I had to lose you to do it.

I hope you can know some small piece of my life. It makes me sad to think that you're missing all I'm doing. It makes me even more sad to think that you're not here to be doing all you should be doing. I'm hoping someday I'll see you again, and you'll tell me you were there with me.

You'll tell me that everywhere I went, you were right beside me, I just couldn't see you. You'll tell me every time I was happy you smiled, and every time I was sad, you saw my tears. You'll tell me that you were sorry you had to leave, but you were proud of what I did on my own.

When you died, I died, but I had to live among the living, and I sure could've used your help.

JUNE 17

The Weight of Grief

Grief is one of the most devastating experiences that any human being can face. It can feel so debilitating and overwhelming.

When you deeply love a person, it sometimes becomes a double-edged sword when you're faced with losing them.

The more you love, the more painful the loss is felt.

Much of your future horizon becomes distorted, shrouded, and hidden. All that remains, for a time, is the dominating awareness and heaviness of grief.

My experience of loss was difficult and painful in the face of my own grief. The weight of grief was particularly heavy for a few years.

Eventually, I chose to acknowledge, accept, and welcome the truth.

Not because I'm crazy, but because I felt ready, in a safe place, to face my feelings of sadness and grief.

Since that time, I have begun to feel most of the weight of grief lifting like shafts of light into a very dark place. I'm sure there will be many moments when grief breaks into my awareness again.

But I feel more able now to agree with the well-worn phrase very much, "It's better to have loved and lost than to have never loved at all."

JUNE 18

Let Things Be Different

Your loved one's death can be one of the most devastating times in your life. Not only will you deal with grief, but if you lost a partner or spouse, you'll also experience a lot of firsts by yourself and you'll need to learn how to navigate the world alone. It'll take time to adjust. Remember, your partner or spouse would encourage you to keep moving forward. Even though they are no longer with you in physical form, they'll always be with you in your heart.

What can you do to embrace life after the loss of your partner or spouse?

First of all, be patient. In times of grief, you may feel the desire to 'speed up' grief. That's a normal response, but unfortunately, that's not really possible. Be patient with yourself and your grief. Set aside dedicated time to be with your grief and try not to rush healing.

When you give yourself time to heal, you'll find that peace might be waiting on the other side of your grief. Allow yourself the time and space to embrace each new experience that comes your way. Everything you do may feel very unknown or different than in the past. Things may not be the same but remember that it's possible to be happy again. The first step in this process is to allow things to be different.

Your loss can bring about a lot of change. You're learning how to live in the world again without the person you love. Instead of fighting the change, try embracing it. It's not easy when grief is present, but it is possible.

Let yourself know that you're safe to embrace change. It's best to ease into new things. Be patient with yourself during this time and take each new experience as it comes. Things may change, but your partner or spouse will always be in your heart. It's okay to feel sad and to miss the one you love in your life, but it's also okay to let things be different.

JUNE 19

Grief Is a Journey, Not a Destination

When I first lost my spouse, I didn't consider that I would grieve forever. I thought after a couple of years things would get better, that the pain would disappear. That obviously never happened, and I'm so glad now that it didn't.

I was recently facilitating a grief support group and sitting in a room full of grieving people who had just lost someone. The conversation was awkward as those around me were struggling to find the words that accurately described the loss of a loved one who was sitting right next to them only a few months ago. Eventually they stumbled through their stories. They had found comfort in those who sat around them, in a community that allowed them to try and find the words.

In each of those people was an individual grief story that would live on in them forever. While the pain will get less intense over time, the memory of their loved one will never leave them.

Grief, like most painful things, leaves its mark on your whole life not just parts of it. It doesn't matter if the person you lost died only months ago or over a decade ago. Grief doesn't fade away.

Each person that's lost is uniquely remembered by the legacy they left behind. Grief is a journey of missing that person and remembering who they were. It's not a destination that ends once a certain number of years have gone by since they died. There will always be moments of sadness and longing for them to be sitting next to you just one last time.

The beauty of grief is that it's a deep reminder of the love that you had. That love never disappeared even when that person did. I'm honored to grieve my spouse. I'm honored to have been loved so well.

Grief is a beautiful journey, not a destination with a clear ending point.

As my journey continues, I'll always be reminded of the legacy left behind.

JUNE 20

Only Speak if It Can Improve the Silence

Without anybody asking, my friend Carol always tells everyone that they can heal their grief by chanting. She then proceeds to tell them how much they would benefit from chanting. Since she has never had a significant loss in her life, I asked her why she does this, and she said, "Because it works!" But I'm not so sure that's true. I tried chanting, and it did nothing for me. When it comes to sharing advice, we all think we're really good at it, and that right there is the problem.

When it comes to offering advice to people who are grieving, sharing is a wonderful idea, but for someone to preach to people who have suffered a loss, that they themselves have not, can be dangerous. The reason is that loss is so unique. Relationships are so unique. Grief is so unique.

The reason this is such a slippery slope is because I'm here sharing my own views with you, so how is this different?

The distinction, I believe, is determined by whether we are asked to share, or if we simply force our opinions on everyone. Carol may believe chanting heals grief, but she has no actual proof. Telling people that it's a fact may cause them to feel defeated when it doesn't work for them.

Unfortunately, advice is sometimes used as a way to 'fix' those that are grieving. The problem is, grief can't be fixed, it has to be experienced.

Don't get me wrong, maybe chanting has helped heal your grief, all I'm saying is sometimes I think we shouldn't talk about something unless someone actually asks us.

Before speaking, ask yourself, "Was I asked?" "Is this necessary to say?" and "Does this need to be said by me right now?"

Because the ego will make us believe we do everything for all the right reasons, but it's not always true.

JUNE 21

I Just Didn't Know

I often feel like I owe an apology to everyone whose pain and suffering came before my own. Before my loss I didn't understand their grief. I didn't know what it felt like to have your heart ripped out of your chest. I just didn't know.

I'm sorry now, that in my discomfort, I may have avoided or changed the subject when they really just wanted to talk about the person that died. I'm sorry I didn't acknowledge their loss and what an impact that must have had on them. I just didn't know.

I wish I had the courage back then to say their loved one's name instead of acting like nothing happened, but I thought it would make them sad. I just didn't know.

I wish I didn't say stupid things like, "everything happens for a reason" and "they're in a better place." That was so dumb. I didn't understand saying stuff like that was only making me feel better and not them. I just didn't know.

Before my husband died, I lived my life without thinking too much about other people's grief. I mean, I felt bad. I sent a card. But I moved on with my life. I wish now that I didn't move ahead so fast. I wish I knew back then that you never move on from your grief. You only move through it.

Today when I'm connecting with other grievers, I say, "I'm so sorry" and ask if I can sit with them in their pain.

I say their loved one's name out loud. I listen. I don't try to 'fix' them. I don't try to solve all their problems. I do reassure them they won't be afraid forever. I tell them that it's okay to not be okay.

I apologize to everyone whose pain and suffering came before my own. I didn't understand their grief and pain. I just didn't know. Now I do.

JUNE 22

Grief Math

Sometimes I just make stuff up. If you've never heard of 'Grief Math,' it's because I made it up.

But I couldn't think of a better name for the questions I now ask myself since my spouse died. Questions like, how long has it been since he died? How old would he be if he was still alive?
What anniversary would this have been for us? How many more years have I lived than he did?

I don't do this because I love math, in fact, I hate math especially grief math. I also don't know why I think about all these questions so much, but I do. My guess would be because grief is forever and doing the grief math is just another part of the process.

I sometimes try to be more optimistic and focus on the positive numbers and questions like, how many years were we lucky to be together? How many times did he make me smile? How many happy memories did we create?

The problem with grief math is it always leads me to that ultimate question, the one that if I can answer it, I'd get extra credit, how much time is enough with the person I love? My answer will always be infinity.

The problem with doing all this grief math is that there's usually no satisfaction in getting the answers right. For example, sometimes I would calculate how many years I had left until I was the same age he was when he died. The fact that I have now passed that age only brings me pain.

I don't think I'm alone in this. I think grief math is something a lot of bereaved people probably do. It's not really something intentional for me, it just became a part of my thought process.

In the beginning, it felt like I was doing my grief math all the time. Counting down the seconds, minutes, hours, days, weeks that I had to live without him.

How I felt about all this time adding up depended on how I felt that day. Sometimes the grief math measured the distance I grieved between myself and the life I shared with him. On other days, it felt more like progress.

I still do the grief math, I probably always will. The only difference is now I count by larger intervals. How many anniversaries or birthdays has it been? How old would he be now? There are some other equations that would only make sense to me, so I won't share those with you.

I can promise you that the exact grief equations depend on your life and the life you shared with that person.

What I can't promise you is that you'll ever stop doing the grief math.

I never have.

JUNE 23

When Sympathy Hurts

I was talking with a member of the LGBTQ community, and she was telling me how her partner of 25 years had died. Shortly after the death of her partner, she received a sympathy card from her partner's sister. She asked if I would share her experience. Although she has agreed to share her story, I'm going to call her 'Beth' to protect her privacy.

This sister included a note in the sympathy card about how Beth should 'seek salvation' and not a single kind word was written, but at one point she did thank Beth for being her sister's 'friend.' This was hurtful because Beth considered her 25-year relationship with her partner so much more than just friends.

On the front of the envelope, she wrote only Beth's first name because she apparently never bothered finding out her last name.

This sister never once asked about Beth in any of the many letters she wrote to her sister when she was alive. She did, however, in the sympathy card ask that Beth send her all the family photos she had since she was 'not family.'

Beth asked me what I thought about all this, and my reply was, "I think the point of a sympathy card is to express sympathy. If you're not going to do that, why send it?"

She wanted to know if I thought she should respond to the sympathy card. She said if she did, her response was going to be a nasty one.

I'll be honest, there is that part of me that thought she should give this sister a good blasting, but two wrongs don't make a right.

I explained to Beth that in sending her back a nasty reply, she would be doing a great dishonor to her partner and their relationship. Just as we don't have to explain our grief to anyone, we also don't need to explain our love.

When someone says something hurtful, insulting, or minimizing to you in your grief, it's tempting to assume the worst and go on the attack. You may be harboring a lot of indiscriminate anger about your loved one's death, and it feels satisfying to have somewhere to direct it.

When you're worn down and vulnerable, I think it's always a good idea to separate yourself from people who you believe will cause you additional pain. I asked Beth if she ever really liked this sister and she said, "No, because she never acknowledged our relationship."

I replied, "Then nothing has really changed."

JUNE 24

Zero Control

"Why did they have to die?" "Why did this happen to me?" Have you asked yourself these questions? I bet you have and like a bazillion times! I think this probably comes from your belief that bad things only happen to people who deserve it.

When you find yourself alone in your grief, you start to believe things like if you had just parented a little better, if a doctor or a medical facility had done something differently, if you just had the chance to say goodbye, if you had just acted sooner, things would be different.

Thinking about these things over and over again is how you try to make sense of the world after your loss. It becomes super important because you think if you can figure out what the cause of the death was, then it will all make sense. Nope!

There's nothing you can do to change the outcome of what already happened, at least not now. So maybe you just think if you can figure out why it happened, you can prevent it from happening again.

You'll probably spend weeks, months, and even years dwelling on 'why.' Either blaming yourself or others until one day you just realize that there is no answer to 'why,' the world is just an unexpected place.

A friend of mine said to me recently, "I still sometimes try to make sense of what happened to your husband."

I replied, "Well, that's because sometimes life just doesn't make sense."

Stop beating yourself up for something you probably had zero control over. Be open to your grief and give yourself a break rather than assuming you're doing it wrong.

JUNE 25

'Grief Police'

When it comes to grief, everyone seems to be an expert. Most people think there's only one way to grieve, their way. They say things like, "Get over it" or "You need to move on."

Everyone suffers some grief in their life, but the way they experience it isn't universal. People take it upon themselves to try and tell you how, where, and when you should grieve. These 'grief police' will tell you how you should grieve and if you're grieving too much or not enough.

No matter how you grieve, the grief police will have opinions about it.

Nobody ever teaches you how to grieve. You just learn it as you go along. You're not taught how to grieve, and so many people tend to avoid and downplay other people's grief. It somehow gives them a sense of control. If they can manage your grief, they don't have to think about their own.

The grief police often think you should grieve in silence. They don't want you to talk about it. If you do talk about it, they want you to make sure you find just the right balance. Don't talk about it too much and don't talk about it too little.

You're never going to please everyone. You're never going to grieve the 'right' way because there's really no right way to do it regardless of what the grief police tell you.

I'm always thinking about what I'd like to say to the grief police. I'd like to sit down with them and have an honest conversation about the realities of figuring out your life after losing a loved one.

Your grief is as individual as you. Your grief is not my grief, and my grief is not your grief. For every loss, there are hundreds of ways to grieve. There's no one size fits all. Grief is an individual journey, and no one can tell you how to do it.

You just have to find the way that works for you and not judge others because they may grieve differently.

I'm always going to talk about my grief and my journey. It's all part of my life and my story.

We each have to move through grief at our own pace and in a way that's comfortable for us. But that doesn't mean we can't be there for each other in a way that's comforting without being condescending, sensitive without shaming, and helpful without being harmful.

We all need and want a safe place to grieve.

JUNE 26

I'm So Proud of You

I want to take a moment and congratulate you on how far you've come. Seriously, I'm so proud of you. You're doing it. You're surviving!

Regardless of how long it has been since your loss, you're breathing in and out, and you're putting one foot in front of the other. You may not think these are really big or important accomplishments but that was before you lost a piece of your heart.

I've learned from my own grief journey that coping with grief is about doing small things and taking baby steps that lead you to that place of being 'okay.'

The bad news is that grief can feel like never-ending work, but the good news is that the work can be done in small doses, and most likely you're already doing it. I'm really proud of you.
You're doing it. You're surviving!

I know you might be thinking you don't deserve my praise because grief can cause you to compare yourself now to the person you were before your loss. So, if you're doing that, you're losing sight of your everyday accomplishments like just getting up in the morning. Stop doing that, because if you keep doing it you'll never notice how far you've come.

There are some things that you may never do like get over it or go back to normal. But I think even just reading this book means you're working on attaining some kind of comfort and relief from the pain you're experiencing.

So, that alone proves you're doing it. You're surviving!

I'm so proud of you, and I want you to give yourself some credit for the steps you've taken in your grief up to this point. No matter how bad you feel or how much you think you're struggling, I bet you can be proud of yourself about at least one thing in this moment.

You got out of bed today, right? Who cares what time it was, you did it! You got dressed, right? Who cares what you're wearing, you did it!

You're reading this book, right? Even if you don't believe it or agree with it, you did it.

You're seeking grief support, and even if all you do today is read this page, it's a step forward.

I know you would trade any kind of forward movement to have your loved one back, but I'm so proud of you because you're doing it, you're surviving!

JUNE 27

Crying Blocked

I had a member in one of my grief support groups say, "I don't understand why I won't cry since my husband died."

My response was, "It's interesting that you say you "won't cry" rather than you "can't cry." I asked her why she thought that was and she replied, "I think my crying is blocked."

To me, this implied that she was making a conscious choice not to cry. I see this more often than you might think. Being concerned about crying is understandable, but it's important to know that crying isn't always a part of everyone's grief. Not crying isn't an indicator that you're crazy or headed for a breakdown.

There are a lot of reasons some people don't cry including the fear that if you permit yourself to cry, you may never stop. I can tell you from my own experience that there's no such thing as crying too much.

Trust me, I know!

There are 'criers" and there are 'non-criers.' If you don't typically cry, even a major loss may not be the time you start. You may be a person who experiences grief more on an intellectual level than on an emotional level. I know as a child I was taught that 'boys' don't cry. Crying was seen as a weakness, and strong people, especially men, don't cry.

That all went out the window after my loss, just saying.

I've since learned that expressing your feelings openly by crying is a sign of strength and wholeness instead of a sign of weakness. Grief is a wound that needs attention. To work through grief means facing your feelings openly and honestly. It means accepting your feelings for however long it takes for the wound to heal.

It takes courage to grieve, a lot of courage. It takes courage to feel your pain and to face the unfamiliar. It also takes courage to grieve in a society that mistakenly values restraint, where we risk the rejection of others by being open or different.

If you feel your crying is blocked, you may want to re-consider your beliefs and attitudes about what you were taught in regard to crying. Think about what might happen if you permit yourself to let go and cry. You might be surprised how much better you feel afterward.

Feelings of sadness are normal, and it's okay to cry.

JUNE 28

Making an Appointment To Grieve

When you go to the doctor you usually make an appointment, right? You call ahead and set the date and time you want to go. Then the day of your appointment arrives, and you show up and discuss your issues and maybe your medication. This usually takes anywhere from fifteen minutes to an hour, depending on the doctor and nature of the appointment. Then you say your goodbyes and you leave. Now I want you to think of your grief in that way.

Whatever your day is going to look like, carve out space and time to be alone with your grief and make it happen. This is important because if you allow the grief to have its way, it will show up throughout the day without an appointment. It will take over your whole day.

It's never a good idea to walk into your doctor's office and see them without an appointment. Apply this to your grief. Say you had your appointment; you successfully followed all of the steps and are moving on with your day.

If grief shows up outside of its appointment time, turn it away. Acknowledge your grief, but don't allow it to consume you outside of your appointment. It's all about controlling your grief instead of letting it control you.

Sometimes it's a good thing to go to your grief appointment alone. Family members and close friends mean well in trying to assist you in your grief, but they can often be more of a hindrance than a help. If you invite them, you might subconsciously modify your grief appointment in order to accommodate them and their level of comfort.

This appointment is not the time to be making modifications.

If you make an appointment to grieve, you'll be taking the time you need to deal with your feelings and emotions head on. You'll be creating a way to move on with your day. After the grief appointment, it's important to get up and get busy living. Remember, don't let your grief take walk-ins!

JUNE 29

Grieving With Grace

I was doing a speaking engagement a couple of years ago, and when it was over, one of the audience members approached me and said, "You speak about your loss with such grace."

You might think that this was a compliment, and I'm sure it was meant to be, but I think it's really just that society has created this narrative that idealizes the idea of grieving with grace. I'm sure you've seen it in movies and read about it in books. I'm also sure you've had people compliment you on how strong you are and how you're handling things with such grace.

Oh please, give me a break.

You and I both know that people that tell you that you're handling your loss with such strength and grace are just more comfortable imagining that grief is this tidy and temporary thing rather than the really ugly and messy thing you're experiencing.

The problem is that these same people that put all this pressure on you to be strong and graceful make it difficult to be open about all the messy stuff.

Grief isn't always those pictures showing some grieving person gazing out to sea with a single tear running down their face. In reality, your grief probably looks like mine, a swollen, snotty, red face, bending over a picture of your loved one while you cry uncontrollably for hours.

Am I right?

So, I just wanted to remind you that grief isn't always strong, courageous, and graceful. Grief is ugly. It's messy, complicated, and sometimes makes you feel like you're going crazy.

I talk a lot about grief including my own. I consider myself a good person, a nice person, but grief can still make me a little crazy sometimes. That's why grief is messy; it can make you do and say things that you normally wouldn't do or say.

I bet sometimes you just don't want to talk about it because you feel like people would be horrified if they knew just how not strong and not graceful your grief really is. But the reality is that's grief. Facing the ugly thoughts, talking about them, and acknowledging that none of them make you a bad person are important.

I appreciate that person telling me that I speak about my loss with such grace, but I know that isn't always true, sometimes my grief is really messy.

JUNE 30

Growth and Honor

Grieving over a death of a spouse or partner can be devastating especially when you have your whole life planned to revolve around them. Dealing with this terrible pain can feel like drowning.

You're heartbroken and clueless about going on with life while everybody else is expecting you to stay strong. You have no idea how to navigate this new world of grief you find yourself in, and everything seems foreign.

You've entered the world of widowhood. You're a new widower, a role where you're unprepared and unfamiliar. You're in shock and still trying to process what just happened. You're worried about facing the future alone.

The good news is, in time, you'll find growth. This is when your outlook in life becomes more apparent. You're now ready to move forward and get on with your life. You've dealt with those immediate needs that you encountered after the loss, and now you're ready to plan and focus on what you need to do for yourself.

If you're not at this point on your journey yet, don't worry about it. Even if it seems impossible now, the day will come when it becomes possible. There's no rush to get there.

Finally, you'll come to a place of grace. This is when your transformation occurs. It's when you pick yourself up, dust yourself off, and embrace a new chapter of life.

If you're still only living in a place of 'grief' that's okay, that part goes along with growth and grace. The three become a part of you. They're not opposing places.

JULY

JULY 1

"I Surrender!"

Surrendering isn't easy. In fact, it's one of the hardest things you can do. That's because you want control. But sometimes, surrendering is seeing uncertainty as beautiful. You don't have to know what lies ahead in order to move forward.

What does it mean to surrender? What will you do when you surrender? I think it's all about allowing yourself to live in your life just as it is now. To do that you have to focus on the beauty found in your broken situation and in you. It's about finding the light you can bring into your darkness.

It doesn't take away from the horrible thing that has happened to you; it's more about believing in yourself and your ability to make change from it. That takes its own grieving time. But during that time, you can't let it consume you. The tragedy that struck you, the heartbreak that happened, the hurt inside that you can't let go, they're all the things holding you back. It's important you don't get stuck on asking, "Why?"

Instead of viewing yourself as a victim, it's time to be a survivor. Let what hurts you be the fuel to your fire. Your loss doesn't define you. What you've been through doesn't define you. Instead of focusing on why it happened, try focusing on why to go on.

There is a reason you are still here. That reason is everything. When you want to give up, that's when you say, "I surrender," which isn't the same thing. Giving up is shutting down. Surrendering is letting go.

When you surrender, you don't need things to work out a certain way. You accept life as it comes. Surrendering is about releasing your fears and doubts so you can see clearly and letting the light come through.

Don't wait for life to change, to create peace, joy, and purpose. Choose to make the best of what you have in your life, right now as it is, and just surrender.

JULY 2

Yearning

Since my spouse died, there's a hole in the world, which I find myself constantly walking around in the daytime and falling in at night. I still miss him like hell!

I'm not alone because I know so many other people feel the same way. These are normal feelings of yearning after a loss. 'Yearning' is a concept that's hard to pin down. At its core yearning is a deep longing, a strong desire, a tenderness or sadness, but I'm not sure whether I consider it an emotion, an action, or a thing?

I asked Google (because Google knows everything), and it told me yearning can be a noun; I have a yearning for home; an adjective, I have a yearning sadness, and a verb, I yearn for your embrace. I don't know though; I think this definition seems incomplete.

I've been through grief, and grief takes yearning to the next level. For those who've experienced loss, yearning becomes something that can't be characterized as a noun or a verb. It becomes a state of being. Grief is really about yearning and not sadness. That sense of heartache. It's those horrible pangs of grief. After a death, there's often a strong desire to have our loved one back. It takes time to integrate and accept the reality they're gone so we continue to look for them in the places where they once belonged.

We roll over and expect them to be next to us in bed or we pick up the phone to call them after a bad day. Then as our brain begins to catch up with reality and we start to acknowledge they're gone, we struggle to hold on to, remember and recreate the things that were them, like their voice or the comforting feel of their embrace.

The research indicates that yearning peaks at around four months, and if someone continues to experience a strong sense of yearning (along with other grief symptoms) after six months, they 'might benefit from further evaluation.'

This is where I start to have a problem, because eight years after my spouse's death, I still have moments when I want to see him so badly it takes my breath away. But would I still classify this as grief yearning? It's been eight years, the landscape has totally changed, and I fully understand he's gone.

But if it's not yearning, then what is it? Well, one thing I've noticed about these moments of intense longing is that they often occur when I'm feeling low, confused, or lost, and they tend to be connected to happier times, like a form of nostalgia.

The bottom line is, if you spend a lot of time yearning to have your loved one back, that's normal. I can tell you, in time you don't do it as much, but if you do, it's still okay.

We never stop wanting back that which we love and miss.

JULY 3

A Caregiver's Story

One of the most difficult and complex things you'll ever do in life is to be a caregiver for a terminally ill loved one. In my case, it was never a question of if my spouse was going to die, but when.

As a caregiver, the burden that you carry is almost too much to bear at times.

My spouse and I won every battle we fought, and there were many. But, in the end we lost the war. It's heartbreaking having to watch someone you adore, so independent and strong, be ravaged by a savage cancer. That quickly puts life into perspective, and you soon learn to appreciate and cherish every day you have with your loved one, regardless of how bad the day is.

Always remember, a good day for your loved one may be a bad day for you. Your day may start out with you carrying around a heart filled with pain as the end draws nearer, and your loved one is simply happy because they're still alive. They can still see, they can touch, they can smell, and yes, they can still love.

You adjust your mood to theirs and give them what they deserve and need. A good day! As caregivers, even when staring such adversity in the face, you can't deny them that.

In my case I had the rest of my life to heal while he was losing his. And once the final bell tolled, the true grief began. The rest of my story has been documented in both my books, and it still continues.

My grief was driven by the love I shared with my spouse. And I do believe, the more we love, the more we lose, which equals a much longer and more difficult journey through grief. Some people never get over their grief, but thanks to our body's resilience, we learn to get through it.

In theory, the loss of a loved one can create a darkness that penetrates your soul which becomes a measuring stick for your grief. As the darkness slowly departs from your body, a wonderful thing happens. Your grief starts to dissipate, and you can feel yourself stepping out into the light.

What I found amazing and unexpected was I had a strong sense that my spouse stepped out into the light with me. I realized it wasn't him that was keeping me in the darkness, it was me.

You know your loved one wouldn't want you to be sad, so why are you? Simply put, you loved, and you lost.

But in the end, although things can never be the same, you do get better and once again find your purpose in life.

JULY 4

Fireworks

Before my spouse died, the U.S. holiday Independence Day, or as we call it here in the states, the 4th of July, was one of my most favorite holidays. We always lived on the beach and would host a big cookout with fireworks to follow. But after my loss, the holiday became very complicated. As a Grief Specialist, I'm always telling people that maintaining annual traditions can give them a lifeline of continuity in a time when their lives have been demolished by death.

On one level I truly believe this, but on another level, as a survivor of loss, I also know things will never be normal again. The first couple of years after my loss, only at the last minute did I remember to buy hot dogs, potato chips, dip, and soda, mostly because people expected me to do that. But my heart wasn't in it.

I think for some people that are grieving a loss, carrying on with past traditions (as if nothing has changed) hurts more than it helps.

In the first year (or two) after my spouse died, I felt raging jealousy and resentment for those going about their days as if everything was okay because to me it wasn't. I couldn't bring myself to hang any of our traditional decorations that we bought over the 20 years we were together.

Here's my advice to you, acknowledge that this holiday will be different (if not downright difficult) for you. Don't feel bad passing on that invite to the barbecue or celebration.

Ask yourself this question before doing anything or making any decisions, "Will doing this make me feel better, or will doing this make me feel worse?" The answer will help you to do what's right for you.

One more thing, while you're doing whatever it is you want to do on this national holiday, please take a moment to reflect on the gift it is to be able to celebrate as you wish.

JULY 5

Living in the Wake of Suicide

My sense of safety was shattered when I lost my grandfather to suicide. I was young and didn't understand anything that was happening at the time. I just knew I loved him, and he was gone.

I now work with people that have lost a loved one to suicide, and it's still an ongoing process for me to fully surrender to the fact that no one, no matter how smart, how loving, how determined they might be, can keep someone alive.

Did you make mistakes? I don't know, maybe. You might've said the wrong thing. You might've turned them away one night without realizing there would be consequences. You might've underestimated how much pain they were in.

You aren't responsible for that systemic failure, no matter what mistakes you did or didn't make. You were failed, too, because you were made to feel responsible for your loved one's life which is much too heavy a responsibility for any person to carry. You're not a crisis professional, and even if you are, you're not perfect. You're only human. You loved them the best way you knew how, but you may continue to ask and wonder, "Why did they die, and yet I'm still here?"

This is the one question nobody can answer. To try to reckon with that question is a reminder of how deeply unfair it all is. I don't think there is anything I can say that will change the injustice of losing someone this way.

But what I've learned since my grandfather took his own life is that grief is a powerful teacher. It's challenged me again and again to recommit living a life imbued with meaning. To give my heart away freely and readily, to speak truth to power, and most importantly, to let the life I lead be a living dedication to this person I loved so, so much. I've learned to live alongside my grief, to let it transform me as radically as possible.

Each moment I find the strength to do what's right, to be brave and relentless in fighting for a more just world, or to simply let myself laugh without feeling self-conscious, I become the living and breathing altar of everything my grandfather stood for: compassion, courage, and joy.

I won't pretend to have a good answer for why your loved one is gone. I've looked for the answer for myself, and I'm not any closer to finding it than I was all those years ago.

But I can tell you, both as a survivor of loss of suicide and the loss of a spouse and parent, that life is unquestionably precious, and I believe that more fiercely than I ever have before.

You're still here. And whatever the reason might be, you still have the chance to do something extraordinary with this life. Fight for your own life the way you so desperately wish you could've fought for theirs.

You are just as worthy.

JULY 6

After the Funeral

Just after someone dies, there's a lot of busywork to do. Contacting friends and family, getting accounts in order, planning the funeral. But after you take care of all that 'stuff' and the well-wishers start to fade, you find that you're just left with yourself, alone with your grief. So how do you find happiness in this new world you've been thrust into?

After the initial fury that comes with laying your loved one to rest, it's normal to feel like your life has come to a complete halt while everyone else's moves on. You've been forever altered, yet the world doesn't change its plans or pace on your account.

People have babies, get married, buy houses, go on vacation, post happy events on social media, and here you are left to pick up the pieces alone. Despair and isolation dominate your thoughts. You don't know how to talk about your feelings, yet you feel disconnected from anyone who tries to ask. You don't recognize your life or any of the relationships in it. You feel utterly alone, confused, and lost at sea. You sit in your house alone and think, "What now?"

When you feel this kind of initial sadness and displacement, you have to remember that there are sparks of hope within reach. Other people that love the person you lost will bring up happy memories that make you smile, but you can just as easily recall them on your own.

You'll find that you're capable of feeling temporary breaks in sadness, if not genuine, occasional joy. The more you allow yourself to feel and experience good things, the more room you'll make for other encouraging thoughts to carry you along.

I'm not saying you'll feel the same kind of happiness you did before your loss, but the emotional and practical upheaval that comes with death will feel a little more bearable. Grief is a part of life, but that doesn't make it any easier.

JULY 7

"I Understand"

Two simple words. If you lost someone you love, you've probably heard them many times. But, they can heal or hurt, depending on who says them.

I think there are two categories of people, the 'griever' and the 'non-griever.' If a griever says, "I understand," most likely they do. If a non-griever says, "I understand," most likely they don't.

I'm not putting down the non-griever, I just think there's certain things only the griever understands.

I'm sure you'll agree with me, that if you lost a spouse, child, sibling, or parent, it doesn't really help when the non-griever says, "I totally understand how you feel. I lost my job four years ago."

Maybe this is why you might find more comfort in the words, "I understand" when the griever says it, especially if they have experienced a loss similar to your own. At a time when there is so much uncertainty, and so few things that make sense, there's an opportunity for support and validation when you connect with other grievers and feel understood.

If you're a griever, you want to talk with those who get it. Because while so much of this experience is foreign to you, the griever, it may seem even stranger still to the non-griever.

Here's what you know, you know how it feels to be exhausted and unable to sleep. You know why you want to be alone even when you're feeling lonely. You know how hard it is to decide what you're going to do with your person's 'stuff.' You know how difficult it is to smile when all you want to do is cry. You know how small tasks can become huge obstacles. You know how much you want your person back and how you don't want to go on without them. You know you would give anything for one more touch, one more kiss, one more chance to say, "I love you." You know that grief is very complex. You know that you'll miss your person, forever.

So, what do you do about the non-griever? How do you make them understand, they don't understand? How about sharing all this information you have with them?

Use it to help educate your friends and loved ones. These non-grievers really do want to help, support, and understand.

You can't blame them for what they don't know, and you have to forgive them for what they can't understand.

Someday the non-grievers will become grievers, when they experience a loss of their own, and that's when they'll be very fortunate to have you by their side.

JULY 8

Signs

My friend died, and she loved butterflies. She was like one too, beautiful, optimistic, soft, and friendly. When she died, I happened to see a butterfly in my backyard, and it landed on my sneaker. It reminded me of her. Now, whenever I'm out in the garden and see a butterfly, I know she's with me.

There's long been a parallel drawn between the transformation of going through a personal grief journey and the transformation of a butterfly. From egg, to caterpillar, to chrysalis, and the formation of a beautiful butterfly, the journey is nothing short of amazing.

The grief from losing a special person in your life can also be thought of in this way. It's a unique process to go from the pain of loss, to being able to celebrate that person, and what was important for you together.

No one can tell you how long that journey takes because everyone grieves in their own way. Your loss stays with you but transforms from devastating pain to acceptance of the loss, then on to strength to move forward with your life. The journey through grief is a transformation to a future where you can celebrate the amazing person you lost, and the impact they had on your life.

To me, releasing a butterfly represents freedom from the pain of grief. I see the symbolism as moving forward from the past and embracing a future in which my friend is remembered and honored.

If you're suffering from the loss of a loved one, you may have seen signs that bring you comfort. Feathers, dragonflies, pennies, stars, shapes in the clouds, or maybe even butterflies.

My unique experience with a butterfly, made me feel a strong connection to my friend, it was like she was communicating with me. That brings me comfort. If you've had a direct sign and communication from your loved one, I hope it brought you feelings of relief, joy, and comfort.

JULY 9

Until Death Do Us Part

I'm often reminded of my wedding vows. "Do you promise to love and cherish each other until death do you part?"

I think this should be changed. I think it should be, "Do you promise to love and cherish each other until death do you part, and then beyond?"

The standard vow suggests that we made a promise, and then once one of us dies our commitment has been fulfilled. We're done. We finished our obligation to love one another.

Not True!

We continue to love each other. Maybe not in a physical sense but certainly in a spiritual sense.

Nothing has changed. Love is not temporary. It doesn't exist for a set amount of time. It's infinite.

So, I think of all those I loved and lost including my spouse and incorporate them into my traditions and carry them into the future with me.

My commitment to love will never end or be fulfilled.

There isn't really anything we take with us when we die, except all the love we've collected while we were here, and that love has no end, it has no expiration date.

JULY 10

Finding Your Self-Confidence

You've lost a loved one and now you're losing yourself too. Unfortunately, this is a very common side-effect of loss.

A significant loss can shatter your self-esteem, leaving you to pick up the pieces and put yourself back together. Maybe you feel you could have done more to prevent the loss, that you somehow failed the person who is gone. You may feel incomplete or 'less than' without your loved one. If he or she made you feel special and loved, you may not feel those things now.

So, what can you do?

Start by cultivating relationships with people who affirm who you are and are honest with you. By this I mean the friends and acquaintances who help you grow. Those who try to do too much for you aren't really helping you in the long run.

Stop putting yourself down. Grief can make you become your own worst enemy.

Frequent self-disparaging remarks are a sure sign of low self-esteem. Saying things like, "I never do anything right!" "I'll never be happy again." "I can't go on alone." If you find yourself doing this, try writing down a list of self-affirmations.

Even when you don't feel good about yourself, you can decide to act in ways that are good for you. Instead of withholding what you feel from other people, tell them what you think, how you feel, what you want.

Remember that no one is perfect, and life is hard sometimes. We all want to do what's right, but we all make mistakes.

You deserve to be yourself, so be your own best friend!

JULY 11

Dear Grief

Today I woke up, and it occurred to me that eight years is a long time.

But I still never should underestimate your power. How you make my chest tight. How you bring tears to my eyes.

You see, words are the only way for me to make sense of what I feel. To make sense of you.

They say a lot of what we do is in our words, deeds, and actions.

I'm not new to my relationship with you. I know that you're a roller coaster. I never know what to expect when you're around. Many would not consider you a friend, grief. But I do.

I consider you a friend because you're an emotion and experience that has been with me for eight years now. I've gotten to know you well. I don't want to forget you because I'll never forget him.

You taught me to be patient with people having a bad day, whether they can express that or not because we all have silent battles to fight. Every single one of us. You taught me to reach out to people. You taught me to express myself and to find my voice.

You are what lead me to writing, and I know that I'm grateful for that.

You taught me to continue to use my voice and know that the impact spreads farther than I might imagine.

You made me realize that you are a very good teacher. I found that out when I decided to make you my friend instead of fearing you. I'm glad I let you in. I'm committed to our relationship.

I don't claim to know it all. I never do. You taught me that even when you do all of the right things, go to therapy, remember your loved one in positive ways, cry, rest, pick up new hobbies, you can still turn up and throw everything out of order.

So, grief, it's been a long journey, one that I know will never end, but I'm confident that neither will my relationship with my loved one. Death ends a life not a relationship.

I shouldn't let you take me by surprise after all this time, but in the same respect I'm still getting to know you. Maybe you'll always just be that ever-changing dance between sadness and joy.

JULY 12

It's Not Permanent

After my spouse died, I was a year out and still crying all the time. I thought to myself, "Will I ever feel not sad again?" I knew the answer was yes, I would.

Not only because I've been through loss multiple times, but because nothing in this life is forever. It's hard to look up from the darkness of grief in search of the light you can't see yet.

But I promise it's there, and while your life will never be the same, you'll experience joy again, and eventually, when you think of the person you lost, the memory will bring more smiles than tears. If you can't find the light, don't be afraid to ask for help. Speak to a friend or family member, find a grief counselor or support group.

Facing our own mortality is never comfortable. My spouse's death was another brutal reminder to me how short this life is and what legacy I want to leave.

Take advantage of every day that you have in this lifetime. Grief provides you with a selfish opportunity to be introspective about the life you want to live.

What do you want to do more of in your life? Do more of those things. What makes you unhappily wish away days? Get rid of those things.

Think about who you want to be remembered by, and how they will remember you, and focus on being that person and living that life. Remember that the horrible way you feel now isn't permanent; grief is teaching you what's important and what's not.

When our mind is wrapped up in work, bills, responsibilities, and so much more, it's easy to go through the motions of life. Sometimes the days become routine, and one rolls into another. We've got things to do and little time to get it all done.

It can be challenging to quiet the chatter in our head, to look at the person in front of us, and to speak, listen, and interact with them like they matter. Often with strangers and even more so with the people we love.

They're the ones we take for granted. Sometimes our grief blinds us to their presence. They forgive us time and time again. But is that what we want?

If you died today, what do you want those closest to you to know? Do they know how you feel about them? How much they mean to you? Do they understand how important they are to you?

Tell them! Leave nothing unsaid.

Love like today could be your last because you never know if it is.

JULY 13

Finding Peace

I was walking on the beach and wishing that my dad was still here. As I looked out over the ocean, I realized that he's not really gone, he's just changed. He was there on the sand, in the air, in the wind, on the water, and most of all in my heart.

I realized that what I was trying to cope with was not a loss but a change.

I've never really liked change. I tend to resist it. I'm always trying to stay in my current state of comfort and security because change is hard! Life is a constant change, like the loss of someone you love. When someone you love dies, they change, then life changes and you have to change.

My dad might not be a person in the sense of a human being anymore, but he is a part of the world somehow. I don't know how, but I know he is.

I believe that the people we think we lose transform into something else and move on to the next stage of life. They're still here but not in the same way as before. I think my dad is in everything I've learned from him, and he's also in my heart and memories.

In my mind my dad isn't gone, he's just changed into something I can't understand and that somehow brings me comfort and peace. Everything has changed since my dad died. Nothing feels the same. After such a traumatic change, the only way I can really cope with it is to change myself.

I knew when my dad died nothing could bring him back. I just have to keep moving forward. I know I can't go back.

I have to accept the change because if I don't, I won't ever find peace. My life feels broken, but it isn't, it's just different.

My dad isn't gone, he's just different. Instead of wishing my dad could come back, I'm accepting the change, and that's helping me find peace.

JULY 14

Fake It Until You Make It

You've heard the phrase 'fake it until you make it.' It's a phrase used to inspire you to accomplish a seemingly insurmountable goal.

After my spouse died, many people offered me advice about how to cope with grief. Some argued the importance of taking care of myself along the journey. On the other hand, most suggested that the only way to 'get over' death was to 'fake it until I made it.' Like somehow if I just pretended that everything was okay, after a while things would be okay.

Now when I look back on that advice, I can see its absurdity. At the time, however, I applied the method for a while in hopes that I'd quickly bounce back from my devastating loss. But what happens when you 'fake it until you make it' until you can't anymore? Despite my best effort, grief worked its way into every aspect of my life. Concentrating became increasingly difficult. Memories flooded my mind at every turn. Sleep evaded me, I felt like I couldn't breathe, and my chest felt as if a brick sat firmly on it with no relief in sight.

I tried to fake it; I really did! Fake smiles. Fake focus. Fake listening. Fake laughter. This is what so many told me would help. It's what I thought I needed. It's not true! All my faking did was land me in the doctor's office, with him saying, "Everything looks just fine." But things were far from fine. "What's the problem?" I continued to ask myself. Little did I know that the answer to my question would be found in a hospice chaplain's office.

Months after my spouse died, I sat across the room from a hospice chaplain who listened to depths of pain I'd never shared with anyone else. Session after session I resisted grief. It wasn't me. I hated it. So, I faked my way through week after week.

After a dozen or so sessions, I continued to feel exhausted. I finally admitted to her how terrible I felt. I shared, and she listened. Then one day she leaned towards me in her chair and gently asked, "What would it look like if you relaxed into the pain of your loss?" In other words, "You won't be able to fake it 'til you make it with this one."

I'd love to say that in an instant, I dropped the veil I'd worked so hard to hide behind and surrendered. What really happened is I became angry. I mean, how dare she ask me to do something so impossible! But, it became clearer as my stress continued to mount, I could no longer fake my way through grief.

This compassionate and caring hospice chaplain taught me, over the course of several sessions, how to FACE IT until I made it.

How to relax into the pain of my grief. Sit with it. Express my feelings in the midst of it. She taught me that faking it, was keeping me from 'making it.'

JULY 15

The End of the Beginning

People always say the first year after a major loss is the worst. True in some cases, untrue in others. But what I want to talk about is my second year and how it was different from the first. Not better, just different. I hope if you're not there yet, it will inspire you to keep moving forward.

In many respects the second year of my new existence felt very different to the first. I long since learned not to utter the phrase 'time is a great healer' to the newly widowed because it's such a cliche that it can't help but sound trite. I vividly remember how much I myself resented hearing it from others in the very early days.

The rawness fades. I found that I could smile again. Once or twice I even found myself about to burst into laughter before checking myself as if unsure whether it would still be disrespectful at this point. I became more easily caught up in other things, slowly returning to my old interests, even beginning, hesitantly, to pick up books again. I love to read, and I was unable to do that in the first year. I began to read every book on coping with grief that was ever written.

I noticed that my life was growing around the loss. I met up with other widowers, not for therapy any longer but simply the social aspects.

Things were undeniably better. Not all right, not back to the way they were. That would never be possible again. But much easier than the early days. I knew that I had made so much progress.

What time did provide was the comfort of distance. The events of the first year seemed to belong to another life, another person. They were never more than seconds away from the forefront of my mind, recalled dozens of times a day, but they felt even more unreal than ever.

My mind still struggled desperately to try and understand what had happened. That he was really gone, and I was alone. I became a little more used to his absence but came to accept that I would never be able to process his death. I would just in time learn to live around it and incorporate it into my new life.

In the second year I was no longer able to look at a date on the calendar and remember what we did on that day the previous year. That was a tough one for me. That was what almost made the second year worse for me.

I think it was in the second year that I actually made it through a whole full day without crying. That was huge! I knew then for sure that at least some healing was evident. It was in the second year that my true battle began. The long journey of grief on the one side and hope and renewal on the other.

JULY 16

Healing Takes Time

Everyone's journey through grief is unique. The initial days, weeks, months, and even years after someone's death can be challenging mentally, physically, emotionally, and spiritually.

When someone you care about dies, it affects all areas of your life. It's important to know grief is normal, healthy, and essential for your well-being. Grief is the tool your mind and body need to heal and recover from sadness and loss.

When someone you love dies, it may seem like your life is overcome with grief. It may seem like grief has total control of you. The road to true healing can sometimes be challenging. Remember there are no rules to follow when it comes to healing.

Some days you may wonder if you'll ever experience joy again. You might feel that, for you, early in the morning and late in the evening are often the most challenging times of your day. The good news is that you can get to a place of peace after your loved one has died.

Your healing journey is what will lead you there, but healing takes time. It's important to know it's not something that happens immediately. Allow yourself time to develop emotional acceptance of your loss and time to find what you need most to heal. It's important to remember that life will get better.

You'll never forget your loved one, and they'll always be missed. Little things will remind you of them. While on your grief journey, be reassured that your pain and sadness will become less intense.

You'll smile and laugh about the good times again. In time, the love you still have in your heart will lead you to a place of peace.

JULY 17

Overload

If you're feeling overwhelmed by too much loss, you're not alone. Loss and unwanted change are unavoidable parts of life, but sometimes you might experience a disproportionate number of bad things. Sometimes the losses stack up too high creating a sorrow that seems too great to overcome.

In the face of too much loss, it's normal to feel devastated, exhausted, or hopeless. It's normal to feel paralyzed and overburdened. Let me assure you that the overwhelming nature of your grief is a normal reaction. What is abnormal is the unusually challenging life situation you are in right now.

There is hope.

By familiarizing yourself with the basic principles of grief, you're already taking a big step toward healing. You see, grief responds to awareness. When you educate yourself about grief and mourning, you're making the experience more understandable and bearable. It becomes something you can work on rather than something that simply happens to you.

I've been a grief specialist for many years, and in my own life I've encountered a great deal of personal loss of my own. It might help you to know that grief overload is a fairly common, though indeed painful, circumstance. At one point or another in your life, you'll probably find yourself dragged under by too much loss. Maybe you even feel like that right now.

Even if you've coped with grief effectively in the past, you may be finding that this time it's different. This time it may feel like you're struggling to survive.

What I've learned through my own losses, is that over time, through active mourning, you can survive.

I did and so will you.

JULY 18

Journaling

My journal was my best friend during my lonely process of grief. Grief turned me into a depressed mess, which made me feel like an outsider. It's a common experience.

As you probably know, one of the most surprising things about grief is how alone it makes you feel. Only those who have grieved will be able to understand what you're going through.

Your friends and loved ones will offer as much comfort as they can give, but they've got their own lives to live, and nobody wants to hear your sad story over and over again.

Writing in my journal provided me comfort and relief at a time when nothing else did. My journal became my lifesaver and my best friend. It was the only place where I could speak my truth and where I could safely express all of my emotions.

My journal was always there for me to listen to the same story over and over again, without judgment, until I was finally ready to move forward.

Journaling allows you to tell the story nobody wants to hear.

Writing in a journal allows you to hold onto your memories and record your story. I found it incredibly comforting to have my journal always by my side. Sadness catches up with you in the airport or waiting for the bus. Being able to scribble in my journal got me through some rough times.

Writing everything down allows you to share your pain. It doesn't make the pain go away, but it allows you to see patterns in your thinking and to focus on the positive.

By writing down your feelings, it can help you to make sense of what you can't understand, and in the process, help you to find healing.

JULY 19

Changing Your Environment

It may seem strange, but several people have told me that changing their physical environment has helped their emotional state.

It got me thinking about how we should all from time to time look around our environment at home and at work. Many times that can reflect our emotional state. A cluttered, untidy, or dismal environment can often reflect a state of mind. But the opposite is also true.

Change usually happens from the inside out rather than the other way around. The more you do to enhance your environment, making it cheerful and pleasant, the more your emotional health will be positively influenced.

I know everyone is different, but I found that after my own spouse died, and I was left alone, that I had to carefully arrange the surroundings in my home in order to better cope. I put a lot of things away because they made me sad, and I had to add some things because they made me happy.

I had a giant empty wall that was on the stairway going upstairs, so I turned it into a 'memory wall.' On it, I hung pictures of all the people that I loved in my life that died. I decided that would be the only place those pictures would be instead of scattered throughout the whole house.

There's no definite point at which the grieving process is complete. Can I ever say, "I have completely healed from the loss of my spouse"? No! But I think one of the secrets to surviving is to redefine yourself. This includes moving on from old roles and establishing new ones. Increasing your confidence in yourself as it becomes easier to talk about your loss. Being able do things without being plagued by painful memories and images. Finding ways to reach out to others and not being afraid to have fun and even laughing again.

When you're able to do these things, that's when you'll realize you're healing. But it does take time. For me getting through the first year was a big event. But once I got through that, I felt like I didn't have to look back. I could look forward to seeing what I could do with what I had left.

So, I asked myself "What am I going to do with the rest of my life?" I wanted to do something significant, but I wasn't exactly sure what that would be. Not yet. But, for the first time in my life, I could do whatever I wanted to do, and I planned to make the most of it.

I decided to not only change my environment but also my life, and why not?

JULY 20

Staying Afloat

They say that grief comes in waves. (I don't exactly know who 'they' are, but I'm assuming they suffered a loss.) But it's true. The emotions come and go just like the waves in the ocean. Some waves come strong catching you off guard. They can hit you really hard making it difficult to stay afloat.

You might understand intellectually that these waves will keep coming, but some days they hit more forcefully, more fiercely than you ever imagined possible. Just when you thought you might be able to predict the next set, a random unexpected wave comes rushing in knocking you off balance and sweeping your feet out from under you. Sometimes I feel it, the sadness all over again.

I've been feeling the waves again since the recent loss of my father. His death has resurfaced a lot of similar memories of my spouse's death. My boat suddenly feels unsteady again.

Sometimes I feel really angry that the universe keeps taking away the people I love the most.

I'm sure tomorrow I'll be okay, or I might go back to feeling angry, who knows? I might feel tired. I might feel joy. I might feel nostalgia and gratitude for the prayers that were answered. I might cry or I might laugh. That's the way the waves go.

Or there might be no waves at all tomorrow. It might be flat and still on the horizon, a day to sail easily in calm seas.

I've learned to live in the day. So today I might do well, or I might fail, but I know there's grace for both.

When it gets stormy, I know I'll stay afloat because I've learned not only how to adjust to the waves, but more importantly, how to accept them.

JULY 21

Emotions

I wouldn't call myself a perfectionist, and I'm definitely not an over-achiever. I was always that kid in school that was happy with a "B," I didn't strive for an "A." It was just too much work.

Even though I can be a bit lazy, I've always viewed myself as a person who generally functions pretty well in the world. I was never the smartest kid in school, but I always did well. I've never been the most social guy, but I always hold my own with friends and strangers.

I like being good at what I do, and I like trying new things. I always want to do things without asking for help. I always want to do everything really well.

But when grief turned my life upside down, I think some subconscious part of me felt a pressure to do that well too. I had no idea what it meant to do grief well. I just thought that it made sense that grief was just another new thing I should at least try to do well. In trying to figure it all out, I bought into a lot of myths about emotions that didn't really help me at all.

Emotions aren't good or bad. Emotions are our brain's natural reaction to external stimuli. Yes, some are easy and pleasant while some are difficult and tough. But that doesn't mean they're good or bad. Emotions just are. We feel them for a reason, and it's important that we're open to that.

The problems arise not when you have difficult emotions but when those emotions turn into behaviors that are problematic. Sometimes you can get "stuck" on certain difficult emotions, and when that happens, it can impact your behavior in a way that negatively impacts your day-to-day life.

It's easy to put on a happy face and tell everyone you're 'fine' when you're struggling. But consider the people you trust the most and push yourself to be honest with them about the feelings you have, even the bad ones.

JULY 22

Mourning a Child

I never had any children, so I don't know what it feels like to lose a child. I do know what it feels like to lose a spouse, but I still feel like the loss of a child is the ultimate tragedy.

No parent can be prepared for a child's death. Parents are simply not supposed to outlive their children. It's so important to remember that how long your child lived doesn't determine the size of your loss. The loss of a child is profound at every age.

You also grieve for the hopes and dreams you had for your child, the potential that will never be realized, and the experiences you will never share. If you lost your only child, you may also feel that you've lost your identity as a parent and perhaps the possibility of grandchildren.

The pain of these losses will always be a part of you. Yet it still amazes me how parents that lose a child still find a way forward and begin to experience happiness and meaning in life again.

But most parents that lose a child have an especially difficult time. Even as time passes, their grief remains intense, and they feel it's impossible to return to a normal life.

People always expect that grief should be resolved over a specific time, like a year, but it's not true. The initial severe and intense grief you feel will not be continuous. Periods of intense grief often come and go. Over time, your grief may come in waves that are gradually less intense and less frequent. But you will likely always have some feelings of sadness and loss when you think of your child. Even years after your child's death, important events will trigger your grief.

Significant days such as graduations, weddings, or birthdays are common triggers. At these times, you may find yourself thinking about how old your child would be or what he or she would look like or be doing if they were still alive.

You should expect that you will never really 'get over' the death of your child. But you'll learn to live with the loss, making it a part of who you are. Your child's death may make you rethink your priorities and the meaning of life. It may seem impossible, but you can find happiness and purpose in life again.

The important thing to remember is that your child's life changed your own. They showed you new ways to love, new ways to find joy, and new ways to look at the world.

The memories of joyful moments you spent with your child, and the love you shared, will live on and always be a part of you.

You may be surprised at some of the amazing support you'll get from them, maybe support you never even expected.

JULY 23

Loss of a Sibling

A child's loss of a parent or a parent's loss of a child leads to a grief that is generational. But losing a sibling creates a particular kind of 'horizontal' grief in which shared histories and futures are shattered. This creates uncertainties and insecurities that are often unacknowledged or misunderstood.

Often when a child dies, the main focus of sympathy and support is given to the parents. The surviving sibling or siblings may suffer from long-term depression. Because of this reaction you may hear of these surviving siblings being called forgotten mourners.

If you're an adult who has lost a sibling, especially one who lives far away, you might feel like you're forced to mourn alone with much of the support directed towards the grieving spouse, children, and parents. If you're a senior who lost a sibling, you might feel like there's a lack of good support as our society tends to accept death more when it comes at an older age. But the reality is that sibling loss is painful at any age.

If you lost a sibling, you may suffer from survivor guilt. You might suffer from feelings of failure to protect your sibling or failure to be supportive of your sibling when they were alive. You might feel fearful about how their own families will manage without them. Siblings don't always have the best relationships, so if you didn't have a good relationship with your own sibling that died, you may have guilt over past tensions that can surface even if your adult sibling relationship was strong.

Sibling loss is different because your sibling will always be connected to you through shared memories, in family discussions, and in memorials. Remembering your lost sibling doesn't have to be always sad. Maybe you can remember that time your sister permed your hair, or your brother taught you how to row a boat. If you can remember and laugh at the good times you shared growing up, it can be very healing.

If you're grieving the loss of a sibling, I encourage you to mourn the loss. It's important and significant. There's no magic technique that will make the grief go away. There's no defined right way to grieve or length of time that you should be expected to move on. Moving on with your life doesn't have to mean forgetting your sibling. In fact, allowing yourself to hold your grief in a special place in your heart can help you to be okay.

There are many ways to create a living memorial by turning your grief into something positive, including continuing your sibling's charitable work your sibling did, establishing a fund in honor of your sibling, or maybe even just being a good listener for another person going through a similar loss. Remember your sibling by pursuing the happiness your sibling would want you to have, and live life for you both.

JULY 24

Make Life Better

My goal in life is to walk along with you after your loss and tell you that I know you'll survive.

I know in the beginning that's just too difficult to believe.

But I also want you to know, not only can you find happiness, but you can also reinvent yourself after your loss. I know this is true because I did it.

After my spouse died, the most devastating realization was that my life had changed forever. I started to think about what I wanted my life going forward to look like. What was my blueprint?

I had the opportunity to completely reinvent myself. Where I lived, where I worked, who my friends would be, and who I was spiritually.

It would be an adventure. I wouldn't take it alone. I wouldn't leave my loved one behind. No, I would take him with me.

You, as a survivor, can take this terrible thing that happened and use it to think about all the areas of your life. You can decide which areas you want to change and which areas you want to keep. You can stay open to all the possibilities life has to offer you. You can make life matter.

Most of all you can learn to be okay with not having all the answers. I've learned to be okay with the fact that sometimes I won't have an answer to every question I have about my loss.

Once I came to accept that, I was better able to accept the reality of my loss. My spouse died. Why? I don't know. Why does a young child die before their parents? I don't know. Why does death take millions of lives? I don't know. There will always be unanswered questions. That's just the mystery of life. I just know that I don't want to spend the rest of my life looking for the answers to questions that don't exist. Life is too short, and I don't want to waste it doing that.

I don't think you should spend the rest of our life being miserable just because the person you love died. I don't believe that they would want you to feel sorry for yourself and to make them the reason for your pain. I think instead they would want you to move forward in a positive way and live a life that brings you happiness. They would want you to heal. You can do this by thinking positively and choosing to be optimistic about your future. Living in the present can make moving forward much easier while honoring the past and keeping their memory alive.

As you walk this grief journey you can remind yourself that even in the darkest moments, you can find the presence of light and love. You can head in the direction of that light and be grateful for the love you receive along the way.

You may not have had the time with your loved one here on Earth that you had wished, but you were blessed that they chose to spend the rest of their life with you.

JULY 25

Survivor's Guilt

Just when I think I've said everything possible about guilt, I'm reminded about another aspect of guilt, survivor's guilt.

So, what the heck is survivor's guilt? Survivor's guilt is exactly what it sounds like - a sense of deep guilt that comes when you survive something. Pretty simple, right?

But what makes survivor's guilt especially complex is that the experience is so different for everybody. The bottom line is that the simple definition is just feeling guilty that you survived when the person you love died and that you don't deserve to live when they did not.

In some cases, this includes feeling you could have done more to save them, and in other cases, it's feeling guilty that another person died saving you. Regardless of what the circumstance is, usually you just feel guilty because you think you could or should have done something to prevent it.

I've done this, we've all done this, but if you really think about it, the whole thing defies logic. I think the reason we do it is because we would prefer to blame ourselves for things outside our control than to accept the fact that we really don't have any control over who dies and who lives.

Then add to that people believing your survivor guilt isn't rational, so they try to minimize it by telling you not to feel guilty which can be really frustrating.

The big question centered on survivor's guilt is usually, "Why?" It might be "Why did they die?" or "Why did this happen to me?" It's really common to feel that you weren't worthy of survival.

Rational or irrational, survivor's guilt is normal. It isn't a sign of unhealthy grief, despite the fact that some people might make you feel that way.

My advice to you is to just accept the way you feel. You for sure aren't alone! Survivor guilt is much more common than you might realize. Finding a support group or other space to connect with others experiencing similar feelings can really help to make you feel less crazy or isolated.

Just don't get stuck too long in the place of asking "Why?" If you're asking that question over and over again, remind yourself that there most likely will never be an answer. Maybe it's better to focus on the meaning you can create from your survival. Whether it's big or small, try to find a way to create something from this second chance.

I know this is going to sound really sappy but try to embrace life instead of feeling guilty about living it. I didn't know your loved one, but I'm pretty sure if they love you as much as you love them, they will want you to enjoy the life you've been given.

JULY 26

Heaven

Here's a question that someone asked me, "I'm not trying to derive personal comfort from this question; I just honestly want to know: Can people who are in Heaven look down and see us (their loved ones) on Earth?"

Honestly, I don't know why this person thought I, of all people, would know the answer to this question. But who among us would not like to know? Who has not asked this question and wanted to know, especially those of us who have lost loved ones and think about it?

Ultimately, I have no clue. I don't think anyone really knows for sure. At least, we don't know to what extent they might be able to see and know all that happens on Earth.

Here's what I personally believe, I think that my loved ones in Heaven do see the suffering and misery, as well as the good on Earth, but I think they see it in a perfectly spiritual way that considers everything they now know in order to make sense of it. They understand now what we're still incapable of understanding here on Earth. I think they have transcended to a higher level of 'being' and so, they will rejoice for the goodness they see and weep for the sadness.

But again, I have no clue. Sometimes I just like to think of life as a race. The people we love that died finished the race, and now they're standing on the side of the racetrack and watching us. And we can take heart from that because, in essence, they would be saying, "Hang in there. You can do this. We made it; you can make it too." And I find that very, very encouraging.

Maybe we should be careful of spending too much time thinking about who's looking down on us from Heaven and instead just focus on being a good person, not just because someone we love might be watching, but because it's the right thing to do.

JULY 27

Returning to Work

The death of a loved one can be devastating, and while many companies provide bereavement leave, the leave is often only three to five days. Some people may be fortunate to take more time, but many of us have to go back to work well before we're ready.

Grief can be even more isolating because people don't know how to act around you when you go back to work. Many of my coworkers just acted like nothing happened at all and expected me to do the same. It was weird.

When you go back to work, you may be surprised by the support you get or even the lack of it. You'll see different reactions from your colleagues. Some will offer help; some will ask stupid questions, and some will say nothing at all. So, what are some things you can do to make going back to work less stressful?

Don't force yourself to share information if you're not ready. Just because your coworkers ask you questions, doesn't mean you have to answer them. You might want to talk through the details of what happened, but if not, simply say, "Thank you. I appreciate your questions, but I'm not able to answer them right now."

I couldn't talk about my loss in work because I would cry, and I didn't work in an environment that crying was really an acceptable thing to do. So, you may not want to talk about things at all or at least not in the middle of a workday. Make your wishes known to a trusted coworker who's also a friend and enlist their help in communicating with the rest of the workplace.

You already know grief is exhausting, and there are days when you might feel capable of doing a good job, but other days you're just too tired. If possible, give yourself space to grieve by using any personal time off for grief days. (These are like sick days for people who are grieving.) Use those days to cry and grieve your loss. Take care of yourself by going for a walk, relaxing, meditating, or anything that brings you comfort.

Before you return to work, think of a private space where you can go. My car was my sanctuary. I would go to the car on my lunch break and get all my crying out.

If you go back to work after a major loss, you're going to feel different. You'll still be in a fog. You may forget things and make more mistakes than you usually do. Write down things that you usually don't bother to and make a checklist. It will help keep your unorganized grief brain a little more organized.

Going back to work while grieving is difficult, but let's face it, everything is difficult when you're grieving. It can be hard on you and also on your coworkers. So have a plan that includes taking care of yourself and find the time to make room for your grief.

JULY 28

Party of One

Grief creates exclusion, especially among our friends and family. I don't ever want to come across as someone who doesn't understand or who dismisses how hard widowhood can be. Believe me, I'm not that person. But I also think there's a different side to our changing friendships that we don't often think about.

I've thought for years how lucky I am that most of my friends didn't abandon me when my spouse died. I gave them all a lot of credit (which they deserved) for sticking by me when the going got tough. But I think for a long time I wasn't giving any credit to someone who was the most important part of keeping my friendships together. Me.

This is going to sound strange, but I think there's a certain training process you have to put your friends through when you lose your significant other. 'You' have to show them who you are now. You have to give them time to get adjusted to who you are becoming. Instead of being upset that they're not calling, you have to make the effort and call them.

You probably don't want to hear this, but I really think there's a certain amount of time after you become a widow or widower where you almost have to insist that your friends stay your friends because they don't know what to do. They need to take their lead from someone, and I hate to tell you this, but you're that someone.

Many of your friends have never been through this before, and many of them haven't even been through this with another friend. They don't know what to do. You're the only one who knows what you want and need. So, why are you waiting around for them to make the effort?

What I'm about to say is going to sound incredibly unfair, but I firmly believe that it's true. When you become widowed, you have to make more of an effort to be a friend than you ever did before.

I'll tell you why. Because they don't know what the heck to do with you. They don't know what to say. They don't know how to act. They don't know if you want them around or if they're an imposition. For a while, it becomes your duty to be as detailed as possible in saying what you want and need. You can't dance around it. You can't hint. And you can't wait. You have to call someone, anyone, and say, "I want to go to dinner tonight. Will you go with me?"

Try starting slowly. Believe me I know what I'm asking of you is not easy. I'm asking that you, in your exhausted widowed state, add yet another thing on your list of things to do. But I'm also suggesting that you have a little more control of this part of widowhood than you might think. In good and bad times, no one wants to go through losing a good friend.

And that good friend is you.

JULY 29

Losing a Girlfriend or Boyfriend

I often write a lot about the loss of a spouse. The reason for this is that it's the loss I know best and understand the most on a personal level. But, what if you lost a girlfriend or boyfriend?

Although the loss of a spouse and the loss of a girlfriend or boyfriend are similar, they still come with some of their own unique emotions and feelings.

Unmarried companions can face the same grief and desolation that a husband or wife does at the loss of a partner. But the suffering of a girlfriend or boyfriend may be minimized by others who assume it shouldn't last so long or hurt so deeply, as in, "Well, it was only your girlfriend/boyfriend."

Grief is a normal, healthy response to a loss no matter the relationship, and things get murky if the depth of grieving becomes connected to how long a relationship endured or whether it was legally binding. For example, the loss of a girlfriend or boyfriend never seems to be taken as seriously as the loss of a spouse. Why is that? Do we have to be married to grieve? No!

Everything about losing a girlfriend or boyfriend is confusing. The first question you may ask yourself is, "Am I single?" Technically, yes. But, in your heart and mind, they're still your girlfriend or boyfriend. You may still feel tied and committed to them.

Even though you may want to rush to heal, part of you wants to just hang on to every moment you spent together. The whole situation just seems so unfair. You never got to see what the future would look like, together. A wedding, buying a house, having children and grandchildren.

All the events of a future together have been stolen from you.

I can assure you that your life will never be 'normal' again. You can't forget someone you loved so deeply, and you can't replace them. Regardless of the status of the relationship. Love is love.

If you're young, it's even more difficult to explain to people how you feel because they expect you to be able to just move on and start again. It doesn't work that way. You still have to take the time to process your grief and all the emotions that come along with it.

Yes, there will be joy again, but it takes time. Time to process the loss, accept the change, and grow from the grief and pain. You may find love again. Perhaps just a different love.

While it may seem all sorts of sad and unfair right now, you will find life, and even love, after the loss of a girlfriend or boyfriend. You just have to be willing to leave your heart open to the prospect.

They would want you to live and live well. The best way to honor their life is to value yours.

JULY 30

Comparing Hurts

There's an old proverb that goes like this, "I was unhappy about having no shoes until I met the man who had no feet." I use this proverb to point out to you how wrong it is to compare your grief to anyone else's, or for them to compare theirs to yours. Why? Because it hurts!

While this proverb may be helpful to you to value the things you have, it doesn't really apply when it's used to compare losses because it ignores a basic emotional truth which is that all grief is experienced 100%, and there are no exceptions!

The fact that all grief is experienced at 100% doesn't mean that all grief is experienced at the same level of emotional intensity. But, when someone meaningful to you dies, it means that the grief you feel will be based mainly on the absolute uniqueness of your one-of-a-kind relationship with that person.

After the loss of my spouse, a good friend told me she understood exactly how I felt because her dog died. Another good friend told me he could totally relate to what I was going through because he got a divorce. These losses didn't compare to mine at all, at least not in my heart and mind. These people may have said these things to me with good intentions but comparing these losses to mine robbed me of my dignity because they could never know how I feel.

It's important to understand that every relationship that has ever existed between people is unique. Because of that, when you compare one relationship to another, it automatically robs dignity from the person who is now made to feel as if their loss isn't as big for whatever reason. It also negates the basic truth that all grief is experienced at 100%.

No one can say their grief is bigger or smaller than yours, or that their relationship to the person who died was better, or worse, than yours. When you look at it that way, you can see how dangerous and wrong comparing grief can be. Since all relationships are unique, so is each person's grief.

There's no hierarchy of grief that can accurately say that a particular loss is worse than all others. Grief relates only to how you process your feelings and to the nature and meaning of your one-of-a-kind relationship with another person. No one can work on your grief except you. Period.

No matter how much someone cares for you or about you, and no matter that they may have had a similar experience as you, they can't do your grief work for you.

Then there's another really important reason why people should avoid comparing grief. It hurts!

JULY 31

Take 'My' Advice

When my spouse died, I received a lot of advice. I found people don't know what to say. They just kind of say the things they have been conditioned to say during these times. It came from many different people, most of them had never lost a spouse. The advice came from good intentions, but it was empty. Not at all what I needed in that moment.

When someone would tell me it would be okay, I was angry. They would say everything happens for a reason. I should look at the bright side, he didn't suffer for long. That made me REALLY angry! Six months wasn't long? It sure was for me, so I can only imagine what it felt like for him. Then they would say, "Give it time. Time heals all wounds." Guess what, it doesn't!

I started judging my grief. It made me question everything I was doing, and I felt like I was doing it all wrong. That made me even more angry. Then I suddenly realized something. I finally understood what I needed to do. It all made sense to me. It was like turning a light on in a dark room.

Do you want to know what it was?

I realized my grief was only about ME. The grief journey I was on was all my own. Nobody could tell me how to do it. I had to do what was right for me. It wasn't my job to make other people feel better. I just couldn't worry anymore about how they were feeling. I know this sounds kind of terrible, but there's an 'I' in GRIEF for a reason.

It was my spouse that died. It was all about him and me. You see, I had to figure it all out on my own just as everyone else did. It was the only way because it was MY spouse that died!

Everybody has their own grief journey to take, and each one has to follow it and figure it out on their own. It seems kind of selfish, I know, but it's also pretty simple.

Since my spouse died, I've changed the way I talk to someone that has experienced a major loss. I never tell them I'm sorry because I know that's the worst thing I can say. When they tell me someone they love died, I just say, "That really sucks!" Because it does! Then I tell them I'm thinking about them and praying they survive. Because I really am!

I tell them I'll throw them a life ring and pull them to shore before they drowned in their grief. I tell them death sucks, and love is all that matters. If I feel the urge to share advice, I simply tell them their grief is unique to them. They have to do whatever is right for them and not compare themselves to anyone else. I tell them to just follow their heart. I tell them not to worry about what anyone else tells them.

This advice would have saved me so much pain.

AUGUST

AUGUST 1

Climbing Out

It's been eight years since my loss. That number is really hard for me to fathom. Until I sit and think about it. These eight years have been an eternity. My life back then feels like a different world.

This grief journey of mine has not been pretty. There were times where I wasn't sure I was going to survive. Life didn't feel possible, and I felt like I was withering into nothing. I feared there would be nothing left because everything was flowing out of a gaping wound in my chest. I was a hollow shell.

I couldn't stand looking in the mirror and seeing my dead eyes staring back at me. Who was this guy? He felt so empty. And behind the emptiness was terror. I was terrified to the core.

I remember spending most of my time walking the beach and crying. I often was confused about where I was and what my reality was. Sometimes it took my breath away. This really happened. I spent the first year in shock trying to comprehend what the hell had happened.

I couldn't handle the weight of the panic, depression, or loneliness. There was such a void left behind by my spouse; he was my world. It was unbearable. So somewhere along the way, I found the strength to seek out help. A part of me insisted on finding help. I couldn't let this be what happened. I couldn't do that to the person I loved.

Believe it or not, part of me is grateful for this journey. I have learned about myself and life on a much deeper level. I've climbed a mountain that eight years ago looked unsurmountable. I think I have made my spouse proud.

I've learned how to deeply cherish life in a way that I couldn't before. I've gone on a crazy journey of self-discovery, and I appreciate what I have found along the way. My priorities changed. My interests expanded.

I'm still in the process of finding myself. This is me finally taking the time to have faith in myself and abilities to truly follow my soul's desire: to help people. I want to help people heal and climb the mountain of grief with me. I don't want them to be alone.

There's so much pain in this world, and I'm being provided the opportunity to be a light and relief to those on their own journeys. I couldn't be more grateful for this gift. It's challenging, but it's worth it. I'm pretty sure my spouse is proud of me and is cheering me on. I'll carry that support in my pocket for the rest of my life. I'm trying to build a life worth living, even if there's still a part of me that feels out of place without my spouse by my side, but I intend to keep climbing.

AUGUST 2

The Doorway to Endless Love

I believe every once in a while our loved ones walk through Heaven's door and visit us in a dream, just to remind us of the love that still exists from a distance.

It was six months after my spouse died. The days leading up to that were empty and long. Then I finally had my first dream. The dream changed my grief in ways I still don't fully understand.

In the dream, my spouse came and sat down by my bed and said, "I've been to the end of time and back and you know what? I still love you."

When I woke up, I just sat on the edge of my bed in wonder as to what just happened. What was that? Whatever it was, that day the color came back into my life and my love of grief dreams was born.

This experience touched me deeply, so I went to speak to my hospice chaplain who had a strong interest and knowledge in dreams about lost loved ones. Through her, I found that this dream experience was not uncommon after a loss. Many bereaved individuals have these positive dreams that can comfort them through their grief journey. She told me there are positive dreams, and there are these profound dreams (like mine). It's almost as if the dream itself was the catalyst for inner change.

One of the shifts that occurred in my grief after this dream was the feeling of love and peace I felt in the dream. It reminded me that although my spouse was dead our love was still alive.

I believe the love in my dreams is much different than the love I feel when I'm awake. It may be because there's so much worry, fear, and anxiety going on in my waking life that it can only occupy so much of my being. In my life, the concept of love is limited by my experience of it.

I've come to understand as the years go on, my concept of love has changed. The more I reduce my waking day stress and become more present in life, the more this love grows. If the feeling of love can be experienced in a dream, why can't it be experienced fully in waking life?

My first grief dream gave me a glimpse that this state of being is possible. My goal continues to be to get to that place of love and stay there.

I believe that when we have these grief dreams, it's the time when the thin veil between this world and the next lifts, just enough for our loved one to reach through, to let us know they're still watching us, still loving us, and still waiting.

AUGUST 3

Death Is Not the End

It's not an actual scientific fact, or even something I researched extensively, but I believe that death is not the end. It's just something I personally believe in.

I don't think there's anyone that hasn't seen, or at least heard of, the movie *Ghost*. I always loved Whoopi Goldberg's ability to connect Demi Moore with Patrick Swayze after he was killed. The thought of communicating with our departed loved one is alluring. No doubt about it!

I watched that movie again after my spouse died with a whole new perspective. I believed it much more, or maybe I just wanted to believe it much more. It was suddenly more important for me to do that.

So why do I believe death is not the end? Because I think when someone you love dies, it just means they exist in another way, in another dimension that's non-local, non-geographical, non-physical looking.

I think in some ways we have access to that dimension. Every day. Every moment. I don't have to wait for my spouse to contact me, I just contact him. I think he likes when I do that.

I think our loved ones that died want us to say 'Hi" and let them know how we feel. They want us to talk to them, and not only share our sorrow, but our happiness as well.

Okay, I know all this may sound strange. I know that. But I think that death is just a word we use to describe the end of someone's physical life. Not the absolute end of them.

I've had signs from my spouse, and I talk to him all the time. I know he listens. I know when I'm sad, he's sad, and when I'm happy he's happy.

So, I try my best to be happy.

AUGUST 4

Tides

Who doesn't love a nice, relaxing walk along the beach? I know I do! To look at the ocean and admire this massive body of water. It extends as far as the eye can see and is filled with so much life that we can't even comprehend its magnificence.

My favorite thing to do is wake up in the mornings before anyone else is up and walk on the beach. It's so peaceful and quiet. The water is still and clear. As the day progresses the ocean seems to become more active. The tide comes in and goes back out, waves crashing on the sandy shore. I could stand there forever and enjoy its beauty.

Grief is like the ocean and the tides. Imagine a time when you were standing on the water's edge just watching the water come in and out. It just barely touches your toes and then retreats into the sea. The next wave might hit a little higher, just above your ankles. But then it barely makes it to your toes again.

As you turn to look at something, a wave comes in much harder and higher, and it hits your legs mid-shin. It doesn't knock you over, but it causes you to get a little off balance, not to mention the sand that seems to be sinking under your feet. As the tide rises, the waves get a little bigger and the water a little deeper. Before you know it, the water hits you in the waist and knocks you over. The next wave may go over your head. But stand there long enough and the tide will eventually recede, and the water will once again barely hit your toes.

Like the ocean, waves of grief come and go. At first it feels like the waves are crashing over your head, but then, eventually, the grief begins to recede. The grief will most likely rise again in some form or other but enjoying the calm and being thankful for the times when grief isn't too bad is an important part of the healing process.

It's easy to feel guilty for being okay, but it's a positive thing when you make progress after a devastating loss or difficult experience. And everyone will experience the waves of grief in a different way.

Sometimes, I'm still sad and wish things were different, but I believe my grief has receded to a point where it's almost non-existent. Almost! I've accepted my loss and realized that being devastated isn't going to change anything. So, the debilitating tears and emotions are now gone, for the time being at least.

The waves still come sometimes; I think they always will. I wish I could plan for the waves, but I remind myself daily that I just have to ride the waves out and trust that that one day we'll be reunited. I can live with that!

AUGUST 5

Keepers of the Lighthouse

I love lighthouses. I always dreamed as a child that someday I would grow up to be a lighthouse keeper. I would live in it and direct all the lost ships to shore.

I live in New England on the coast, and there are a lot of lighthouses. It makes me think about how although I never did end up a lighthouse keeper, I am working very hard to direct people that are grieving work their way towards the light.

There's this concept of post-traumatic growth that happens after a major loss. That instead of being weighed down by a terrible loss and its fallout, we eventually rise from it, and better yet, change for the good. That's pretty much what happened to me. I think in many ways my loss has made me a better person.

But I have to be honest, I admit that I would probably not choose to have gone through that trauma to gain the growth. It's not like I have a choice to go back and start over. Being a lighthouse keeper of grief was not my career of choice. It was thrust upon me.

However, that growth was actually the silver lining of my loss. I'm grateful for what I have learned, grateful for the people who held me when I could not hold myself, and grateful, especially, for the people who loved me enough to teach me to be a lighthouse keeper of grief.

What I learned on my grief journey was that as a member of the club nobody wants to join, I had a responsibility to be the light for those entering the club after me.

Will you be a lighthouse keeper of grief? It's easy. You already have all the training required; you suffered a devastating loss. Now all you have to do is shine the light for those walking the dark road of grief behind you.

What helped me through my darkness was knowing that there was a chance of light. That light was shown to me, in part, by other people who had navigated the same journey before me and survived.

Many of the flashes of peace I experienced through the most intense grief, I owe to my lighthouse keepers. And so, I have decided that I needed to be a lighthouse too.

Perhaps sharing our darkest days is not being brave or confident, but I believe it's courageous, and more than that, it's an act of compassion and empathy.

When we're lighthouse keepers, we shine the way for others, so they can navigate, and land more gently and more safely than they would if they felt like they were completely alone in the darkness of grief.

AUGUST 6

Morning Tears

Grief feels like a constriction of the heart. A choking. A gripping of our most vital life organ that threatens to annihilate everything we know to be true about love and hope. Grief grabs us and pushes us into a place of collapse. We move forward because we have no other option, and grief follows us. Never letting us forget what we lost.

Waking up in the morning after a dream of my loved one can still leave me drowning in tears. It's depressing. It makes me question whether or not I should be doing the work that I'm doing. It makes me wonder whether or not I'm 'still broken.'

Sometimes it bothers me, scares me, that I still have dreams of my spouse dying. Like I should be better by now. Like if I'm dreaming about it, I still need fixing.

I don't work with grief because I'm 'above' or 'beyond' it. I haven't transcended grief. I work with grief because I continue to live and experience it. That's my truth. The maddening and universal truth of grief is that it doesn't really end. It just gets different with time.

I can say everything there is to say, read everything there is to read, and do everything there is to do, and still have dreams about my spouse dying. This may happen to you as well. When it happens, the grief and pain you feel will be as raw and as fresh as the moment you found out your loved one was gone.

Don't believe anyone who tells you can totally heal from grief. (They're probably selling something.)

So why do I do the work that I do? What's the point of talking about grief if we can't fix it?

Because I truly believe we can coexist with grief. Society has taught us our whole lives that we shouldn't be experiencing grief or pain. That it can be fixed or solved or get better with time.

But what if we let ourselves grieve? What if we allowed ourselves to still wake up crying? Even after years? Even after decades? What if we allowed ourselves to sit with grief and make it our own so much that we see it as another expression of our multi-faceted selves?

That's why I do the work that I do. That's why I keep speaking on grief and the nature of loss. Because I believe that grief, while it's our darkest, heaviest layer, is a vital layer in learning what it means to be human.

The truth is, I'm not broken, damaged, or unqualified, and neither are you. So, allow yourself to wake up to those morning tears. Allow yourself to question whether or not you'll ever be whole again. Grief doesn't break you. It just asks you to grow and feel more. Grief doesn't mean you're broken. It just means you're living.

AUGUST 7

Wishes

There's always a look of complete terror on people's faces when they ask me about my spouse, and I have to tell them he died.

The conversation usually continues with a long and awkward apology by which I try to assure them that I'm 'okay'.

I wasn't very good at this conversation for a long time, but it's been a long time now, and I've learned how to address these inevitable encounters with grace. But I do still dread these occasions so much. Not because it's painful to acknowledge that my spouse is no longer here on Earth with me; that fact I face every day anyway. What makes it really hard is the fact that people feel so ashamed for bringing up someone who's died.

One of the hardest parts of grief is that you feel so alone in it. It can seem there are so few people you can talk to about it. It can be hard to understand someone's deep grief if you've never truly experienced it yourself. Most of the time, it's hard for those of us grieving to understand too. But all I want people to do is acknowledge it with me, as best they can, and with an open heart.

I wish they knew that if they do ask, sometimes it may be sad, and I'll want to cry. Sometimes, I'd like to talk about how much better I'm doing. Sometimes, I don't want to talk about it at all. I just wish they wouldn't run away from the conversation.

I wish they knew they don't have to quickly change the subject when it gets brought up and look at me sadly as if they've broken my heart all over again, and that grief doesn't only exist on the inside. I wish they knew they could talk about my dead person because it actually helps my healing. I want to talk about him.

Only when they understand these wishes, will they see my heart is healed.

AUGUST 8

Getting Back to Life

After my loss it was like I was sitting in a dark cave and couldn't decide if I even wanted to leave it or not. I didn't know what the world would look like without my loved one. The life I had was over. I didn't want a new life. I wanted the life I had.

It's kind of a job hazard for me when I talk about the realities of grief to non-grieving people. It's never too long before someone says, "Well, yeah, but eventually you have to get back to life, right? You have to eventually get over it."

Get over it. Get back to life.

Get back to life. Have you heard that phrase from people outside of your grief? Even people who truly love and care about you might be pushing you to get back out into the world, live your life. They may even tell you that you have so much to live for.

People who often say these things actually do have a life to go back to. They may be deeply impacted by the death of the one you love, but if their family is intact, if there's no gaping hole in their daily life, they just aren't going to be affected the same way you are.

I don't necessarily mean that you had to live with the person you've lost in order to be the most impacted by their death. Not at all. What I mean is that, for many of us, the people we've lost were such an integral part of every single day, every single facet of our lives, there really is no 'normal life' without them.

There's no part of our universe, our daily lived existence, that they didn't touch. There truly is no life to get back to.

Eventually, perhaps, new things will begin to grow around the crater that has erupted in the center of your life. The hole itself will remain. I don't mean that as a downer, either. I mean that a central loss, a loss that shifts the axis of the universe, is not something that simply shrinks over time.

Getting back to life can't always happen inside grief. Instead, we can come to ourselves, to each other, with kindness and respect for what cannot be resumed.

We will not return to the life that was. That's simply not possible. What we can do is bow to the damaged parts, the holes blown in our lives. We can wonder what parts of ourselves survived the blast. We can come to ourselves, and our irrevocably changed worlds, with kindness and respect.

That's the real work of grief, to show up with kindness, every day, many times a day. Somehow, if you don't see it as fixing your grief, or getting back to life, it makes it all just a little bit easier.

AUGUST 9

The Empty Chair

When working with those that are grieving, one topic that inevitably comes up is what to do with their 'stuff': clothes, medicine, eyeglasses, etc.

You can split a room on this topic. One half who are holding on tight to their loved one's belongings, keeping the toothbrush where it was left, shoes where they were taken off, and medications on the countertop. The other half says they have a hard time looking at these belongings, as they feel they are a constant and sad reminder of the person who is no longer here.

There's no right or wrong answer in this debate. But what happens when it's not so simple, and you're finding it difficult to move forward?

A grieving widow was telling me about her struggle after the loss of her spouse. It had been several months since he died, and while she said she was coping well in a lot of ways by keeping busy, she recognized that being at home was a real struggle. She found herself staying out as long as possible, driving the long way home, anything to not go home. This isn't unusual, especially for those who have lost a spouse. The quiet and loneliness of the empty home can sometimes be too much to handle.

She asked, "What do I do? I can't even sit at my dining room table because I can't stand to look at the empty chair?" My answer to her was, "If you can't stand to look at the empty chair, sit in it."

Part of what is so challenging about being home alone is having to constantly face all the places your loved one is supposed to be. You can actually make this easier by changing your perspective, and I mean this literally. These places that we are assigned to in the house happen so organically and usually with no talk or planning, and yet they are so firmly cemented they seem almost impossible to change. But they aren't.

When I said this, she kind of looked at me with a blank stare. I told her to just give it a try and sit in his chair instead of her own. The next time I saw her, she smiled and said, "Thank you, it worked!"

No, it didn't take all of her pain away, and she wasn't finding herself anymore eager to get home. But, when she was there, instead of sitting at the table in her seat, looking where her husband was supposed to be, she sat in his chair. She said it somehow made her feel better. More connected to him, rather than disconnected.

This simple practice isn't just about filling the empty spaces, so we no longer have to look at them, it makes us feel closer and more connected to the places, times, and memories we shared with our loved one.

AUGUST 10

Why Am I So Mad?

Anger is a common and expected emotional response following the death of a loved one. I was so mad after my spouse died. I was angry at the world.

In life, we often get angry when we can't control what's happening to us. We have no control over death, and so it's normal to feel anger. But it can be one of the most confusing feelings to experience at such a time.

People expect to feel sad, lonely, or tearful. But feelings of anger can leave people feeling anxious and as though they're somehow not normal.

You may wonder why and what you've done to deserve the loss, that you weren't a good enough partner, mother or father, or even that you're being punished for something you have or haven't done. It's possible you may find yourself taking out your frustration on family and friends or feeling overwhelmed with a deep sense of resentment.

Your anger might be directed at the person who's died for leaving you, or at friends, family, medical people, God, or even yourself for not noticing they were unwell or not encouraging them to go to the doctor sooner.

Anger can be experienced in many ways throughout the grieving process. Some people who've been bereaved can talk easily about their feelings of anger. Others may initially experience it as envy or resentment of others for still having their partner, mother, father, or child.

Many people question why their loved one died, and yet the world is filled with so many bad people.

So how do you make sense of it?

Anger can be thought of as your brain trying to make sense of what's happened. The death of your loved one often needs to be accepted emotionally as well as logically, and this may involve recognizing feelings of anger and then exploring and working through those feelings.

If you're unable to express your feelings in a way which feels safe, feelings of anger may increase. Sometimes, if you express anger towards people who don't understand, it might seem to them that you're pushing them away. This in turn can lead to increased feelings of anger and isolation.

It's good to remember that feelings of anger don't take away from the positive feelings you have for your loved one. They're there because you cared for them.

AUGUST 11

I Can't Remember What I Forgot

I talk a lot about my loss. I don't do that for sympathy. I just do it because by telling you about my journey, I'm hoping I can guide you along if you're behind me on the road of grief. I can let you know about some of the potholes and even some of the peaceful stops along the way.

I still think about my spouse that died and the things I miss. That's the thing about the road of grief, the further you travel it the more it takes on different twists and turns. Just as I'm starting to feel better and moving along at a good and healthy pace, a new and strange emotion arises and causes me to stop.

I always say our grief evolves and grows with us as time goes on. Sometimes that means walking along smoothly and sometimes it means tripping and falling down. The potholes I was telling you about. That's what's happening for me. I'm starting to feel so far away and disconnected from the past that I suddenly have an intense yearning to go back.

I can't remember what I forgot. I want to refill my memory with all the things I feel like I forgot. Just the small things. For example, I forgot I always liked to smell his hair, but I can't remember what it smelled like.

As heartbreaking as this all is sometimes, I also have those peaceful stops I told you about. I like a lot of things about my current life. When you find your way to a place of peace, you will too.

But that doesn't mean that sometimes I don't wish that I could turn around and go back. I'd do it in a heartbeat if I could. The thing is that chapter is over, and I'm now living a whole new chapter in a completely different story.

I accept that my person is dead; I accepted that a long time ago. But that doesn't stop me from not really accepting that the past is out of my reach. That's why I keep trying to remember what I forgot. Like a dog with a bone, I keep chewing at it.

I know if you're early on in your grief, you are probably thinking this is only making you feel worse. That's not my intention. Remember, there's no guarantee you'll ever feel any particular way in grief, including the way I do.

Don't ever feel bad doing what you have to do to keep the memories of your loved one alive. No matter how much time has passed.

I didn't even care that everyone in the store was probably staring at me, as I was smelling every bottle of shampoo trying to find that smell I forgot.

AUGUST 12

Stop Beating Yourself Up!

You're sitting at your desk at work and suddenly realize you've been staring at the wall, lost in thought, for the last hour, and you're late for a meeting.

You're driving home and drive right through a stop sign that you dutifully stop at every day. You put dinner in the oven, and almost two hours later when you smell something burning, you realize you forgot to pull it out. You get up and walk into another room to do something or get something, and by the time you get there, you have no idea what it was.

Sound familiar?

How do you manage the complete inability to focus that can come with grief?

After a death, constant and overwhelming distraction is one of the most common pieces of evidence people cite when explaining that they think they're going totally crazy. So, before I go any further, let's clear one thing up, grief and concentration don't mix well. That's not a sign that you are losing it. I promise!

Struggling to concentrate is very normal soon after a loss. It's simply a sign that your brain is completely consumed by something painful, overwhelming, and life changing.

If the inability to focus keeps up for an extended period of time or is interfering with your life in an unmanageable way (for example, you're at risk of losing your job or you can't care for your children) you should seek professional help from a therapist right away. Otherwise, a basic tip will probably be enough to help you over the hurdle. Though I certainly don't believe time heals all wounds, I do know that time helps a lot with this grief and concentration thing.

It takes time for your brain to adjust to a new reality and the completely different world that exists after your loss. There are emotions you are processing, fears and anxieties, secondary losses, and countless other things your brain is trying to manage, but that does get easier with time. In the meantime, I have a tip for coping with grief and concentration.

Here's my tip, stop beating yourself up!

Seriously. I know it's hard when you have always been a focused, fabulous, functional person. But grief is the worst, and it really messes with your brain. You aren't a failure for being distracted. You're a normal, wonderful, griever who is just doing your best to cope.

So, in those moments when you've lost all focus, try to give yourself some permission and space to know it's okay. You're still a fabulous person, and it might just take some time and a little work to get that focus back.

AUGUST 13

It's All Good

I worry about anything and everything. When I would worry my spouse would say, "It's all good." Somehow this always calmed me down.

He requested I inscribe, 'It's all good.' on his gravestone to remind me not to worry after he was gone. It's there now for eternity, and yes, it does remind me not to worry.

Do you ever wonder what the person you loved and lost would wish for you? What it is they left behind?

I think they would be moved by your tears but saddened by your sadness. They would want you to miss them, and, at the same time, they would hope for their memory not just to be a source of pain for you. They would hope for you to remember that behind this pain, there was joy and moments of complete happiness. They would want you to continue to be happy.

I believe a person really dies when the last person whose life was touched by them dies. So, when you think about it, they have so long still left to live. They continue to survive within you.

The conversation with them goes on without end in your own mind. They will be with you through many things that have not yet happened, through so many days filled with joys and sorrows. You will take them into your confidences. You will hear their voice, and they will advise and console you. Death can't rob you of this because they live inside you now.

You'll never forget them. You'll live tomorrow and the next day. You can live on and still be faithful to everything they meant for you.

They left behind love, and love wants what's good for the other; love wants there to be more love. They'll follow you through the rest of your life. No one can separate you from them. You may miss them so much, and yet they're still here.

AUGUST 14

A Second Chance

All of us have romantic predicaments, but I think it's worse if you're a widow or widower. We seem to have even more. Should we search for someone else to love? If we do find someone, while still loving our late spouse, how can these two people we love reside together in our heart?

For us widows and widowers, is loving again worth the effort of having to adjust to another person, and is widowhood the proper time to fall in love again?

These are tough questions. They're also not questions for everyone. But if you've at least given it a thought, I'd like to share with you some of what I learned on my grief journey as a widower.

Whether you're a man or a woman, romantic love forms an essential aspect of our lives; without love, life may seem worthless and devoid of meaning. Romantic love is a central expression of a good, meaningful, and flourishing life. Without love and desire, many people feel that a large part of them is dead.

Is the human heart large enough to encompass more than one romantic love? There's a ton of evidence that this is possible, and much of that evidence is in the form of widows and widowers. You'd be very surprised how many members of the support groups I facilitate include widows and widowers who are grieving the loss of their 'second' partner. These second time members tell me that although their late partner is physically absent, their love for them remains, and it even grows. It wasn't diminished by their new love for another.

Now if you're shaking your head, what if I asked you if the love you shared with the one you lost was worth the pain you have now, or would you have preferred to never have loved them at all to avoid it?

The death of a partner places you in a new situation, and widowhood has unique aspects. The case of a widow or widower's love for a new person is different from that of a regular love affair. This is especially so if at the time of the death, you both shared a profound love. In this case, your love as the 'survivor' does not die with your partner's death.

But the love you have for your late partner will actually increase. Although a new love might physically replace the previous one, from a psychological viewpoint, you might feel like you now love two people at the same time.

'Second love' is different, but it's very good. It requires the ability to open your heart again without feeling guilty about that. You'll always miss the one you love and lost, but a heart is flexible and can hold the love of more than one person at the same time. Your reason for being is love, so gather up all the love you can, while you can, because in the end, it's all you take with you.

AUGUST 15

If You Can't Be Happy, Be Kind

A close friend called me and said, "I've got a favor to ask. A couple of friends were at a grief workshop you spoke at last year, and they liked what you said."

"That's very nice," I said, "so what's the favor?"

"Well, one of them is dying, and I was hoping you could visit with him. He's not said anything in a long time, and he won't talk about anything serious, and I thought, well, maybe he'd talk to you."

I'm never afraid to sit with someone that's dying. I do it all the time working with hospice patients and being a grief specialist. I always think it's one of the most important things I do. It's an honor to sit with someone in their final hours. To be able to be present for someone in their most intimate moment is a gift, especially if they have nobody else there for them.

The dying man and I had a long conversation. He seemed very open to talking, so I was glad about that. We talked about death as being nothing or maybe something wondrous. We discussed whether love is stronger than death. We complained about how sometimes life isn't fair, and death sucks, especially if you're not ready to go yet. It was a nice visit. I told him I would like to come back if that was okay with him. He agreed.

A few days later I got a call from my friend telling me the end was near, so I rushed over to see him again. He told me he was tired and ready to go. He told me all about what he would like to have done for his funeral service. He had already picked out his place of burial and his headstone. I asked him what he wanted written on the headstone. He said, "If You Can't Be Happy, Be Kind".

I wondered about this strange choice of words, but he explained it to me. He said, "Everyone will be coming to see me there, and I know they won't be happy. I don't want them to be sad, but at least if they have to be sad, I would also like them to be kind. I hope that they will be kind, not only to one another, but to everyone."

I will always remember this man and his final wish. I hope that, in the midst of your sorrow, and the bleakness of what you're facing, you can find a way to be kind. Being kind can be a great way to relieve the burden of grief.

You can take this terrible event that has happened to you by spreading kindness. In doing this, you step out of your own sorrow long enough to take the wisdom you now have and share it with others. So maybe this dying man had a message we all need to hear?

If we can't be happy, at least we can be kind.

AUGUST 16

It Goes On

Robert Frost said, "In three words I can sum up everything I've learned about life, it goes on".

The problem is that after someone you love dies, life does go on, but it's not as simple as it sounds. When you're submerged in grief, it doesn't seem like you could ever possibly move on and learn to live without that person.

The last thought in your mind is that life is ever going to go on, and that things are ever going to be better. The truth is, it never really gets easy, but instead, you just start to learn to adjust to this new life. Then you have to figure out how to move forward and survive.

Not all at once does this happen, but slowly. Slowly you start to pick up the pieces of your broken world and put them together in a way that starts to give you some purpose and meaning again. One day, you find yourself crying less than the day before. Another day, you even find yourself laughing, smiling, and finding genuine joy and happiness in daily life. One day, the pain has subsided more than you ever could have imagined. Eventually, you're genuinely living life again.

Life doesn't give you an option when the person you love is taken from you. You don't get to pick and choose who leaves your life, when and how it is going to affect you. One day, your world gets flipped upside down, and you have to figure out how to continue on.

After a while, everyone around you goes back to their own life. Life is continuing to move and happen everywhere you look, and no matter how much it feels like yours is at a standstill, it's still happening whether you like it or not. People start asking about you less. You stop being everyone's first priority and you go back to being just another person with another sad story.

Then you start to realize that you don't have any other choice but to carry on too. Everyone else is doing it. It's time that you go back to work. You have to start leaving the house again. You have to get dressed and go out and do all the things life demands of you. You have to live again.

Let's be honest, what other choice do you have? What would your person want for you? Would your loved one want you sitting in the house crying all day while you could be out and living your life? I think they wouldn't want to see you like this. It just wouldn't make them happy.

Don't you agree? Life goes on, and this includes your life. Yes, the person you love died, but you're still here. Yes, it's going to suck without the person you love by your side, but the world still holds all the opportunities, experiences, and most of all love, that it has to offer you.

You're still living and have every chance to make the rest of your life whatever you want to make it. Do it for them, but also make sure to do it for yourself.

AUGUST 17

When Your 'Ex' Dies

Grief is messy and ugly on its own. When it's the death of an ex, those feelings become even more complicated, regardless of how the relationship ended. It can stir up a lot of emotions you didn't expect and leave you feeling extremely heartbroken all over again. The experience could be extremely isolating.

I'm always committed to never telling you to move on, and this goes for grieving an ex as well. Love isn't something that dies with the body, it's an emotion that lives on within you.

One of the most important things to remember when grieving a loved one is to acknowledge your feelings and remember that it's okay to love that person even if you didn't love all parts of them.

Any negative feelings you had about the breakup were about the person's behavior, and they don't minimize the things you did love about them. You don't have to feel shame for grieving someone who broke your heart. Love is love, and even though you may not have been able to co-exist or make the relationship work, that doesn't mean you stopped loving that person.

A common problem that with grieving an ex is that no one expects that you'll be impacted by your ex's death, so others don't reach out with condolences and kind words the same way they would if you were currently dating or married. This is when you might start feeling isolated.

A good way to find support in this situation is to reach out to mutual friends you shared with your ex in order to find comfort in conversation with them. These people knew the special relationship the two of you shared and will be more likely to understand your grief. You should never have to sit alone with these overwhelming emotions.

One aspect of your ex's death that may have been complicated was navigating the events afterward, like the wake and funeral. Maybe you didn't feel comfortable going, or that it would've been awkward for their current partner. So maybe you didn't go at all. Whatever choice you made may have left you feeling guilty, sad, or full of regret. If you did go, maybe you felt sorrow over what might have been.

Remember, the love doesn't die because your ex passed away. Using that love as a force for good, instead of caving to the notion that you should move on, will help not only you, but everyone else that love ends up touching.

AUGUST 18

My Year of Firsts

In her book, "The Year of Magical Thinking," Joan Didion said about the first year, "People who have recently lost someone have a certain look, recognizable maybe only to those who have seen that look on their own faces. I have noticed it on my face, and I notice it now on others. The look is one of extreme vulnerability, nakedness, openness. It is the look of someone who walks from the ophthalmologist's office into the bright daylight with dilated eyes, or of someone who wears glasses and is suddenly made to take them off. These people who have lost someone look naked because they think themselves invisible. I myself felt invisible."

In the first year, from the moment my loved one took his last breath, the clock started ticking. Slowly, a distance grew between me and him. The moment he took his last breath became a kind of marker, measuring the distance in the space that was left by his dying. There were now 365 days for me to endure. This would be my 'year of firsts.'

I went through the first year almost without knowing it, but I was painfully aware of every moment. Much of it I don't remember, some of it I can't ever forget. I felt invisible. After he died, all I could see was a long, lonely future stretching out in front of me without him.

Places I would have to go, things I would have to do, alone. There were so many days I didn't think it was ever going to get better or that I would even survive. Every event that happened that year, birthdays, holidays, family vacations, all became a traumatic event. Everything was sad.

Social media became my worst nightmare. I had to see everyone else posting pictures of happy times with their spouse, while I was trying to survive the first year without my own.

For me, it wasn't so much the big events that kicked me in the heart but the small ones, like picking up the mail addressed to him, finding an undiscovered love note he hid in my lunch bag, and realizing the oil needed

325

to be changed in the car, and he always did it. He wouldn't be doing it. Not that year or ever again. Despite all this, life was going on around me as if nothing had happened. It was going on even though I felt like I was standing still.

Then when the one-year anniversary finally arrived, my year of firsts was over. I completed what everyone told me would be my worst year. The problem is when the first year was over, grief was still my companion. All the people that told me I would feel better after the first year were wrong.

You see, in the first year each day I could look back and reminisce about what I did with my loved one on that day the year before. Now I could no longer do that.

Wherever you are on your grief journey is where you are and where you should be, and nobody but you can know which year is the worst, and that's okay.

AUGUST 19

One Is a Lonely Number

One of the very worst things about losing someone you love is being alone. If this doesn't exactly apply to you, and you're still surrounded by people that love you, consider yourself lucky. But if you are one of those people that lost the one person you love and have been left behind, you know all too well what I'm talking about.

The problem with grief is even if you're in a crowded room full of people that love you, still you may feel like you're alone.

With an overwhelming sense of missing the one you love comes the crushing awareness of what you have lost. You would give anything to have them back. This feeling can be so strong that you actually lose sight of all the other people in your life that you love and that still love you.

The loneliness may even become something that you find comfort in sometimes because being by yourself means you don't have to deal with other people or the pressures of everyday life. This need to be by yourself is normal and can actually be helpful in giving you the time you need to cry and figure out where you're going from here.

Sometimes you might feel like it's just too hard to be around other people because they can't understand what you're feeling and going through. This feeling of loneliness is intensified because your world has stopped, yet all around you everyone else is going about their business as usual. So, what do you do to cope with the loneliness?

Try to think about who is supportive to you in your life. This can be family, friends, neighbors, co-workers, church, support groups, or even pets. Spend time with people who are caring and make you feel comfortable. Talk to people with a similar loss, who won't judge you or your grief, and will allow you to talk about the person you lost.

Be honest about how you're feeling. If you feel bad, tell people you feel bad. Don't be afraid to express your sadness, fear, and anxiety. Don't just always say you feel okay if you don't. If you need help, ask for it no matter how simple the task may seem.

You have every right to miss the person who died. Accept that feeling that way is normal.

Find a place to be alone with your grief. Go to that place and have a good cry. Go to that place anytime you need to let out all the feelings and pain. Go to that place when you're missing your loved one so much it hurts.

Grief is a place of loneliness. Grief is a place of sorrow. Grief is a place of isolation. Grief is a place to visit when you need it but not a place to live. If you want to find your way out of the loneliness, go to that place of grief whenever you need to, just don't stay there.

AUGUST 20

My Place of Grief

"I know how you feel." People said that a lot to me after my spouse died. I knew they meant well, and that they were just showing compassion, trying to be with me in my pain, trying to stop the suffering they could see I was going through. Sometimes they would even tell me about their divorce or how they lost their job. They would offer these stories to show me how much they had in common with my loss. But they didn't know how I felt. They couldn't.

Yes, they had a divorce, but their spouse was still living and breathing. Yes, they lost their job, but you can't hug a job or snuggle next to it in bed. I was sorry for their loss; I just didn't understand how it was the same as mine. Losing the someone you love isn't the same as losing your car keys no matter how terrible that may seem.

I had a unique relationship known only to me, so that made me the world's only living expert on the subject. They didn't know the countless stories we shared, the private jokes that only we could understand, the songs that belonged to us, and all the special memories we created together. They didn't know the way I felt when he was alive, the feeling that everything would be okay, and how I lost that for good. They didn't know what it was like to be me, and how different I felt when he was gone.

They didn't know these things, not because they didn't want to, but because they simply aren't qualified to know. As much as people who love me want to sit with me and grieve alongside me, there's a place they can't go, they can't go all the way into the grief with me. They can't go to my place of grief. When I'm fully feeling my loss, I'm alone in that place; no one else can share that place with me.

That's the terrible and profound isolation of loss, the absolute loneliness of being in a crowded room, or a busy sidewalk, or a restaurant filled with people, and still feeling totally alone. People I love have no idea. On the surface, I seem to be among the living and fully in the moment. I appear to be participating, but I'm alone. That's when I go to my place of grief.

When I go to my place of grief, it's a place where no one else can go. It's the place where I feel closest to my spouse, the place deep in my heart where I leave the world behind, and I get to spend a few moments with him.

The place where everything and everyone else falls away and he is present with me again. I get to be with him again, and I remember the things that only I know about him, and about us, and about myself. The loneliness of that place is comforting.

And then, after I spend the time I need, I move slowly back in the world and take my place here among the others who don't understand, who have said to me, "I know how you feel," knowing that they too will someday go to a place where I can't follow them.

AUGUST 21

Falling in Love When You're Falling Apart

What happens if by some crazy twist of fate, you find yourself falling in love while you're grieving? Nobody plans these things. It often just happens that you're lucky enough to meet someone that you can bond with, perhaps over a shared experience of loss.

For people that lost a partner or spouse, there's such a fear of starting a new relationship. The problem with grief is it causes your thinking to be so limited. "If I love someone else that means I'm being disloyal to the one I lost." "If I love someone else that means I'm letting go of the one I lost and people will think I'm not sad anymore, or that I don't care anymore."

Some people never want to enter into another relationship just to prove that nobody can ever 'replace' the one they loved and lost. It really has nothing to do with replacing the person, and everything to do with having the capacity to love more than one person.

Some people are hesitant about entering into a new relationship because they're not sure they would be able to handle another loss.

I know you might be thinking, "I will NEVER love anyone else!" I get it. I've been there. You may think you'll be unable to see through the fog of your grief, but truthfully, the heart has a great capacity for love. It has boundless room to hold more than one love.

The love you have for someone who dies is often idealized and strengthened after their death. When you lose someone, you tend to remember only the good things about them which makes it pretty difficult for any new relationship to live up to the memories of the person you lost.

It's inevitable that comparisons will be made, and perhaps the new love doesn't seem as strong as the old relationship. But all relationships are different. It's another person in another time with different life experiences.

If you're lucky enough to find someone who cares for you, then don't be afraid to build on that relationship. Remember, a relationship doesn't have to be romantic. You can love many people; that doesn't mean you want to be romantic with them.

It's your life. Do what's right for you, but don't close your heart to love. Take up the challenge and have the confidence to build a new relationship. It could just be a new friend who loves and supports you on your grief journey.

You might even be one of the very lucky ones who have not one but two great loves in their life.

AUGUST 22

Three Stops on the Journey

Facing your grief over the loss of a loved one can seem like a frightening journey into a foreign land of dark corners and scary terrain. You may wonder how you'll survive the days ahead. In the first days of shock and sorrow you might feel like you're walking on a barely lit unfamiliar road of grief. You may feel very alone regardless of whether or not you have companions alongside you.

But then in time, some days the light shines through and the shadows around you feel less frightening. With the passage of time, sometimes weeks or months, you actually move back into ordinary daylight. The journey begins with disbelief and hopefully completes with acceptance of your loss and moving forward in life.

There's no timetable for how long grieving persists. But as a road map for the journey, it may help to notice three stop signs of grief that you move in and out of for some time.

The first stop is shock. Death always feels unreal, expected or not. You react by feeling shocked and numb. At first you may be unemotional and able to manage your life pretty well. You're basically hanging on the edges of your pain, but you don't fully feel it yet. You're in a perpetual fog.

The second stop is mourning. You may feel flooded with feelings like sadness, anger, longing, loneliness, and regret. The intensity of your feelings may scare you. Your heart, mind, and body are all impacted. You just don't feel like your 'normal' self. You can't concentrate or focus. Your mind races, and you find yourself obsessing over the life and death of your loved one. This stop is the most difficult as it's hard to find your way back to who you were. You can't hide anymore from the reality of your loss. You might feel like all you do is cry all the time. You can't do any of the things you liked to do before your loss because you can't concentrate. The pain of your loss may feel endless. You may feel hopeless to move beyond your feelings. It's important to remember this is a stop that won't last forever.

The third stop is reinvesting in life. In this final stop your sense of loss diminishes; you'll have more energy and more interest in your life. You'll begin to move forward toward the possibility of new friends, new activities, and new pleasures. Your attention will move into the present time instead of being preoccupied with who you lost.

You'll make these stops, but you won't stay there. Eventually you need to give yourself permission to keep walking forward, to live fully, even though your loved one is no longer here.

The best memorial you can give to your dead loved one is to live a great life in their honor.

AUGUST 23

Missing Me

I remember after my loss a friend said to me, "I miss you" and I replied, "I miss me too."

When I experienced my loss, I also experienced a loss of my identity. It's weird how that happens. I know now it's a huge part of grief. But at the time it was yet another aspect of grief I wasn't prepared for, and it hit me hard.

What I lost was the piece of my identity based on my relationship to my spouse. In a matter of seconds, I went from being married to a widower. Do not pass go; do not collect 200 dollars. I asked myself questions like, "If I'm not a husband, what am I?"

I realized that my outlook and perspective on the world was deeply connected to my identity, and it was really shaken by my loss. When I was married, and part of a team, I was comfortable being a happy person. I believed that the world was a predictable and safe place. Then death shock these assumptive beliefs I had about the world, leaving me feeling more negative, pessimistic, and I wasn't able to engage with other people or activities the way I always did before.

In time I learned this was all a normal part of grief. But here I was with no identity, so now what?

Like so many things in grief, trying to go back to how things were before your loss just isn't possible. Part of regaining a sense of self after your loss is accepting that the identity you had then is going to be different now. It's important to remember that different doesn't mean bad. I don't like change. I think most people don't like change. We all have ideas about how life is supposed to look and who we're supposed to be. When life doesn't turn out that way, it can be easy to assume that no alternative will ever allow us to have a sense of well-being.

Though there will always be a deep sense of grief around the people and things in life that we lose, this doesn't mean there won't be other things that bring a sense of purpose, joy, and contentment and that will slowly become part of your identity.

The whole notion that you have to let go of the one you love to grieve your loss isn't true. The person you lost, the person you were, those are things that will still be a part of you as you go forward. A continued connection to the person you lost is actually a very healthy part of moving forward.

I refuse to be defined by my loss, so I've changed my perspective from a negative one to a positive one, and the rebuilding of my identity was born from an awareness of changes in myself. Of course, I will always be sad because of my loss, but I'm also happy about the new relationships that were born out of that loss.

AUGUST 24

A Curious Heart

I like to walk on the beach. Sometimes when I'm doing that, I see what looks like a beautiful shell, but when I reach down to pick it up, I realize it's really just seagull poop.

Grief is like that too. You can see it as an experience that will change you for the better or you can see it as only something really terrible. The beauty of the process is really in the experience of how you look at it.

If you look at it really closely, you might see that perhaps it's not all bad. Grief can make you become a more caring, compassionate, and empathetic person.

Grief hurts, but you don't have to get stuck in it and only see it as a bad thing. Grief is actually your friend now. Your constant companion. It took the place of the person you love. It's there to help you through and to remember the love you have in your heart.

If you gaze at grief with a curious heart, what at first appears desolate can become a place of hope. I think the real key to finding beauty in the process of grieving is to have a balance between the bad and the good. Both can help you heal.

For example, my spouse and I would always walk the beach and collect seashells. He would always be the one to hold them all in his pocket. If I found a shell, I gave it to him for safe keeping. Doing it alone after he died was so painful and sad. So, I bought a jar, and I wrote "Memory Jar" on it. I started to bring the jar with me and began to fill it. Filling that jar gave me a purpose. That jar is now full. The shells remind me of my walks, the walks with him, and the walks alone. I see the beauty in that jar when the sun reflects against the glass, and it has a calming effect on me.

It's the beauty of that jar, and what it means to me, that reminds me there's still beauty in grief, and it's not all just seagull poop.

AUGUST 25

It's Hard To Say Goodbye

How do you say goodbye to someone you love?

Even if they died, it's almost impossible to say goodbye. To me, it just seems so final. But saying goodbye to someone might be important to you. You may feel a strong desire to say a final farewell. You may have been one of the lucky ones that got the chance, or maybe you were one of those people that missed the opportunity because of an unexpected death, or because you were feeling uncomfortable accepting that the end was near.

If you didn't get a chance to say goodbye or are still struggling with whether you want to say goodbye or not, expressing a farewell can actually help you heal from the loss. In many ways it can bring peace and comfort to you.

As Winnie the Pooh said, "How lucky I am to have something that makes saying goodbye so hard."

If you didn't get to say goodbye to the person you love before they died, you might be feeling greater pain about their loss. If so, find yourself a private, quiet location. It could be in your house or a place that was special to both of you. Bring an object or photo that symbolizes their life or your memories together. Take this moment to say anything you need to say even if it's 'goodbye.'

I'll be honest, I never wanted to say goodbye, and I still haven't said it. Instead, I said, "See you on the other side."

If you continue to struggle with guilt or anxiety over not saying goodbye before your loved one's death, think about a happy memory of your loved one or visualize them forgiving you.

I think it's not really all about saying goodbye; maybe it's more about how to hold onto the love, until you meet again.

AUGUST 26

Life After Trauma

Someone you love died. Trauma enters into your life, destroys the world as you know it, and then leaves you wondering how to put things back together.

In the wreckage of your loss, you're consumed with feelings of fear and sorrow. Naturally, these emotions lead to anxiety. You start to worry about the future and how to discover the best path for moving forward.

Grief is your own personal response to loss. If you find yourself crying unexpectedly, waking up in the middle of the night with anxiety, or carrying what feels like a very heavy sense of sadness, this is what grief feels like, and it's perfectly normal. These emotional and physical experiences are a sign of how meaningful your loss is. The greater the loss, the more grief you feel. The more grief you feel, the more you loved the person you lost.

If you've experienced trauma, then you've also experienced grief, and probably even anxiety. These often go hand in hand. Sometimes the trauma is the loss of your own self. In an instant, your 'before self' seems to have evaporated, leaving your 'after self' grieving who you used to be.

If you surround yourself with the people who will sit with you in your grief and support you, that'll be when you'll begin to integrate the loss into your life. Avoid the other two types of people you will encounter: people that don't hurt you, but they also don't help you, and people that make you feel worse when they're around. Seek the first type of people; they will sit there with you and be supportive.

You also have to learn to support yourself. If the death of your loved one was traumatic, you could be suffering from PTSD, and avoiding it is not the answer.

While you can't go back to who you used to be, and you can't reclaim the loss you went through, you can move forward towards becoming a stronger, more resilient person, and even lead a purpose-filled life after trauma.

AUGUST 27

To Mom, With Love

You're gone. I'm sad because I'm no longer blessed by your presence. You're dead, and a piece of me is dead too. You slipped away quickly. You slipped away before I could get all your insight, your knowledge...and your memories. You slipped away before I could tell you everything.

You died with things left unsaid, because let's face it, there is always more to say. Always more hugs to be given. Always more memories to make. Always more left to say, to know, to wonder.
In your absence, I look for answers to the questions that pierce my heart and soul. Sometimes in the middle of the night, sometimes while I'm in line at the store, sometimes while I'm driving down the road, these questions pop up and remind me of the harsh reality of your death.

You aren't here, you can't answer, so I won't ever know. But it doesn't stop me from asking.

Did you know how much I loved you? A love so deep, so pure, so effortless that it occupies a part of my heart and soul.

Do you know how much you changed my life? Do you know you still inspire me even though I can't see you? Do you know you were more than a mother? You were the best teacher, friend, counselor, nurse, and so many other things to me. Do you know what an empty space you left in my heart?

Did you know you were my hero?

If not, I'm telling you now. Wherever you are, whatever you're doing, I want to say, Mom, I love you and miss you more than any words can say. You hold a piece of my heart that can never be replaced by anyone else, and your light shines bright in my soul.

Your absence hasn't changed your importance, to me you will always be the biggest influence in my life. Always and forever.

AUGUST 28

50 Shades of Anxiety

Do you ever think about things that scare you? Even if you're a really fearless person, I bet you can think of one thing that scares you.

I'll tell you mine.

I've always been really frightened to speak in front of people. This is kind of ironic, since now part of my job is to get up in front of large audiences and speak about grief and loss. If I think about it, the thing that scares me about speaking in front of people is usually the thoughts I have right before doing it. That's what causes my fear and anxiety. I know you know what I'm talking about. Even the bravest people feel fear and anxiety. I guess they just know how to navigate the experience better than I can.

Think about a time when you experienced the thoughts and sensations of fear and anxiety in your grief. Using a personal example, I remember feeling total panic and anxiety when my spouse died. How would I ever manage to go on alone? How could I ever be happy again? Who would take care of me if I got sick? Who would hold me when I was sad?

I felt like I was going crazy. I think a lot of my anxiety was based on the fact that I had very little confidence in my ability to cope with the emotions that were born out of my loss. I had to learn.

Grief and anxiety can make it difficult to take care of yourself. So, if you're not sure where to start in managing anxiety after your loss, go back to the basics. Take steps to improve sleep, eat healthy, and exercise your body. Spend time with family and friends who give you energy and support. Engage in your favorite activities and put things on the calendar you know you'll enjoy. When daily tasks start to feel more manageable, your anxiety has a greater chance of receding.

Working through grief and anxiety should never be something you have to do alone. Talking with a counselor about the loss and gaining tools to manage symptoms can also help prevent complicated grief or the development of an anxiety disorder. Be sure that you check in with your doctor to make sure that physical health issues aren't also contributing to your level of anxiety.

I'll be honest, I still experience anxiety when I have to speak in front of large groups of people, and I still grieve my loss, but I know the steps I need to take to manage my anxiety and navigate my grief.

With the right self-care and support, you can gain back your sense of control after a loss. Life may not feel manageable now, but with time and the right tools, you can begin to sculpt the life you want for yourself. It's normal to feel anxious about experiencing new emotions, grief triggers, and painful memories because you now know bad things can happen.

AUGUST 29

What You Don't See

The thing about grief is that other people tend to forget you're doing it. Or they think that after a week or two, you should be over it. But you and I know it doesn't work that way, right? We have to somehow strike a balance between the act of grieving and our total lack of control over it, along with the will to continue living life and making plans.

But grief is a tricky thing. There's an array of thoughts and emotions I continue to face in my grief that's somehow invisible and unfamiliar to everyone else. The only people who can understand this are those of us who have experienced a tremendous loss. After my loss, for months I felt like everything I said and did was foreign to the outside world. It was like I carried this invisible, massive boulder, cradling it between both my arms, trying hard not to drop it. I was really just striving beyond everything else to keep a tight grasp on this boulder, praying that at any second, the whole thing wouldn't fall and smash my feet.

How do you explain to people who have no idea what you're experiencing that it's been several months and you're still crying yourself to sleep? That you're always sad? How do you show them what you had to witness with your own eyes or explain to them why you still just want the person you love to come back? Well, you can't.

I'm not trying to blame people for not understanding, but I'm arguing that we have to get better at supporting those who are struggling. When someone we love dies, it's not just their death that we struggle with, it's also the regret of all the things said and done during the time in which they were still alive. And it's in all the things you can't say or do now that they're gone.

It's not just about the last interaction you had with someone, it's about all of it. It's about the lifetime of good memories.

I'm finally at a place where I'm at peace with the fact that my loved one is gone. When someone you love is taken from you suddenly, your brain has a way of doing whatever it does when you experience a traumatic event, it holds onto it tight and constantly floods you with thoughts of it.

So, I'm still going over the events I witnessed and applying the fear to other people in my life. Will more people I love die? Will my dog die? Is my own life at risk of being cut short?

The death of my spouse crushed me. It left a hole in my heart. I'm still trying to figure out how to fill that hole or whether it can ever be filled.

Maybe nothing's ever really gone? I don't know. But what I do know is that I'm still trying to reconcile the fact that every day is just another day without my loved one in it, and that will never change.

AUGUST 30

Walking Right Through It

It's important to journey through the grieving process. You have to grieve. If you think you don't, grief tends to follow you until you do.

I remember when my best friend died three years after my spouse. I was incredibly saddened by her death, but I found her passing to be easier. Was it because it was my second big loss? Was I better at this? Did I love her less? I don't even think I can answer any of those questions, but it proved to me that each loss has its own journey.

I miss her just as much as my spouse, but the pain of her passing was not as great. I also think part of it is because her death was a surprise. I knew my spouse was going to die. I just didn't want to believe it. But her death was unexpected, and yet I still felt numb but not as crushed.

I think it's important to let grief have its way with you. Let the emotions happen. They need to be expressed and often not at the most convenient moments. Sometimes little things will trigger a memory, and you'll be overcome with emotion. That's okay!

It's important to remember that you have to go through the difficult center of grief to journey to the other side in the healthiest manner possible. You can't go around it. You can't go over it. You can't go under it. You have to walk right through it. I can tell you from experience that it will get worse before it will get better, but if you grieve thoroughly and well, you'll feel better. The pain will be less sharp.

You'll learn to live in a new way and find the only direction the road goes is forward.

AUGUST 31

Getting Unstuck

There are some experiences of grief that are beyond all others. Two that come to mind are the death of a child and the death of a spouse.

I have some good friends that have experienced the death of a child. The extreme grief of such a great loss causes stress on the structure of the entire immediate family. In some cases, the grief has brought the parents and siblings closer together, and in other cases, it has broken them apart.

I have personally never lost a child, but I have experienced the death of a spouse. The grief of losing him was like me losing part of myself. For me, it was extreme grief.

I had a great romance and friendship. We were drawn ever closer to each other. After twenty years of being together, we instinctively knew each other's moods and could communicate on a non-verbal level. Life without him seemed impossible to imagine.

When he died, I felt I had lost everything. I was afraid to be home and face the loneliness. But eventually I had to. When I was in that empty house, I screamed in agony. Banged my fist against the wall. I felt pain in my chest like my heart was going to stop.

In public, I was able to pull myself together somewhat, but my sadness was always evident. I cried every day, sometimes in public, but mostly when I was alone. I'd go to bed crying and sometimes wake in the morning crying.

After a year of seeing me grieve, my family and friends started to think it was odd that I was still not recovered from the loss. So, for their benefit, I started to pretend that I was better.
It was all an act. No more did I break down in public, but I was nowhere near recovered.

I had to get unstuck.

I decided I had to make a more active effort to somehow recover. I did some deep soul searching to find what was keeping me from moving forward with my life. In a moment of clarity, I realized that I was afraid to let go of grief because that would mean I was letting go of my love for him. It seems irrational that I was hanging on to grief in order to feel love, but extreme grief can throw common sense out the window.

I knew that he would always be in my heart whether he was alive or not. So, every time the sadness came, I reminded myself that nothing could diminish that love. I could never lose him completely. The awareness that love transcends death was a turning point. The sadness lifted, and the grief softened. I finally came to acceptance. Friends say to me now, "You've changed."

Yes, I did change. Grief broke me down and rebuilt me. My grief journey gave me a new outlook on life, loss, and love, especially love.

SEPTEMBER

SEPTEMBER 1

Friends in the Aftermath

When I went through my loss everyone knew about it, whether I wanted them to or not. It's like I was wearing a sign that said, "Caution: Widower!"

All my friends and family would look at me funny. You know that look that says, "Are you okay?" They had that look on their faces like a deer caught in the headlights, so I would just say, "Sure, I'm okay," just to let them off the hook.

They looked at me funny and said stupid things. They checked on me constantly or they completely ignored me. Some of them had no idea what to do, so they did nothing. Some tried to help, but only offered what I didn't need. Some of these people thought they knew what I was going through, but they didn't.

The one thing all these people had in common was they knew about my loss. In time, many of these friends and family drifted out of my life. Maybe it was my fault for changing? The loss of someone you love does that to you. Maybe they just got sick of trying to help me? Even I didn't know what it was I needed other than my person back. Maybe they couldn't relate to me now that I was grieving?

So new friends came into my life. Most of them never met my person that died. Though part of me missed the safety of the friends and family who knew everything that had happened, there was a relief in being surrounded by these new friends who were strangers to my loss.

There were no weird moments, no awkwardness, no looks at me like I might suddenly burst into tears at any moment, no unwanted advice. Though I felt totally consumed by my own grief, something about being away from everyone who knew gave me control over something again.

As time went on these people became my new lifeline. Many of them had also suffered a major loss. They knew how I felt. They understood my pain.

They understood my grief. It felt good to be around people that 'got it,' and me. Everything about my current life is the way it is because my person died, and to the outside world I'm sure I look just like every other guy. Only I'm not. These new friends know this about me. They understand.

I didn't know how I would ever be able to find new friends, but I did. I didn't know how I would ever find people who hadn't been part of my anguish and loss, but somehow I did that too. I discover new friends who only know me in the 'aftermath,' and when I meet these new people, I at some point tell them about my loss.

I've learned to say words out loud that I never imagined I would have to say. I help these new people meet my person for the first time through my stories and through my memories.

SEPTEMBER 2

There's No Getting Over It

Everyone will expect you to eventually stop grieving at some point. Right? They think it can't possibly be healthy to grieve someone you lost for too long. Wrong! You'll grieve the one you lost forever. Why? Because love is forever. So, do you know why you'll never get over 'it'? Because 'it' is the one you love.

What you learn to do is live with the grief. The pain, visible or not, stays with you forever until you take your last breath. You may wonder how long the grief will last. The truth is that healing comes slowly, but it does come.

Nothing can replace the person you lost, and yet gradually you will find you are able to continue with life and start to feel happy at times while remembering the one you love and lost. Grief comes in waves; you will have dark days when it seems as though nothing can ever be right again. But there will also be better days when the pain eases, and it is possible to begin to hope and believe in the future again.

Some people find it easier to show their feelings than others, but nearly everyone finds at some stage that it helps to talk. So, talk about your loved one every chance you get. This can be to friends, relatives, or by seeking professional help. There's no magical, invisible wall clock that's ticking, pressuring you to get over 'it'. You're allowed to take as much time as you need to heal.

Don't think that you have to get back to 'normal,' that will never happen. The pain you feel when you miss them is never going to go away, but that's okay. You'll never get over it, because 'it' is everything you loved about the person who died. It's all the memories and time spent with them.

You don't get over it, you carry it.

SEPTEMBER 3

Losing John

Experiencing the death of a loved one is always painful, but there's a special kind of grief associated with the loss of a child. It cuts the heart in a way no other loss can. It reminds us of something we spend most of our life trying to ignore, trying not to believe, that death can take anyone, at any time.

Whether you lost a child or not, and I have not, I think we still begin asking really big and overwhelming questions. I know I do. Like is there a God? If there is a God, how could he let something like this happen? I sometimes feel bad asking these questions, but I can't help it.

When I was very small, I had a friend named John. He had Down Syndrome. He was my best friend. John died when we were both only eight. I asked my mother why he died, and she said, "John was special, and God takes all special children to Heaven."

Hmm? Now I know my mother meant well, but this was probably not the best response to give to a very sensitive little kid. I was happy John was in Heaven, but I worried about myself. If God took my friend John and not me, did that mean I wasn't special? Maybe being special wasn't such a great thing to be if it means you have to die at eight? Sure, I wanted to go to Heaven, but I also wanted to grow up first. The whole thing just didn't seem fair.

We moved away shortly after John died, but I've often thought a lot about him, and now as an adult I also wonder about John's parents. Where does something like that leave grieving parents? I suppose John's parents were never the same after that. After all, he was a pretty special kid and a great friend. Losing John must have been really horrible for them.

I heard years later that John had a heart condition and some other health issues. In the end he was in a lot of pain. I wonder if his parents found comfort in trusting that John was not only free of all pain but also in Heaven. Maybe it left them with a deep sense of hope that death doesn't have the final word.

I think when death takes a child, parents are left not only with pain and grief but with unfulfilled hopes, the broken promise of memories that were never made, and with the sadness of knowing what could have been but never will be. I bet that's how John's parents felt.

I hope that when I die, I go to Heaven, and I hope I see John. Maybe the thought of that is what has enabled John's parents to survive all these years? I sure hope so, because I was really sad losing John, so I can only imagine how sad his parents must have been.

I have faith that all parents will see the children they have lost again, and when they do, they will rejoice with their children forever and ever, I hope that's how it is for John.

SEPTEMBER 4

Finding a Purpose

Do you feel like you not only lost your loved one, but also your purpose in life? This is a totally normal and common reaction to a major loss. So, the question is, how do you find your purpose again?

First, you have to decide that you actually want to move forward, and that you're ready to see what might come next. I always say this is when you get to the point in your grief journey when you realize you have two choices: getting to work on living or getting to work on dying. I hope you will chose 'living'.

Like most things, the first step is the hardest. While you might say you're tired of being sad all the time, and you're ready for a change, you would be surprised to know how hard moving forward can be. And it's not always for the reasons you'd think. Moving forward may feel like leaving your loved one in the past. It may feel disloyal, or you might worry if you're not actively grieving it means you're not actively expressing your love either.

The dark place of grief can become a surprisingly comfortable and familiar place to be. Moving beyond it can feel like a step into the unknown. That unknown could be a place filled with disappointment or rejection. Or perhaps taking that step is simply more work or energy than you actually feel you have to give. Grief is a place to go to when you need it, just don't stay there.

When you think you may be ready (and remember, there's no right or wrong answer to when this is) then the real work begins. This can be a wonderful time of reflection and research. A chance to search for what's out there, to talk to other people and find out how they're spending their time. What is meaningful to them, and how are they finding purpose.

It can be a chance to do the thing you always wanted to do and never had the time. It can be the cause that you always believed in, or it can be helping people who have suffered in ways you can relate.

To really find purpose and to make the next step forward in life, there's one thing I think helps more than anything else, getting out of your own head. Getting out of your own head and finding a way to help others can be one of the most meaningful and productive things you can do. By taking the focus off yourself and turning it to someone or something else where there's a need will be one of the most soothing and healing ways you can spend your time.

Spend some time today thinking about finding purpose and what comes next. If you don't have interests of your own, that's okay. Think about your loved one. What was meaningful to them? Can you feel closer to them by finding a way to honor them or by being part of something they cared about? If you can't do it for yourself, then do it for them.

SEPTEMBER 5

Grief Is Love

Grief is hard to conquer and even harder to understand. It's a painfully strong emotion that takes over the entire body. But grief does have its roots in love. It's easy to think that grief and love are worlds apart from each other, but in some ways they're more similar than you might think.

We all enjoy being loved. While grief hurts, love is something we welcome, and it fills us with warmth. The death of a loved one brings the loss of that warmth in the way we aren't used to experiencing it. Their love for us becomes a memory rather than something we can experience in a physical way. This creates a hole in our heart that can make us feel really empty inside.

So how can we say that grief and love are similar? We don't really grieve the loss of something we don't love. When someone you love dies, it can feel like the pain of losing them is all there is. You might feel like you'll never fill that hole in your heart.

But the love you shared with your loved one doesn't just disappear because they're physically gone, it merely changes. It changes into memories of your life with them, into the way you share what they taught you with others, into the countless ways you remember them and include their memory in your life, on special days and every day.

The bottom line is there are no rules to grief. We can only surrender to it and let our hearts break open for it. We don't work through our grief and return to who we once were. It doesn't work that way. There can never be a return to the person we were before our loss. We're broken and shattered by our grief. We can never look the same or be the same. We lose a piece of ourselves, an important piece.

So, in our grief, the only thing to do is to give our love a place to go. We can love with the things we say, love with the deeds we do, and love with the actions we take.

We can love one another so fiercely that our love is spent, that our chests are no longer hollow, that the lump in our throats hurts a little less. Love for those who hurt the most, who have lost the most, and then love them even harder. Because the truth about grief is that it never leaves. Grief lasts as long as love lasts, forever.

I know you may not believe me because right now your grief seems like a nightmare. I'll admit that some days I don't believe it myself.

You may be feeling really isolated, sad, and alone. I want to remind you, that underneath the stress, frustration, anger, disappointment, despair, guilt, loneliness, and sorrow of grief, quite often there's love.

SEPTEMBER 6

You Have the Compass

The two most common questions I'm asked about grief are, "What's normal?" and "How long does it take?" These most asked questions are usually just a cover-up for, "When will this pain, suffering, loneliness, longing, yearning, or (fill in the blank) stop?"

The misconception is that if you can stop the pain then you have successfully found your way through your grief, and now you are all done. Not true! What actually happens is you suddenly realize you don't know what you don't know about the whole grieving process.

This then leads to the third most common question I get asked, "How do I navigate grief?" There's usually no cover-up for this question, just the burning need for an answer.

When it comes to grief, nobody hands you a map, compass, or a guide, right? You're pretty much drifting on uncharted waters with no sight of land then add to that a hole in your boat and no oars. Grief is really just a journey of time. Not in the sense that 'time heals all wounds,' that's just not true. It's more a journey over time that includes action, presence, and a plan.

Navigating grief means planning out your next destination. Whatever that looks like to you.

You can decide when to walk, rest, turn back, or push through all the rough and difficult moments. This is how grief works. It's a process. Different for everyone. Each destination unique. When your loved one died that was a detour, but you can decide if you'll take that detour life handed you.

There will be different directions to go in, but you can choose to make and take your own route. You determine who and what you need along the way. You learn your lessons. You might find unexpected gifts but not when you are in hurt and pain. And decision-making while in the fog of grief can be overwhelming.

You can decide to release the pain of your grief as you hold on with love, hope, and connection to your loved one. When you plan for a trip you prepare for it, right? Well, it's the same thing with grief. Grieving your loss is the preparation for the rest of your life.

Grief isn't easy. Grief isn't pretty. But neither is what you're experiencing right now. You can choose to do something about your grief and navigate your course toward healing. Your definition for what is normal is likely to change. But it's possible to find that on the other side of grief you become more of yourself, rather than less, without your loved one.

You're the expert on your grief and on your life; you already have the compass you need for navigating your grief. It's all about you. To find yourself, you have to ask the right questions and answer them from your own heart. Once you do that, you'll begin to visualize and create the life that lies ahead.

SEPTEMBER 7

Year #3

You've heard a lot about grief in the first and second year, but what about the third year? What does that look like?

Most of the challenges you face during the first year after the death of a loved one could fill a whole book, so I won't go into them. But in a nutshell, it's all you can do to cope with the seemingly endless emotions like shock, pain, confusion, anger, regret, sadness, you name it, you'll feel it.

In the second year you're trying to understand where your loved one went, how you're going to go on living without them, dealing with all the grief, finding a way to create a new life, and dealing with how much you miss them.

So, what about the third year?

The third year of grief seems to be a year of transition with only one new challenge, beginning to rebuild your life. You still have times of sadness, still miss your loved one, still yearn for them, but these feelings are not as prominent as they once were in the first and second year.

You may no longer feel that moving forward is a betrayal of your love because you understand that you had no choice in the matter. You had no control over the death, and you have no control over the fact that life keeps going on. You're still trying to figure out who you are now that the person is gone.

Although this transition between your old life and your new life seems to be a time of being stuck, you're still rebuilding your life day by day, becoming who you need to be, which is a sign of hope for the future, even if you're really not yet feeling hopeful. Whatever the challenges are you have to deal with in the third year of grief, you'll meet them as you did all the other challenges in the first and second year, with courage, perseverance, and strength. Because you have no other choice, right?

SEPTEMBER 8

Permission Granted

I started writing about grief and loss to help other people. It's just a way for me to share what I've learned on my own personal grief journey. I really just wanted to let people know what the view from a widower's eyes looked like because maybe they could relate.

Then people started to ask me questions. But I wondered, would they actually want my advice?

I heard from widows and widowers, parents who lost a child, and children who lost a parent. All kinds of people, and all kinds of questions.

One widower asked, "I lost my wife, she died a year ago, and now I want to move, but I'd be leaving all of our friends and the cemetery where she's buried. Do you think I should do it?"

A widow asked, "I got offered a new job. Before my husband died, I would have taken it. Now, I feel like I shouldn't because I need to be home with our young child. But this new job would be better money. Should I even be considering it?"

Every time I answered these questions, I gave what probably seemed like a very frustrating response, I'd say, "It depends." Because of course it does. I mean, in the first example, how far are you moving, and do you have a support system there? And in the second example, what are all the pros and cons with this new job?

I can take a guess, but obviously all people aren't the same, and all situations aren't the same. I can only say what I'd do if it were me. But the thing is, they aren't really asking me what I'd do. They're asking me what they should do. I'll be honest, I don't have the answers. But I think that's okay because I don't think people are asking for an answer. I think what they're really asking for is permission.

If you're wondering what the right thing is to do, I'll answer you with, "It depends." Because I think you do know the answer. And if you actually know what you want to do, but are just feeling unsure about it, then I have another answer for you: "Do it!"

I'll give you my permission. That's stupid to say, of course, because you don't need my permission. But maybe you just need someone's permission. And if that's the case, I'll give you mine. I'll say, go for it. Follow your heart. Take the risk. I'll totally support any decision you make, right or wrong.

I'll be the first to admit, I don't have all the answers, but neither does anyone else, right?

So doing it might not be a good idea, but it also might change your life for the better.

SEPTEMBER 9

When Feeling Better Feels Wrong

My relationship with grief has changed immensely over time. No matter how bad my grief has been, especially in the early days, I've never truly wanted it to go away.

Do I regret why it became a part of my life in the first place? Hell yes! But if my spouse was going to be dead, then I was going to grieve.

I know this sounds crazy because people are always telling you that you need to resolve your grief. It's kind of hard to explain, but even when my grief was extremely painful, I didn't want to escape it. I guess at the time, as terrible as grief felt, it also seemed like my memories and connection to my spouse existed within it.

My grief became an ongoing vigil allowing me to stay focused and devoted to my spouse's memory for as long as his death mattered to me. I didn't really care that other people seemed to be forgetting.

After my spouse died, I felt like my love was defined by my pain and suffering. My spouse's death was devastating, so it was only right that I should feel devastated for a really long time.

For me, feeling okay seemed like getting over it or moving on, which I wasn't ready to do. Not only did feeling better feel impossible, but it also felt wrong.

I mistakenly believed that my grief and pain had to end before I could feel better. I didn't realize that getting over it and moving on weren't even a part of the grief process. I didn't know that a person could bring their loved one with them as they move forward in life. I didn't know that my grief would eventually become a part of my being okay.

I didn't know a lot of things, and if at the time you had told me all the things I didn't know, I wouldn't have believed you. These are realizations I had to come to myself. Just as my words here can't make these realities any truer for you. I get that.

Just because you have positive thoughts and feelings, it doesn't mean that you're somehow okay with your loved one's death. This thought process is normal when you're grieving.

If you're not open to these concepts now, give it some time.

Obviously, you would never have chosen for your loved one to die; this grief journey was forced on you.

So, any growth you have from this point on is just your way of coping with the only choice you were given, to survive.

SEPTEMBER 10

Death Is Random

I bet when you think about the person you loved that died you say, "It isn't fair."

I think that fairness is in the eye of the beholder. I'm guessing that you're angry at the unfairness of the circumstances of your loved one's death. I totally understand your pain.

Why do some people die young, and others live to be 100? Why does a plane crash and some live and some die? Why do some people get cancer, and some don't? Why are some babies born healthy and other babies die? Why do bad people live long, and good people die young?

I always think it's unfair when someone dies before their time. I can never seem to explain the unfairness away. I don't like when people say, "It was part of God's plan." Well, it wasn't part of my plan, and it hurts like hell.

Another one that's not helpful is, "They were in the wrong place at the wrong time." Chances are they were in the place they were supposed to be going about their day just like the rest of us. But unlike the rest of us, the unthinkable happened. Many times death is random, unpredictable, and it just isn't fair.

Grief is so unique to everyone, and everyone's process of it is different. For me, it came down to accepting my spouse's death. Why did the circumstances unfold the way they did? What if any one of my actions or choices was different; would it have changed the outcome? Why did it have to happen to us? Was there some reason?

The questions of 'why' haunted me and took up all my energy. I looked everywhere to find the answers to all these questions. I read books, joined groups, went through counseling. I asked those questions over and over again…and yet I just never could find the answers.

I finally realized that even if I had the answers, my spouse was still going to be dead. So, I made the choice to stop asking why. My spouse died, and I couldn't change it. So, what was I going to do to honor his life and memory?

I've heard of many wonderful ways people turn their pain into ways to honor their loved one's memory. Some have created large foundations in their loved one's name to help others. Some just do simple acts of kindness.

No matter what the act or activity, focusing your efforts on finding a way to honor your loved one can provide meaning for a death that appeared to have none. It can help shift your focus from despair to love, from anger to acceptance.

I know it will never change the fact that their death was unfair, but it can help you begin to heal.

SEPTEMBER 11

Between Happy and Sad

There are times when I'm happy, and times when I'm sad, and then the times I spend between them both.

I write a lot about grief. I try to teach people how to live life to the fullest how to live in the moment, and how to embrace the unknown, even after a significant loss. This takes time and work. It requires a leap of faith and opening your heart. It's making life changes that you never wanted to make.

It's a risk.

There are moments you'll be happy and moments you'll be sad. Then there are the moments you live between happy and sad.

These are the days when someone asks you, "How are you?" You'll struggle to figure out whether you're happy or sad or maybe just 'okay.' This might be when you feel like you're living without any purpose and have no goal to pursue. The days when you're 'just living.'

The moments of living between happy and sad are the days you aren't lonely but not feeling happy, and you can't claim to feel sad. You're not depressed, but you're not calm. These are the times when you're neither happy nor sad, just empty.

You don't feel anything. You want a shoulder to cry on and an ear to listen, but at the same time you want to be alone.

Living between happy and sad can be uncomfortable. But being uncomfortable can be a great motivator for making every moment of life countable. It can force you to achieve something bigger than what you've got.

It can give you the courage to build a new dream to pursue, and that makes life worth living again.

SEPTEMBER 12

The Last Goodbye

I've suffered the loss of some significant people in my life, and sometimes I still get hung up on the fact that I didn't say goodbye to them. It might seem insignificant, but I think a proper goodbye provides a sense of finality.

I think there's a special kind of comfort in acknowledging, and even accepting, that I would never see them again. That last goodbye is like a summation of events and a period at the end of the story, right? It seems like at someone's bedside, in their final hours, that goodbye represents the farewell of a lifetime of moments together.

Now, whenever I leave any of the people I love, I make sure to give them a hug, and I make sure I say goodbye. I just don't think I could bear the weight of missing anyone else, especially if I forgot to say goodbye.

Looking back, I don't really think I forgot to say goodbye, as much as I just didn't want to do it. I didn't say goodbye because I didn't want to upset them. Saying it would have been acknowledging their deaths. It would've looked like I was accepting it, that it was fine, but it was absolutely not fine.

Then I wonder if saying goodbye would have given them some kind of peace at the end or made them feel more comfortable? I guess I'll never know.

I really doubt any of these people I loved ever pondered whether I loved them or not. I just wonder if by saying goodbye, I could have let them know how much I really did love them.

Maybe it really isn't important that I forgot to say goodbye. Maybe it was me that needed to hear it from them, then I would have been surer they were okay with it and were accepting that it was the end of their journey.

The real question is, would saying goodbye have changed the course of my grief or lessened my pain? Probably not.

SEPTEMBER 13

I Feel Your Pain

You don't know me, but if you've suffered the loss of someone you love, I feel your pain, and I understand what you're going through. I don't know your personal and unique pain, but I know the pain of losing someone you love.

If you're reading this, I think of you when I'm struggling, knowing somewhere out there you're struggling, too. I'm very aware of how much your world has changed and how much you've suffered. I know you're wondering, "Where do I go from here"? I know that you feel that life isn't worth living without your loved one.

I won't be the one that tells you that you should keep your chin up or fake a smile. I won't be the one that tells you that you should be over it by now. I won't be the one that tells you how you should grieve. I'll be the one reaching out my hand to help you up.

I know that you'll never have a 'normal' day again. But today, I hope that you do whatever you want to do. If you want to drop to your knees and cry, I hope you have a soft rug. If you want to stay in bed all day, I hope you have warm blankets. If you want to sit in silence, I hope you find peace in the moment. You see, I know what happened to you isn't fair, and I'm so sorry.

I'm sure you have some people who've quietly slipped out of your life, and although their absence hurts, I hope you have found other people who support you even if you're broken. I hope you'll consider me one of those supportive people because I feel your pain, and I understand.

In the weeks, months, and years ahead, you'll begin to put the pieces of your life back together. The scar will remain, but you'll be able to live again. I can tell you it's not easy, but I can also tell you that if you take my hand, I'll take the first steps with you.

I feel your pain, but I also know there's a future out there for you.

SEPTEMBER 14

Gathering Love

If you've lost a person you love, nobody can ever replace them, but it's not a matter of replacing, it's about opening your heart and adding to the love that's already there.

Nobody can ever replace your loved one in your heart nor should they. But to forever close your heart to others would be no longer living life. We all need love. Isn't that why you loved the one you lost in the first place? Our hearts are capable of all kinds of love.

Does a mother or father who loses one of their children no longer love the others? Does a husband or wife who loses their spouse and remarries no longer love the spouse that was lost? Would your loved one want you to be sad and close your heart forever or be happy and leave your heart open to let love in?

You have the option to honor your loved one by sharing the love you had for them, and they had for you by remaining open to love. Not just romantic love but love for life and others. The other option is to close your heart and live the rest of your life in a sad and lonely state just waiting to die so you can be with your lost loved one again.

If you had been the one who died, what would you want for them? Would you want to look down and see them in a self-imposed prison of sadness and pain, or would you want to see them happy and living a full life?

Keep your heart open because love has no limits. Your heart will always search for a way to express your love to someone. It can be as simple as opening your heart to a family member, friend, or even a stranger.

Live the rest of your life with a heart that's open, joyful, and full. Be willing to give and receive all the love your loved one would wish for you. In the end, all the love you've gathered in your heart is all you take with you when your journey here is over.

SEPTEMBER 15

Silent Grief

There are circumstances when you're forced to hide your pain or vulnerability. Our society lives most of the time with its back to death and loss, in a hurry to turn the page and return to a time when everything was 'normal.'

But for you, nothing is normal.

This silent grief can make you not know what to do with your feelings because you feel compelled to move on. This is very common if you lost a loved one due to suicide, a subject that remains taboo in our culture. You may be more likely to develop silent grief when you can't find support from others to share your suffering from your loss.

Sometimes silent grief is caused by a lack of sensitivity from those close to you. For example, the loss of a pet also can lead to silent grief because the people around you don't understand your deep pain, and they encourage you to turn the page as soon as possible.

There are many other losses that have to be lived in silence because they don't generate emotional resonance in those around you, such as the loss of a pregnancy, the failure of a professional project, or even the loss of a job.

When people tell you, "It's over, don't cry anymore" or "Be strong, he/she wouldn't like to see you like this," the message that comes to you is that your pain isn't understood. Other people may decide to walk away thinking that this will make them less of a nuisance, but in this way they leave you alone with your grief.

Overcoming a loss, whatever it is, is difficult. Trying to overcome it alone can be a daunting task.

I believe the solution for silent grief is finding people that are willing to listen to you. Emotional validation can work miracles, facilitate acceptance, and give you a more objective perspective on the situation.

When you can express yourself freely, and someone listens to you in a respectful way without judgment or haste, there's a rearrangement of the feelings and thoughts related to your loss. Therefore, you can continue to advance in the grieving process.

Grief is hard, it takes time to find a place for it, and a little understanding goes a long way.

SEPTEMBER 16

I Want To Live

I talk a lot about surviving grief, but I think there's more to it than just surviving. I don't want to just survive; I want to live.

I try to look at my experience with loss as strength. I know when bad things happen, they can be painful to go through, but as I go on without the person I once had, I'm becoming stronger.

By reaching out to other people I've learned I'm not alone. I share my story and ask questions about how other people got through their loss. It reminds me that if they can do it, I can too.

Sometimes my loss opened me up to new experiences and possibilities. I felt really guilty at first for having those thoughts, but then I realized there was nothing wrong with looking for ways to improve or change my life after my loss.

When someone you love dies, it's almost automatic to focus on the pain. But by focusing on the good times I had with the person I lost, I was practicing gratitude for those experiences.

When a heart has suffered a big loss, it can be very difficult to even have the desire to live and seek out ways to be happy again. I experienced that.

It took all my energy just to survive! That was never easy. Some days are still better than others, but I refuse to give up.

But surviving for me also had to have a purpose, and I needed a reason to keep moving forward, and when the time was right, I decided I also wanted to live.

I know that things will never be the same, but I want to live, and that has brought me its own sense of happiness.

SEPTEMBER 17

When 'We' Becomes 'Me'

Do you want to be happy again or keep drowning in your sadness?

Grieving over a death of a spouse or a longtime partner can be devastating, especially when you had your whole life planned, and it revolved around them. Dealing with the terrible pain and loneliness is overwhelming, and you may feel totally clueless about going on with life. So, how do you go on after the loss of a partner or spouse?

It starts with having an attitude that allows rebirth. It will take time, so be patient with yourself. In time, you'll feel the sadness, anger, and fatigue fading away. You'll start to regain interest in others and the world around you. It's about moving forward with grace, and that starts with changing your thinking from "there's no reason to go on" and learning to stop saying "never."

Your brain can make you believe what you want to believe. If you consider having a life after your loss, then your brain will gather the information you need to do just that. Allowing yourself to grieve is important and going to that place of grief is necessary. Just don't stay there.

The healing process may be slow, but you're getting there. You're free to express your emotions in your own way. Rediscovering 'you' starts with taking care of yourself. Find ways to stay active and fill your time with activities that you enjoy.

Widows and widowers have all moved forward. They've been doing it for all time. Going through the loss of a partner or spouse is a personal battle but know that you're not alone because one half of every couple will one day be left behind.

So, heal at your own pace, but allow yourself to fill your mind with positive thoughts. Negative thoughts will stop you from moving forward, but positive thoughts will help you find ways to fill the void.

SEPTEMBER 18

It's Okay To Be Happy

After a significant loss, negative feelings can often be all-consuming, which is why it's okay to search for small moments of happiness wherever you can find them.

Grief is hard, and it takes time to find a place for it. Even though you may feel sadness associated with your loss, you can also feel joy. But sometimes when you do feel the least bit of happiness, you can also automatically feel guilty about having those feelings.

How can you feel happy when someone you love has died? Impossible…right?

It's important to first face the reality of the situation by identifying all the bittersweet emotions of losing a person you love…while at the same time appreciating the value of life. It could be anything from the laugh of a child, the nature around you, or even a kind act from a stranger.

Whatever it is, embrace it even if it's only temporary. These are the moments that will get you through your grief.

Remember that your grief is fluid and changing all the time. Feeling sad and happy are emotions that will come in waves. They become part of your everyday life. This is normal.

When you get stuck in your grief, there's no fluidity and it remains unchanging. Having feelings of happiness and joy can ease the pain, even for a moment, as it helps to move you forward.

It's okay to be in a place of sadness when you're missing someone you love…just don't stay in that place until you get stuck. How you navigate the pendulum of sadness and joy will make all the difference in your grief journey.

It's okay to be sad, but it's also perfectly okay to be happy.

SEPTEMBER 19

My Pain Takes a Backseat

I recently told a friend that I didn't want my old life anymore. My old life is the life I had to live after my spouse died, and that's a life that was full of grief and pain. My previous life didn't exist anyway. When I look at pictures from that life, they're just reminders of what I used to have but don't anymore.

It's funny; in the beginning after I lost my spouse, I was afraid the pain would leave. It was almost like I'd lose him if it went away.

Now, I'm still carrying the pain, but it takes a backseat to my happiness. But like I've always suspected, grief has a life of its own. I don't control it, and it doesn't listen to me. There came a time when all of a sudden there was a definite shift forward. A sense of 'getting on' with things.

I can tell you from my own experience that this wasn't always easy. I could decide that I was going to move forward in a positive way in my life, and still, it could feel like I was pushing a giant elephant up a stairway. And then, the thought would pop into my head just like it did after my spouse died, "How do I get through the day, let alone the rest of my life?"

Then the answer came to me. Get twice as strong, and then get stronger than that. Sometimes that thought makes me feel very tired, and sometimes I feel ready. I want to feel ready.

It's strange how much grief takes out of you in just trying to function every day, and for me, I think the reserves that were depleted during my spouse's illness, and then further smashed into smithereens after he died, have now been fully replenished. For a long time, I felt that it'd be much easier to sit around, waiting to die, and never doing anything.

It seemed like an option. But then I realized I still wanted my life to mean something, and that was a positive sign to me.

SEPTEMBER 20

Life Doesn't Make Sense

"Why did they have to die? Why did this happen to me?" Have you asked yourself these questions? I bet you have and like a bazillion times!

I think this probably comes from your belief that bad things only happen to people who deserve it. At least that's probably how you felt until the person you love died.

I often do an inventory of my own quest for "why?", along with that of the thousands of grievers I've seen grapple with this question over the years.

When you find yourself alone in your grief, you start to believe things like if you had just parented a little better, if a doctor or a medical facility had done something differently, if you just had the chance to say goodbye, if you had just acted sooner, things would be different.

Thinking about these things over and over again is how you try to make sense of the world after your loss. It becomes super important because you think if you can figure out what the "cause" for the death was...then it will all make sense. Nope!

There's nothing you can do to change the outcome of what already happened, at least not now. So maybe you just think if you can figure out why it happened, you can prevent it from happening again.

Don't get me wrong, sometimes that's kind of true, like when there's a very clear source or cause for a death. There are things that if done differently in the future could change the outcome for someone else. There are lessons learned from so many losses, to stop smoking or to avoid risks like drunk driving.

You'll probably spend weeks, months, and even years dwelling on why, either blaming yourself or others, until one day you just realize that there is no answer to "why?". The world is just an unexpected place. I still sometimes try to make sense of what happened to my spouse, but now I know that's just because sometimes life just doesn't make sense.

I hope that you'll try to stop beating yourself up for something you probably had no control over.
Start by becoming aware of how some of your thoughts, especially those guilt and blame thoughts, may be coming from this want to put an order to things.

Be open to your grief and give yourself a break rather than assuming you're doing it wrong.

Remember, there's no right or wrong, especially when it comes to grief, and you had no attachment to the outcome. So don't let the quest for 'why' take over what's left of your life.

SEPTEMBER 21

Never Feeling the Same

Will I ever feel the same? This question is a very normal and natural response to loss and an understandable part of the grieving process. I can tell you that the answer is NO. The death of a loved one marks you with a scar and inevitably changes you. It's just about the worst thing that can happen to you, and the feeling of losing who you were makes coping with change even more difficult. It tragically leaves you never feeling the same.

Grief is change, and change can be hard. It changes your life, your daily routine, and the plans you had for the future. Most of all, it changes you; however, some of the changes aren't necessarily bad.

The worst part of a major loss is that sense that nothing, including yourself, will ever be the same again. You'll spend so much time wishing that life would go back to the way it was before your loved one died. You want to go back to the person you were before the loss.

In my own personal experience, I was forced into once again being single after many years of being a couple. So how could I ever go back to being the person I was before my loss?

Before my loss I was part of a team and that was over, forever.

So, maybe a better approach to all of this is to focus on all the ways these changes that were thrust upon you impact you in a positive way. After a loss, your personality may change. You may become more impatient, less tolerant, angry, isolated, anxious, and afraid, just to name a few. But these changes are only temporary in the early stages of grief.

I know if you're in the early stages of grief, you'll find this hard to believe, but there comes that day when you'll wake up and realize you're starting to feel better about yourself again. This doesn't mean that you're not still grieving. Even if you're crying every day, you can still be healing. In time you'll come slowly out of the fog and feel a bit better.

I would trade anything to have my loved one back, but maybe that's why some of the changes that happen after a loss are good. You have a deeper understanding of what's important and what really matters. You become more compassionate and understanding when you hear that someone else suffered a loss.

You've survived the worst possible thing and have become stronger and more resilient.

No, you'll never be the same again…but you can choose to embrace the roles you've been given because of your loss.

You can forever be someone who can help other people walk this long and painful road of grief.

Maybe by doing that you can learn to grow and heal along with them.

SEPTEMBER 22

On Being Lonely

In a recent grief support group, someone asked "Is it normal to feel completely alone?" The overwhelming answer was 'yes' from the other members. As the Facilitator, I didn't focus on providing a direct answer. It wasn't that I didn't have one, it was just that I wanted to see where the conversation would go.

I could tell the participant was speaking from her heart, and it felt very empty. As I observed other responses, I took notice of the overall group. Everyone felt deeply alone.

Even in times of being surrounded by many people, it's common to feel misunderstood…and not be seen for what's really happening to you. We all know how special it is to have someone who completely understands us. We all have a deep need to be seen for who we are….as vulnerable human beings. We all need to know that we matter and that we're loved. When that doesn't happen, we suffer.

We all have those special people in our lives that help us feel whole or complete. They mean everything to us. When they die, we long for them to return. This causes pain. There are healthy coping strategies that can help you feel more supported. It sometimes fills a void when you need to feel more known, seen, and loved.

Have someone to talk to that's been through the same experience. Not just a friend with a listening ear, it also really helps when you feel understood.

Never allow anyone else to run your grief. Do it on your own time and in your own way. As time goes on, you may still miss your loved one, but the grief changes and it will become more manageable.

Most of all be kind to yourself. If there's something you would do as a treat when you're feeling good, do it as a treat when you're feeling bad.

SEPTEMBER 23

"I Lost a Child, and Here's What You Need To Know"

I was talking with a friend who came to me after losing her only child. She was telling me all the things she thinks people need to know about her loss.

I'll never be an expert on the subject of child loss. I've never had a child, so I'll never fully understand the pain of losing one. So, I'll tell you what she thinks people need to know, including myself. I'll share with you what she taught me. If you've lost a child, then you'll most likely know and understand the pain.

My friend said, "If you see something that reminds you of my child, tell me. If you're reminded at the holidays or on his birthday that I'm missing my son, please tell me you remember him. And when I speak his name or relive memories, relive them with me; don't shrink away. If you never met my son, don't be afraid to ask about him. One of my greatest joys is talking about him."

She also said she wishes people would stop trying to 'fix' her. What I call an 'out-of-order' death, such as child loss, breaks a person (especially a parent) in a way that's not fixable or solvable. They'll learn to pick up the pieces and move forward, but their lives will never be the same. Every grieving parent finds a way to continue to live with loss, and it's a solitary journey.

Never tell a grieving parent it's time to get back to life, that's it's been long enough, or that time heals all wounds. They need support and love, and although sometimes it's hard to watch them suffer, their brokenness isn't going to go away. It's something to observe, recognize, and accept.

My friend told me that there are at least two days a year she needs a timeout. She still counts birthdays and fantasizes about what her child would be like if he were still living. Birthdays are especially hard. Her heart aches to celebrate her child's arrival into this world, but she is left becoming intensely aware of the hole in her heart instead.

Then there's the anniversary of the date her child became an angel. No matter how many years go by, the anniversary date of when her child died brings back deeply emotional memories and painful feelings. Parents who have lost a child struggle every day with happiness just like anyone else that's grieving. It's an ongoing battle to balance the pain and guilt of outliving your child with the desire to live in a way that honors them and their time on this earth.

My friend said everyone needs to know that a parent will never forget their child. And, in fact, their loss is always right under the surface of other emotions, even happiness. She said, "I would rather lose it because you spoke his name and remembered my child, than try and shield me from the pain and live in denial."

I'm grateful my friend shared her feelings with me, and I agree it was all information I need to know, we all need to know.

SEPTEMBER 24

The Gravity of Grief

If you've experienced the loss of someone you love, you know grief feels like you're carrying around a boulder, and no matter how hard you try, you can't seem to shake the weight. Grief can pull you down; it's physically and mentally exhausting.

Looking back, I remember the first night I slept alone in our house. I recall thinking I should've felt sad, but that's not what I remember. It was more like an empty, numb sensation. Honestly, I was sick to my stomach. It seemed like a bad dream.

It took months before I felt anything outside of the initial shock. But then, one morning I woke up, started crying, and didn't stop for over a year. My whole identity was tied to my role as a husband and a caregiver, and at the time, I wanted nothing more than to have it all back.

Eventually, I did move through that difficult period in my life. In fact, almost eight years later, I'm confident that I'm a stronger person because of it. But at the time, it was hard to see the light at the end of the tunnel. It was a struggle just to get out of bed, leave the house, and even do basic things like going to work and interacting with other people. I'd hit rock bottom; my grief was so heavy.

It wasn't until I committed to putting the pieces of my shattered life back together that I started to feel better. Each day, the weight of my grief became lighter. The pain associated with my loss began to lessen.

Life after loss is hard. Personally, I spent so much time ruminating on the past that I struggled to see into the future. But at some point, just like anyone else who's experienced grief, I needed to move forward.

Turning the page to the next chapter of your life doesn't mean who you're grieving is forgotten or any less significant.

SEPTEMBER 25

Moving Forward

The problem most people have with the phrase 'moving on' is that it feels like you're being told to forget about the relationship that you had with the one you love. That's why I always say, 'moving forward.' It just sounds less final. But let's focus on what moving on means. Moving on isn't about forgetting, it's not about being happy or sad, or black or white, it's shades of gray.

It's about learning to live a full and happy life even as you miss and long for the person you love. It's about remembering and honoring the one you love while also embracing the fullness of the life you still have to live. It's about your love and the shadow of your loss coexisting.

Moving on also doesn't mean the end of your grief. There is no end. It doesn't mean suddenly you're done grieving and will never hurt again. Moving on is more about moving forward than being done.

Grief is complex, and your loss becomes integrated into your life. It's not something you get rid of; it just changes over time. You get stronger as you carry it. The edges dull. It starts to take up less time in your life, but it will always be there to remind you of your loss in different ways and at different times. You get to define moving on for yourself. I call it moving forward, and you can call it what you want to call it.

There are no timelines or rules to the grieving process. You'll move through it at your own pace and not one minute faster. The process of grieving is unique. No amount of pressure from others can make you move through your process any quicker, at least not in any kind of healthy way.

Only you can know when you're ready. Only you can decide what it means to you and the loss you experienced. Only you can truly decide what it means to move on or move forward.

Whatever that looks like for you, that will be the right way!

SEPTEMBER 26

This 'Club' Stinks

Eight years ago, I was given exclusive membership to one of the world's worst clubs. January 24, 2014, I went from being half of a team to becoming a widower. I didn't want admittance to that club, and I certainly didn't ask for it. Quite frankly, this 'club' stinks.

It took me some time to come to grips with the fact that I was a member of this horrible club, and no amount of pleading, begging, sobbing, or anger would revoke my membership.

As a new widower, I lived through things no human being should ever have to experience. But one thing I also learned is that those of us who are card-carrying members of our horrible club are some of the best people in this entire world. We've lived through pain and anguish, and so many of us have come out the other side more beautiful than ever before. Grief teaches us many things.

Grief teaches perspective, patience, love like never before, kindness, tolerance, acceptance, appreciation for the present moment, and so much more. Grief is perhaps the greatest teacher known to man, but it comes at a very steep price. I always say that I would not wish my pain on my worst enemy, but I'd wish my perspective on the world. Grief is that powerful.

Through the years, I learned to embrace my membership in the world's worst club. Becoming a widower has never defined who I am, but it has significantly shaped who I have become.

I've made priceless friendships with people who see the world through my lenses. I've changed my life and adjusted my goals.

I've cried, smiled, grown, and I've evolved as a person.

Becoming a widower, gave me strength and the courage to go on.

SEPTEMBER 27

Everything Changes

Do you ever wonder why grief is so hard, and why it lasts so long? It's because grief changes everything.

You probably always thought you knew about your life and the people in it. Then one day someone you love died, and you not only lost them but also your belief that things happen for a reason and that everything works out in the end.

After your loss people expect you to accept it at some point. The truth is that you may never really be able to accept the reality of what happened, especially when you've been given more than your fair share of pain. But I think there's an alternative, how about not accepting it?

Maybe that sounds like a crazy idea to you, and it for sure doesn't fall inside the lines of what all the grief experts will tell you. But that's not me, I usually just tell you the truth.

Maybe you don't have to be okay with what happened. Maybe you're allowed to think that life isn't fair and sometimes things happen that just downright suck. Maybe you're allowed to be disappointed with people and with the way things turned out.

What's really important to remember is that feeling that way doesn't mean you can't move forward. Your feelings of disappointment and wanting the person you love back can still co-exist with hope and faith.

Grieving the loss of someone you love is about change. While it may not be what you expected, and while you may never feel that you can accept the loss of your expectations for life, maybe you can make room for both sadness and hope as you look to the days ahead.

Grief changes everything, and sometimes you just have to embrace that change and accept if for what it is, even if it's not always perfect.

SEPTEMBER 28

A Tangled Mess

Grief is a crazy thing. I thought I was doing good when my spouse died. (OK, the first two years I'll admit I was a complete mess.) Those first two years were especially difficult for me, and I found myself wondering how I would go on without him. But as time went on, I began to realize that I could live without him and not feel so sad every single day.

This may sound strange, but it wasn't until I lost one of my best friends two years later, and recently the loss of my father, that I really began to understand grief.

Saying goodbye is so hard, no matter what you know about loss.

But I realize that grief is a journey. It's not a fluid process by any means. There are stops and starts on this journey as there is with life. One day you feel happy, like you can enjoy life, but the next day you find yourself sad and wondering if you can go on.

I was pretty naive shortly after my spouse died because I thought that grief would end. I guess I thought it was like ending a relationship or a job. I found out that wasn't the case at all. The grieving never stops. I learned that grief isn't a linear or a predictable progression.

Instead, it's very unpredictable and tangled.

After my loss I would think to myself, what is there for me now? How can I go on as if everything is okay when it's not? My friends were all telling me that I should 'move on.'

So, what exactly does that mean? For me moving on would mean forgetting the person I love and lost. It would mean forgetting all our many cherished memories.

I think that when we experience a loss we don't move on, but instead we learn to cope with the loss. We find a way to enjoy life again yet keep our loved one close to our heart.

As much as I hate the term, we find a 'new normal.'

See, I know now that I'll continue my grief journey as long as I'm on this earth. As a result of my experiences with grief, I'm able to better connect with people that are grieving a loss and provide them with support. I find myself more empathetic towards others, no matter what type of grief they may be experiencing, a loss of health, loss of self, loss of a loved one.

Because of my many losses, I've found a greater sense of myself. I've learned to live with saying goodbye.

SEPTEMBER 29

So, What Now?

The worst part about losing someone you love is you also lose your purpose in life, or at least it feels that way. This is especially true if you were a caregiver. I was a caregiver for several years, and my days were always full because I was so busy. My purpose was to get up every day and take care of the person I loved. Then my reward at the end of all that work was my person died. It didn't seem fair, not to me, but now I realize it isn't the life of the person that survives that suffers the biggest change, it's the person who died.

So how do you find your purpose after someone you love has died?

Before finding clarity, direction, and purpose in your life again, you have to first do the work of facing your grief and going through all the hard parts of it.

After the fog lifts, perhaps you don't want to change a thing. Maybe you are content right where you are and don't want to make any changes at all. But maybe after you look at your life, you realize it's missing something important that you enjoyed in the past.

Sometimes when you add these things back in, you feel more fulfilled. You might even want to fill the empty space with new things like a new friendship, traveling to new places, taking up a new hobby, or helping others that are hurting.

To find your purpose again, you have to be ready to have a sense of openness to what life has to offer. It means having the courage to take stock of your current situation and giving yourself the time and space to figure out what changes need to happen.

Only you can make the decision when you're ready to move towards your full potential and find your life's purpose again. It won't be easy, but you owe it to yourself and your loved one to start living again because you're worth it.

SEPTEMBER 30

Embracing the Moments That Suck

I've always been told that the way to find happiness and peace is to live in the moment. But what if the moment sucks?

It's been over eight years since my spouse died, and a year since my father died. What I've learned from both of these significant losses is that to survive, I do have to just live in the moment whether the moment sucks or not.

After my spouse died, I wallowed in my misery for a long time, but then I acted. I didn't want to just feel the pain, I wanted to do something about it. So, I started writing. I wrote in my journal every day. I embraced every moment, and even though my pain didn't go away, it lost its hold on me.

I lived in the moment, even when that moment sucked. I cried until I couldn't cry anymore. Sometimes there were just no tears left. But by feeling the pain, and writing about it, the painful moments passed.

You can't run from the pain when someone you love dies. If you try to bury the feelings of each moment, the pain just grows. But by feeling the pain, the moment passes to the next, and the next may be better. But by learning to embrace the sad moments just as much as the happy moments, I've come to realize that they, like everything, are not permanent.

Sometimes I can even find ways to turn my sadness into a type of joy. By remembering who they were and what they still mean to me, I can still appreciate and celebrate the time we had together. So, when the sad moments come, and the pain of missing the person you love takes over, embrace those moments. Don't avoid them. Think about what they might say and embrace the moment for all it is, even if it's not all you wish it could be.

By embracing the moments that suck, you limit the hold your pain has on you, and you'll find that in time the moments of sadness begin to turn into moments of happiness and even joy.

OCTOBER

OCTOBER 1

A Constant Battle

When you lose someone that was an important part of your life, your first response is to be shocked. You tend to reject and deny what happened. Your brain wants to shield you from the pain that's already present in your heart.

Denial in some way prevents you from suffering the pain and despair that can be too overwhelming.

You find yourself saying things like, "I still can't believe it." This is because there's a part of your brain that wants to keep you in denial. It protects you from being flooded with difficult emotions, until you're certain that your heart is ready to endure the pain.

Then after a few weeks, or even months, your heart starts to catch up to your brain.

As the months go by you start to feel the pain, and you begin picking up the pieces of your broken heart. Then as the years go by your brain begins to focus on the things that you've forgotten about. You start to think about the future and find the willingness to move on with your life.

It's never the case that you're done with grief and become willing to leave it behind. You often stay in between the need for grieving and the desire to move forward.

Your heart keeps experiencing grief while your brain is responsible for returning to normal life.

This whole process takes a long time. It's completely natural that your heart and brain will be in a constant battle, shifting between difficult feelings of sadness, longing, and despair, and a desire and willingness to move forward.

Be patient with yourself because in time there will be more positive emotions arising, as the battle between your heart and brain continues to rage on.

OCTOBER 2

Living With Uncertainty

The loss of someone you love is devastating. It tears down the structure of your certainty and confidence. You can't be sure if you could have prevented what happened and that you weren't in some way responsible for it. Even though you would be the last person to be the cause of their death, these uncertainties seem to haunt you.

The only thing you can really be certain about is that you'll never know what role you might have played in your loved one's death. Even though you may have done everything in your power to prevent it, you may have had no control over the outcome. Maybe you could have prevented what happened, and maybe not. I think you have to accept that you can't know. You just have to live with that uncertainty.

If you're forced to live out the rest of your life being uncertain of whether you could have done something to prevent it, then you'll forever be uncertain about everything else that you do.

Maybe you always saw yourself as someone who possessed fine personal qualities, or you were a good person because you've accomplished this or that. This thought of self-praise can become very hard to sustain under the pressure of your loss.

The truth becomes obvious. The simple fact is that no life is granted any kind of certainty. Not only are you vulnerable, you're also human, and nobody's perfect.

When your perception of what you control is punctured by a loss or grief, you have the opportunity to acknowledge a fundamental fact nobody is safe from what happens in life, and nobody, including you, is in control.

What this all means is that you're just like everyone else, and you now have the capacity, if you work at it, to give others your compassionate understanding from a place of actual knowing.

OCTOBER 3

One Breath at a Time

Grief is hard. It has no concept of time. Healing from it doesn't happen in the minutes of an hour or the hours in a day…it happens one breath at a time.

When someone you love dies, the pain is overwhelming. You have the right to feel anger, guilt, rage, and despair. You have the right to feel it all. You're also allowed to tell the truth about it all, even if not everyone wants to hear it.

You may find that by telling your story you lose some friendships along the way. Some people will offer advice and even say things that hurt. These people don't know how hard it is for you to get through each moment, regardless of how much they think they know about what you should do or how you should act.

You have the right to grieve in the way that's best for you. No matter how long or how short that may be, this journey belongs to you.

When the person you loved died, a part of you went with them, and you're allowed to grieve. You have a right to it, and no one should belittle, deny, or try to take it from you.

Your world is changed. The challenge is how to respond to that change. It may be too difficult to do that in any set amount of time.

Your hurt is real, and to survive, sometimes all you can do is take one breath at a time.

You have that right, and you also have the right to go on living.

OCTOBER 4

Normal and Complicated

If you're crying every day, obsessed with the death of your loved one and completely devastated by your loss, you're experiencing normal grief. If you're staying in bed in a dark room 24 hours a day, not eating and not interacting with anyone else, you're suffering from complicated grief.

Normal (or uncomplicated) grief has no timeline and encompasses a range of feelings and behaviors common after loss such as bodily distress, guilt, hostility, preoccupation with the image of the deceased, and the inability to function as one had before the loss. All are normal and present us with profound and seemingly endless challenges. Over the course of time, with average social support, most individuals will gradually experience a diminishment of these feelings, behaviors, and sensations.

So, how can you know if your bereavement is no longer within the range of normal? Dr. J. William Worden, Ph.D. proposed these four tasks:

-To accept the reality of the loss
-To process the pain of grief
-To adjust to a world without the deceased
-To find an enduring connection with the deceased in the midst of embarking on a new life

These truly are the stages you go through before you find healing. If three or four years have gone by and you are still dealing with the first or second task, you may need professional help to deal with your grief and loss.

There are many types of complicated grief; it can be delayed, masked, exaggerated, or chronic. Self-diagnosis is without purpose. A year after the death, if you feel your grief symptoms worsening, I advise that you seek a referral from your family physician for professional grief counseling or therapy.

OCTOBER 5

Looking for Rainbows

In the book, *The Little Prince*, it says, "Grownups are given-ups."

It's like, as we start nearing our expiration date, we get old as we sit on the shelf, lose our flavor, our excitement for life and our will to live. But, let me entertain this thought. Has life ceased to be a journey to learn from? Grow from? Turned from an adventure to an "Okay, you win," situation?

Yes, it's undeniable; we do have an expiration date. I do and so do all the people I love. (You do too.) I know this to be true, and at times I feel like we're hurtling towards that date way too fast. For me, life used to mean green grass, the ocean, rainbows, and the sparkle of a new morning. But since I lost the person I love, life means loss. Now, maybe, just maybe, I need to be as big as life?

Challenge it. Embrace it. Maybe I need to be the one that stands in the storm bracing myself, grinning as the sharp biting wind stings and blows on my cheeks. Maybe I should dare to celebrate who and what I love in spite of the threat of them being taken away. And if they are, celebrate that I had something that life itself cannot claim. Maybe this is the storm that we are all in. But we aren't smiling or embracing it. We're just enduring it.

I've had thoughts that maybe we need to get angry, we need to allow ourselves to not be strong at this time, we need to open ourselves spiritually.

I know one thing for sure; we need to deal with our grief differently than we have before. We need to stand back and remind ourselves 'we are doing the best we can.' And I'm not perfect, but I'm doing my best.

I'm still here. Still upright and putting one foot in front of the other. Which to me means hope is possible.

I've learned that life sure isn't for the faint of heart. But I'm going to try to not worry about other people dying and continue to look for the rainbows.

OCTOBER 6

What Works for You

After my own loss, one of the things that eventually helped me to overcome my grief and find hope was the recognition that my spouse would not want me to be suffering. I believe our loved ones would want us to remember the good times and to continue with our lives and be happy while celebrating the love we shared. I think an approach to resolving our grief is to identify the emotions we're feeling and be still with them.

Death can test your spirituality. Sometimes during times of grief, you may shift the beliefs you once had for another. You don't have to feel guilty or ashamed about it.

The ocean is one thing in nature that brings me a sense of peace. I can look out at the ocean and hear the silence around me, and I instantly feel calmer. I think how we deal on a spiritual level with our loss is a very personal thing.

If you're struggling with accepting the death of your loved one, prayer and meditation can help you to come to a place of acceptance. You may never understand why your loved one had to die, but by establishing a relationship with a higher power or even nature itself, you may be able to find a deeper peace within yourself.

The journey to healing looks different to everyone. What works for one person may not work for another. That's okay. There's no template to follow. Whenever you find yourself feeling overwhelmed with grief, you can take a few minutes to sit in silence. You can imagine the person you're missing and what they look like and how they sound. Then you can have a private conversation with them. You can say whatever you need to say or just focus on one of your favorite memories. This will help you to release your grief and replace it with positive feelings.

I can't say this enough, but the grieving process takes time. Learning to find ways to feel connected to the one you lost can come in many forms. It doesn't matter what you believe or what you do if it brings you comfort.

OCTOBER 7

The Crying Stops

When my spouse died, I cried so much I had to go to the eye doctor because I was suffering from extreme soreness in my eyes. He said I had 'grief eyes.' I had no clue what that was so when I asked him, he said I had just put a strain on the ducts of my eyes from crying too much. (I partly think he made all that up, but it made perfect sense to me because I just couldn't stop crying.)

Crying starts slowly and gathers momentum, builds in power and force, until it dissipates its energy with a crash, then a whimper. I believe each person feels a release from crying at a different point in time.

You may be overcome with tears if your loved one has just died. So, when does the crying stop?

Here's what I think, and this isn't a clinical explanation, it's simply what I have learned. The crying stops when you accept the nature of death. A sudden death occurs within an hour of the onset of symptoms. An accidental death, as you may expect, is a random accident. But a traumatic death is violent, random, and unpredictable. So, if the death was traumatic, it's difficult to ever accept it. In some cases, regardless of how the death occurred you may cry for as long as it takes for you to accept that your loved one is really gone. This is obviously not easy!

The crying stops when you accept your relationship with your loved one. The relationship may be loving, happy, competitive, smooth, unreliable, or painful. All relationships are unique, so since we all grieve in our own way and in our own time, when your crying will stop depends on your own relationship with the person that died. Nobody can know how you feel. It's your loss and your grief.

The crying stops when you can move forward. Parting with a loved one is a wrenching experience, and there's no easy way to move on. But we must eventually move forward because unfortunately life goes on. We can't control it, and we can't stop it. Time does heal and, as the days pass, you begin to find hope and are grateful for your loved one's life.

The crying stops when you move beyond the pain. Being able to talk about your loved one without crying is one sign of recovery. You lead the pain; it doesn't lead you. Eight years after my loss I'm able to lead the pain. The length of time depends on the relationship and the unique grief experience of each individual that's left behind.

The crying stops when you give thanks and tears are healing.

Golda Meir once said, "Those who do not know how to weep with their whole heart don't know how to laugh either."

OCTOBER 8

Blame

After someone has died, it's often a griever's first instinct to go back and take responsibility for the outcome, all they feel that they could or should have done differently.

Do you do this?

Grief has a way of making you feel suddenly and entirely responsible for another person's life, and I find many grievers fill their every waking thought with regret and guilt.

This next part may only apply to a select group of people, but (and this is important) you know who you are.

This isn't easy to hear, acknowledge, or talk about, yet I know this to be true. It must be acknowledged that there are certain circumstances where the deceased played their own role in the outcome and the way things turned out.

I worry about the potential to be misunderstood, so I want to be very clear. While we never want to 'blame' anyone, especially after they're gone, why do we find it so much easier to put all of the blame and responsibility on ourselves? In the end, does anyone need to be blamed at all?

Life is horribly unfair. Terrible things happen to good people.

Some get saddled with mental health issues and addictions that can overpower and destroy even the best efforts and intentions.

Take some time to consider this. Think about what it would feel like to let yourself off the hook, and to let go of some of the guilt, even just a little.

You may spend a lot of time forgiving other people, so why not also forgive yourself.

OCTOBER 9

Keeping Connected

The loss of a loved one is not something that anyone ever 'gets over.' We may get used to our loved one not being in our lives, but we never get over the fact that a piece of our heart will be missing forever.

So, what do we do if getting over our loss is not a realistic option? We journey through it, eventually recovering from our wounds. But just like other journeys in our lives, we will need directions, supplies, plans, and most of all, support from others.

Unfortunately, most of us go into grief ill equipped for the journey. This is not because we're poor planners, but because whether loss comes suddenly or following a long illness, we are never fully prepared for the absence of the one we love so much or who has affected our life in such a deep and profound way.

When we're in the throes of grief, we need to remember that we're not lost in the deepest depths of a dark cave with no way out. We are surely in the dark, but more like a dark tunnel. If we begin to move forward, we will work our way through the tunnel to the other side to where we can begin to learn to live again.

So often, what perpetuates the oppression of loss in our lives is the belief that we must say goodbye to our loved one. Others around us tell us it's time to 'move on,' to 'let go.' But how can we move on with the thought of our loved one being left behind? How can we come to terms with the fact that we didn't get to have closure or say everything we wanted to our loved one? How do we reconcile the unfinished business?

So, we end up stuck. Stuck between acting on the outside as if we've moved on in order to please everyone else. Yet struggling on the inside with a mix of emotions that we're not able to sort through. We're not able to let go of our loved one because we simply don't want to and because it's simply impossible to do so. Over time this conflict of emotions manages to strangle any joy that comes our way.

Faced with this dilemma, one of the most important things we can learn about traveling this grief journey is that we DON'T have to move on or let go of the person we've lost. If we think about it, when something of sentimental value to us is lost, it still exists; it's just in a place where we are not. Its value remains in our hearts although it's no longer where we can see it or touch it.

We don't have to 'let go' or sever our relationship with the one we have lost. Instead, we can learn how to create a new relationship with our loved one. A relationship that keeps us connected to the purpose and inspiration of the bond between us.

OCTOBER 10

Screaming Out Loud

One of my friends lost her mom. I sent her a message expressing how genuinely sorry I was for her, her family, and all the hard days they were about to endure.

Later she responded and asked, "Does the pain ever get easier?" I hated that the only thing I could tell her was that it never gets easier; we just eventually learn to hide it better. But the heartbreak, that stays with you forever.

And that's the truth. My heart didn't suddenly mend on Day 365. The pain isn't any less just because the people around me feel that I've grieved long enough. I can't just numb my heart or shut off my mind, no matter how dark, painful, and lonely of a place it is. I don't remember what life before my loss felt like, how light and happy my soul was, even if I didn't realize it at the time.

I know now I will never be able to go back to the person I was back then. I've drifted so far from the guy I used to be that I barely remember that version of myself anymore. Grief now lives inside me, indefinitely. It's a part of me. It may continue to change shape, continue to break me in new ways, and continue to change me in ways that I could never have imagined. But it will never go away.

I'm done with the silence. I'm done feeling ashamed for being sad. And I'm SO done avoiding bringing up my loss just because I'm afraid everyone else is sick of hearing it.

I'll never stop talking about how much I miss the one I love or how bad it hurts every time it hits me again that he's gone.

Only those who have lost a piece of their heart will ever understand why we can't just forget someone we love and lost. No matter how much time has gone by. Sometimes we just have to keep inside what we want to scream out loud.

405

OCTOBER 11

Sudden Loss

As a bereavement facilitator, I'm often asked by group members, "What's worse, a slow death or a sudden death?"

My usual response is pretty simple, "They both suck."

There's never a good time or good way to lose someone we love, but if we experience the sudden loss of a loved one, is it harder?

In an effort to move forward, there are questions that the griever of a sudden loss may want to consider: Can I accept that in life, and death, there are some questions that have no answers?

Is it possible to recognize that no matter how much time or energy I search in yearning for 'closure' that I may never get it or find it? Do the residual emotions of a sudden loss like guilt or anger serve a purpose, and can I redirect the attention of that energy elsewhere?

Can I find a way now to express my love and my goodbyes to the person who is gone through a ritual or a type of remembrance? Can I ask for forgiveness, find forgiveness, and live in peace even if my loved one isn't here to relieve me of the pain of any unresolved issues?

Take time with this. Sleep on it. Pray or meditate on it. Take a walk and clear your head. Give yourself permission, space, and time to consider the questions that have been left in the wake of your sudden loss and recognize that letting go of the pain and hurt is not the same thing as letting go of the love and memory of your loved one.

Find people to talk to who get it and be patient for the answers that will begin to reveal themselves.

There is peace to be found in those answers.

OCTOBER 12

A New Tomorrow

Someone you love died, and now you keep hoping or wishing that it wasn't true. You expect them to walk through the door. You wait for someone to tell you it was all a big mistake. You just can't accept that they died, that you'll never physically see them again, or hear their voice, or feel their hugs.

It takes a long time for the reality to finally sink in. In time, you come to know, in both your head and your heart, that they actually did die and aren't coming back. You don't like it, but eventually you know it's true.

Once you accept this reality you can start to actively make forward-thinking choices that help you heal. You'll slowly start to envision a life different from what you had planned, a life that doesn't include the person you lost.

You'll still hurt and feel the pain, but it won't crush you and bring you to your knees. This healing begins slowly and can take a long time. It will involve a rollercoaster of ups and downs.

You'll bounce back and forth between tears and joy, while constantly taking three steps forward and two steps back.

Healing doesn't mean forgetting, it means taking the love into the future with you.

You begin to accept that yesterday is gone, but at the same time you realize you're taking the past into a new tomorrow. You weave your loss into the fabric of your life, and it becomes a treasured part of your story.

There won't EVER come a day you stop missing the person you still love. You'll NEVER forget, so you'll always cry, just not as much.

You'll find your way to a new tomorrow, and although yesterday may be gone, you'll never close the door and lock it behind you.

OCTOBER 13

Why I Do What I Do

I don't work with grief because I'm 'above' or 'beyond' it. I haven't transcended grief. I work with grief because I continue to live and experience it. That's my truth. The cool and maddening and universal truth of grief is that it doesn't really end. Grief doesn't end. It just gets different with time.

You can say everything there is to say, and read everything there is to read, and do everything there is to do, and still have dreams about your loved one. And the grief and pain you feel will be as raw and as fresh as the moment you found out they were gone.

So why do I do the work that I do? What's the point of talking about grief if we can't fix it? Because I believe we can coexist with grief.

Society has taught us our whole lives that we shouldn't be experiencing grief, pain, or darkness. That it can be fixed or solved or drugged away. That we should cry alone, distract ourselves, or 'let it get better with time.'

But what if we let ourselves grieve? What if we allowed ourselves to still wake up crying? Even after years? Even after decades? What if we allowed ourselves to sit with grief and make it our own so much that we see it as another expression of our multi-faceted selves?

That's why I do the work that I do. That's why I keep speaking about grief and loss. Because I believe that grief, while it's our darkest, heaviest layer, is a vital layer in learning what it means to be human. In learning things like empathy, compassion, and love. Both for ourselves and others.

The truth is, I'm not broken, damaged, or unqualified. And neither are you.

So, allow yourself to wake up crying. Allow yourself to question whether or not you will ever be whole again. But remember with that thought, you already are. Grief doesn't break us. It just asks us to grow more. Feel more. Know more. Grief doesn't mean you're broken. It just means you're living.

OCTOBER 14

Never-Ending Grief

I have always loved the ocean ever since I was a child. There's something serene and calming about it. It now also reminds me of the never-ending grief that we experience after the loss of a loved one.

In the eight years since I laid my spouse to rest, I've developed an appreciation for just how unpredictable and, well, amazing grief can be.

I'm not talking about the period of grief when the shock and fog of loss clouds every thought and every waking (and perhaps sleeping) moment. No, I'm talking about the grief that comes after that. After the deceased loved ones' absence is no longer a constant presence. After the acute ache subsides and then, unthinkably, stills. After life moves forward, opening to new experiences and events that include no connection to the person who died.

The grief I'm referring to lays claim to no stage and holds no hope of being put behind. Even on the happiest days, it lies patiently in wait for some quirk of logic to unleash it. A scent. A song. A glimpse of an almost-familiar face. Suddenly, wham, you're puddled in a heap, sobbing, and thinking, "Will I ever stop grieving this loss?" The grief I'm talking about is the grief that's never-ending. This is the grief that never extinguishes. The grief that cannot be gotten through, gotten over, gotten past. The forever-after grief.

If you've lost a loved one, you know exactly what I'm talking about. It sounds merciless, even downright cruel. Certainly, while in its throes, forever-after grief can feel like that. But here's the surprising thing: if you open yourself to it, there's a silver lining that can be quite wonderful and comforting.

Two years after my spouse died my best friend died. I was still processing my grief over the loss of my spouse, but I stood up in a very crowded church and read my friend's eulogy. I think I was too focused on tending to everyone else's grief that I wasn't able to connect fully with my own pain.

That's when my grief got really confused. I would start to think about my friends' children, then think guiltily that I should be thinking about my friend - or vice versa. Or I'd think of one of them and the thought would intrude that, no, I should be thinking about my late spouse whom I'd buried 23 months earlier. It was all so confusing.

But that's when I realized the silver lining of grief. But more like a 'tarnished' lining). Because I had suffered the worst possible loss, I was never going to feel that same intense pain again that I experienced when my spouse died. Yes, I felt pain when my friend died, but now I was familiar with it. I wasn't shocked and paralyzed by it. I find comfort in knowing if I can survive the greatest loss I could never have imagined, I can survive any loss that follows it.

OCTOBER 15

What Surviving Is All About

People want to know how I survived.

I talk about grief all the time and how to survive it but recovering from my loss is never something that comes to my mind. I still get sad when I tell my story. OUR story. It's been several years since my loss, and I feel like I've told my story, OUR story, at least a million times. But it's not just a story. It still matters. It still hurts. It's been a long time since my loss, but sometimes it still feels like it happened yesterday. It still feels like a bad dream, and I never did wake up.

The ironic part is that I'm surprised I survived. When it first happened, I never imagined that I would. But here I am. I'm happy, and I have a very full and good life. It's not a perfect life, by any means, but despite the gaping hole I have in my heart, I'm doing pretty good.

Life kind of grew around my loss. Sometimes it seems like it happened when I wasn't even aware of it. I still miss the life I had before my loss and the person I was back then, but life just kind of keeps rolling along and taking me with it. So, when people ask me how I survived, I just tell them I didn't die like I wanted to at the time, instead, I just kept moving. It just kind of happened, and I'm thankful for that.

The truth is, being happy now doesn't negate the pain of my loss. They don't cancel each other out. I carry both with me. Those two realities share the same space, side by side. They most likely always will. Sometimes it just takes a long time for your heart and mind to carve out a new life after loss. But, little by little, pain and love find a way to coexist.

It doesn't feel bad to me that I survived. I still grieve my loss as I live the life I've been given, and I do my best to never forget the courage it took to keep moving forward when all I wanted to do was go back.

That's what surviving is all about.

411

OCTOBER 16

Joy

My spouse and I used to talk about who would die first. (We actually joked about it.) It was a weird thing to do, but we just figured we had our entire lives ahead of us. Even though we talked about it, we never really thought it would actually happen. It was only something that happened to other people, not to us. If it did inevitably happen, it would be much later in life.

We finally compromised and decided that if we couldn't die at the same exact time in our sleep as we planned, then I would have to go first. I was the one that was taken care of and pampered. I could never go it alone. But I didn't die first.

No one can prepare you for becoming a widow or widower. It's one of the most difficult losses you can endure. Losing your spouse means the loss of the future you planned together. The loss of intimacy. The loss of income. The loss of security. The loss of health. The loss of your social circle. The loss of your best friend and confidant.

There isn't a single part of your life that's untouched by the loss of your spouse. But as time marches on, you find your way from grief to healing. You learn to find joy while living with grief. It's hard to see that in the beginning when the loss feels so dark and raw.

When you first feel joy, you also feel guilty for laughing or being happy when your spouse is no longer able to laugh or be happy. But the joy will eventually come and that doesn't mean the grief goes away, it just means you've learned to balance both.

You've learned to expand yourself to a point where you'll feel more than you thought possible. You've learned how fragile life is and that creates a sense of urgency to live. Carrying grief gives you a perspective on life that others who have yet to experience such a loss will ever understand.

Grief is hard, but you'll find your strength and joy again.

OCTOBER 17

Going Back in Time

Don't you wish you could go back in time? I'm sure you think about that. If only you could turn back the calendar. You would have things go back to the way they were. You would have your person back.

How awesome that would be! But the reality is, unfortunately, it's not possible.

Within the limits of human wisdom, you know what's happened, and you try the best you can to understand it. Not always an easy thing to do. The reality of what's happened may be difficult to accept, particularly in the case of a sudden death.

Acknowledgment of the permanency of your loss may not make its full impact on you for a very long time, and that's okay. There are so many things in life that we fear, and dread, and do everything within our power to avoid. But certainly, at the top of the list is the death of someone we love. We have been made to fear death. It makes us frightened. We feel insecure. Our stable world has suddenly and drastically changed.

But in the weeks, months, and years that follow, you'll begin to put the pieces of your life back together. The scar will remain, but you'll be able to live again. You can't see a hundred days ahead or even tomorrow morning. You just have to have patience and faith to take the first step you can see and trust the next step to show itself, knowing that there are plans, purposes, and a future.

I've been with so many people who have gone through the experience of grieving. I can promise you that you too can emerge from it. When tragedy strikes, many of us find within ourselves resources for coping that we never could have imagined. An inner strength often sustains us.

You know that you're not alone, many others have experienced such a loss. They've survived. I've survived, and so can YOU!

OCTOBER 18

An Ongoing Connection

There are things in life that you get over. For example, a cold, a lost job, or an argument with a friend or sibling. Often, when these things happen, they cause temporary sadness and then you let them go.

There are things we can and should leave in the past for the benefit of everyone. Imagine how much pain and negativity we'd all carry around if we couldn't forget and move on.

I'm not saying that it's possible to get over everything. There are times when doing that just isn't possible. There are times when 'getting over' something is not what you would ever want to do. Like getting over or forgetting a loved one who has died. The only people who believe this is possible are those who have never lost a piece of their heart. Many people mistakenly think that grief is something that can and should end at some point. Not true!

The reality of grief is that it often stays with you until the day 'you' die. But, if you do the 'grief work,' and change your relationship with grief, you'll eventually notice yourself healing. You can do this by changing how you respond to grief and how you learn to cope with it. You'll find hope and healing by doing this.

If you really think about it, grief is one instance where there's a strong benefit to accepting its ongoing presence in your life. It creates an ongoing connection with the person who died.

I know this is true because I did it. I know it's hard to believe if you haven't done it. Because all our relationships are unique, so is our grief. My grief is unique to me. Your grief is unique to you.

I changed my relationship with grief. It no longer controls me. I'm no longer afraid of it. It's not a place I chose to stay in.

Grief will be with me until I die but so will joy.

OCTOBER 19

Nobody Understands

Are you finding it hard getting any kind of understanding from friends and family? Have some of them stopped contacting you entirely? What about the other people that seem to be well meaning, but you feel like they just don't understand what you're going through? Are some people even judgmental and tell you how to grieve, or that you should be over it after a certain period of time?

I suspect that you probably answered 'YES" to at least one of these questions or know at least one person that came to mind. These are the people that don't like who you have become, or they just find it difficult to be around you. Maybe they're just afraid to bring up the subject of your person that died because they're afraid of upsetting you.

It's not really their fault. In our society, death is always swept under the carpet and feared. Nobody wants to die, and they certainly don't want to think about it. If it happened to you, it might just happen to them, so they run and hide. Unfortunately, what this does is make you feel even more lonely and isolated.

When you lose a loved one, people might feel bad for you but have no idea what to do or say. For that reason, they may try to 'fix' the problem with comments that you really don't want to hear. They say stupid things like, "Everything happens for a reason.," "Think positive.," "Let go.," "Move on.," "Don't cry." The list goes on and on. Sometimes they just avoid you because they're afraid of talking to you about your loss because it might make you get upset, cry, or they just don't know what to say.

Then after some time, (usually far from enough), they will expect you to have gotten over your loss and for everything to be back to normal. All this can make you feel isolated and misunderstood. You might feel angry with your loved ones and friends.

So why don't they understand you? It's because they may never have experienced the loss of a loved one; they don't know what to expect and are probably afraid of death and anything related to it.

Grieving is exhausting. Not only are you dealing with all these crazy emotions, but now you have to work at teaching your friends and family how to talk to you and what you need. This is the only way to help them understand the new 'grieving' you.

This might include letting them know that you would appreciate them talking about your lost loved one, and that even if it makes you cry, that's okay. You might want to sit them down and explain how you are feeling and what they can do to help. Most of them have probably never helped anyone through grief and they don't know what you need or what to say. So sad as it may be to have to do it, you have to let them know.

OCTOBER 20

Is Being Happy Really the Goal?

Before loss, when someone asks what you want or how you picture your future as it lays out in front of you, how many times have you said, "I just want to be happy."? What's strange is that in some ways it's such a big request, and yet in the simpler times, it doesn't feel like you were asking for much at all. It's not like you're expecting to be ecstatically happy each and every day, just a consistent and stable amount of contentment would be good.

And then someone you love dies.

Suddenly, being happy, being content, or even feeling just a quiet sense of peace seems to be completely out of reach and not attainable at all. You want to be happy again, but you just can't imagine it happening.

I think we may all be missing the mark. As a you look ahead and take the steps to move forward, don't you need to stop and think about whether being happy should really be the goal at all? Happiness is just one emotion, and it may be what friends and family think you want and what you need. It could even be what you think you want and need. But perhaps a shift in perspective is what's needed instead, along with the recognition that some part of you will always want to mourn the person you lost.

Seek happiness, not in the form you knew before, but in the small things that bring you joy. Find moments where the silence brings peace instead of longing. Look for moments of goodness, in friends, family, and strangers.

Know that you can be filled with both pain and purpose. That you can make room for the good and the bad, and you don't need to set goals that you'll never be able to reach.

When something that brings you joy touches you, even for a moment, celebrate it. Realize that love and loss can co-exist, and that a life lived without a loved one in it will forever be a scramble of feelings and not just one emotion.

OCTOBER 21

Becoming an Expert

If you've read my book, *Surviving – Finding Your Way from Grief to Healing*, you most likely know all about me. If not, then let me tell you who I am, why I'm here, and what I know.

I was in finance for 30 years. I was an Assistant Vice President of a major financial institution. I had a beautiful home, a spouse I loved more than anyone in the world, and a very happy life. I had it all! Then all that was taken away when my spouse died.

Here's what I know. The first year after my spouse died was the hardest. I knew it was going to be because everyone around me told me this would be the case. What they didn't tell me was the second year would be hard too, and the third, and the fourth, and every year to follow.

But that first year was full of so much heartache and so many adjustments. Not just the adjustment of my spouse no longer being with me, but the day-to-day changes that I underestimated. They seem small but end up feeling enormous, like picking up your phone to call or text and realizing you can't do that anymore. These were the things I didn't anticipate. The little things that add up to those waves of grief.

I saw the one-year anniversary on the calendar as a milestone. I would get to that day, a whole trip around the sun without my spouse, and it would be an accomplishment. I was just so ready to feel differently than I did.

And then the day came, and you know what? Nothing felt any different. I'm not sure what I thought would happen; they don't exactly give you an award when you make it through. No pat on the back, and no tangible relief. Kind of a rip-off, right?

So, I took the really bad thing that happened to me, and I turned it into something good. I knew nothing about grief until my spouse died, but on that day, I became an expert.

OCTOBER 22

A Better Destination

I'm eight years into my grief journey, and believe it or not, even with all I know, it's still hard work. Not in the same way it was in the beginning, but definitely different. There's a part of me that feels like I'm 'supposed' to be back to normal. But I'm not. Because things keep changing. New challenges come along that make my loss more real and make it almost feel new again.

I read something early on that said after about 18 months, many people can and do feel back to normal. If you find this same timeline, take my advice, keep scrolling. It doesn't work that way. I was ready to throw a party and circle that date for myself on a calendar. But I found a whole lot more information that said there is no timeline. It only set me up for disappointment to think this whole road was a linear one. It's as winding as it gets.

I think I just got somewhat quieter about my pain after a while. Because it feels like I should, or because it feels easier to pull off of this road for a while and take a break. I get it. I may help other people, but I'm still grieving. I'm still trying to figure out where that grief fits in my life after the initial shock wore off and all this time has passed.

I used to think I needed to be in pain to remember my spouse. Now I know better. That's just not how it works. I can miss him without hurting so much over it. And while the crushing moments are fewer and farther between, the dull pain persists.

I've heard grief described as 'a heavy coat that you can't take off.' But after a few years went by, I was ready to take it off. The problem is it still sits in the back of my closet, and there are still days I see it, and it never lets me forget.

I've gotten to a better destination at the end of my grief. But I suppose there really is no end. It's just a part of the fabric of my life now.

OCTOBER 23

You're Not Alone

In a lot of social conversations happening right now, people are frequently using the word 'isolated.' They're saying they feel more isolated than ever before. As I listen, I empathize. I feel it. I put myself more into their shoes. And there are many times when I do that, I feel incredibly sad. However, if I name the sadness I feel, I notice the conversation begins to shift.

I find that when a feeling is named or owned, it provides a safe space for others to speak to something deeper inside them. They open up to their feelings more, naming their own experience once they know it's safe and that they'll be supported rather than criticized or condoned.

I'm finding more people speak to their loneliness instead of isolation. They mention how things are so quiet in their homes, or when they talk to loved ones, it feels as if no one is listening. They long for a sense of closeness, something that's provided only by a special someone who completely understands them.

I often wish their situations were different and that their loneliness was replaced with joy and connection, but their circumstances are beyond my control, I let those thoughts pass so I can be more present with the person in pain and more present in the moment. I feel truly honored to support someone in a space of deeper emotional sharing.

But there is a way to ease loneliness. Having healthy social connections and feeling cared about helps. It reduces lonely feelings and helps you feel more seen, heard, known, and understood.

I think that's where loneliness is a bit more challenging to people in grief. Losing a loved one can make you feel very lonely. The sense of closeness is instantly taken away. Suddenly, there's a void that came about way too fast, and it makes absolutely no sense. In trying to understand it all, some of the things family or friends will say or do can feel hurtful despite their best intentions.

Grief and loneliness create a need for the world to slow down allowing for empathy, love, and compassion to fill the space and help the healing process. But the world doesn't stop for your grieving. That's why it becomes easier to feel isolated.

Even in times of being surrounded by many people, it's quite common to feel misunderstood and not be seen for what's really happening to you.

If loneliness and grief are causing pain in your life, please trust that there are people and resources available to help support you. My suggestion is to find a support group where the group members have experienced a similar loss to yours. This can make you realize you're not alone.

OCTOBER 24

Worrying

In the aftermath of loss absolutely EVERYTHING feels overwhelming. Everything is a decision. Everything feels filled with the potential for something to go wrong. Why? Because something did go wrong, very wrong.

The worst thing that could have happened has happened, and now it's going to be very hard to have faith or trust that anything could ever go right again.

It's important to remember that in grief, you're often mourning the people who could actually help you with all this stuff, and now you're not only grieving their loss, but you're also having to keep living and doing and deciding without them.

As a result, you may find that worry robs you of sleep, steals your peace, and forces you out of the present and into a future of uncertainty where you'll try to fix and know things that can't yet be fixed or known.

Stopping the cycle of worry begins when you understand what worry is, and what it isn't, and you need to recognize one very important point, worrying and doing aren't the same thing.

Worry is not planning. Worry is not being productive, and above all, worry is not problem solving.

I want you to really begin to think of it in these terms.

Recognize that being an observer of your thoughts and behaviors allows you to look on as an outsider would, and to experience without judgment or labels just how much of your life and thoughts are spent in such an unsettled mental and emotional state.

Ask yourself: is this worry for the sake of worry? Is it something you have control over or not? Are thoughts alone enough to change the course of whatever may or may not happen? Decide what is a worry for the sake of worry and what is something you can actually do something about, and then practice letting it go when you can't.

Turn these thoughts and worries into an action that will clear them from your thoughts. In other words, turn them into something productive, and meaningful. Focus on the present and recognize that you have plenty to do and manage right now without having to travel so far into the future to find even more problems to try and solve.

In the end, it's a shift in mindset and perspective that makes the difference, and a decision you can make to not add more stress or grief to your stress and grief.

OCTOBER 25

Difficult Days

What can you do about difficult days? It's important not to regard them as 'set-backs' because as tough as they may be, they're actually an invitation to come to terms with your loss a little more. But when you ask yourself, as much as I will miss the person, what can I do on that noteworthy day to commemorate their death and celebrate their life? How can I make that day meaningful though difficult? This gives you some measure of control.

Grief invites us to remember, not to forget. To try to ignore the day or pretend that it's just like any other day is unnatural, and actually increases the tension. It takes more energy to avoid the situation than it does to confront it.

Observe the special occasions in ways that are comfortable for you. Feel free to make some changes. Remember, there's no right or wrong way of handling these days. Once you've decided how to observe the time and what you can handle comfortably, let family and friends know.

Allow yourself to feel and to express your feelings. Those difficult days often magnify feelings of your loss. Share your concerns and feelings with a friend or in a support group. Recognize that the need for support is often greater during holidays.

Don't be afraid to have fun. It's natural to feel sadness, of course, but it doesn't have to be all sad. Laughter and joy aren't disrespectful. Give yourself and your family members permission to celebrate the person that's gone.

Try to remember the good memories that you shared with the person. For example, a birthday is a celebration of life, so celebrate it even as you remember their death. Balance sorrow for their death with a celebration of their life.

Celebrate the good times.

Don't allow looking back at the past to spoil what you have in the present. You only have a one of two choices when it comes to grief on difficult days. Do you let the day control you or do you control the day? You can allow the grief to dominate you, or you can try to control it. By doing something, anything, to acknowledge your sadness that they're no longer here while at the same time celebrating the fact that they 'were' here will make a difference.

You can shed tears that they're gone, or you can smile because they lived. Or maybe just do both at the same time. But try to make the difficult days a day to remember what was good.

OCTOBER 26

The Ultimate Tragedy

The death and loss of a child is frequently called the ultimate tragedy. Nothing can be more devastating. Along with the usual symptoms and stages of grief, there are so many issues that make this type of loss difficult to resolve.

The grief over the loss of a child can be exacerbated and complicated by feelings of injustice, the understandable feeling that this loss never should have happened.

The relationship between a parent and their children is among the most intense in life. Much of parenting centers on providing and doing for children, even after they have grown up and left home. A child's death robs you of the ability to carry out your parenting role as you've imagined it, as it was supposed to be. You may feel an overwhelming sense of failure for no longer being able to care for and protect your child, duties that you expected to fulfill for many years.

You can mourn the death and loss of a child regardless of their age. It still feels unnatural to outlive a child. It doesn't make a difference whether the child is three or thirty-three when your son or daughter dies. The emotion is the same. You still feel like you lost a part of yourself.

The search for meaning in a child's death is especially important to you if you're a parent. An understanding of how death fits into the scheme of life is difficult and often unattainable. Faith is a source of comfort for some parents, but others with religious beliefs report feeling betrayed by their higher power. Religious confusion is normal, as is questioning many things that you may have believed to be certain.

One father dealing with the death of a child told me that his faith in life, in general, had been shattered. He had long believed that if you lived your life as a good person, striving to make a positive contribution to the world, life would turn out well. The death of his son robbed him of that belief. This reaction isn't uncommon; losing a child feels like the ultimate violation of the rules of life.

Surviving the death and loss of a child takes dedication to life. As a parent, you gave birth to life as a promise to the future. Now you must make a new commitment to living, as hard or impossible as it may seem right now.

You'll survive this; however, the experience will change you. You'll always miss your child, and you'll never stop wondering what would have been.

OCTOBER 27

Main Street

I remember a few weeks after my loss I had to go back to work. I was driving down Main Street in my small town and crying in my car (always one of the best places to do that) when I noticed nothing had changed. People were walking along the sidewalks, shopping, laughing, and holding hands. Couples were strolling along together, and mothers were pushing their babies in their carriages. The kids were playing, and the restaurants were full of happy people eating their breakfast.

How could this be? Didn't they know that the world had stopped for me? Didn't they realize this horrible cataclysmic event had occurred? Everything was the same for them, yet everything had changed for me. Nothing was the same. Yet there I was, driving down this familiar street where nothing looked different. I was suddenly living in a world I no longer recognized. It was a world I didn't fit into anymore. I didn't belong.

How would I ever feel a part of this new terrain? How would I ever be able to see the world in the same way I saw it before my loved one died? Was it even possible? This must be how Dorothy felt when her house flew out of Kansas and landed in Oz. But that place was colorful and happy (well, except for the witch). The world for me had become dark and lonely. The world had stopped.

As time went on each day I drove down Main Street, it began to become more familiar. The only difference was that I had changed. I would never be the same again. It was as if my life was like a beautiful picture puzzle. But then the puzzle fell to the ground and all the pieces scattered in different directions. I had to put all the pieces together again, and when I did, there was one piece missing. A piece that would be missing forever.

In time I realized that the world hadn't stopped. It had just changed for me. The picture puzzle was still beautiful, it just had that missing piece. Just like Main Street that was so familiar to me had a different feel to it. So did the world without my loved one. But the picture was still beautiful, and the world was still moving. I just had to find a way to move along with it.

But now when I look at the missing piece of my picture puzzle of life, I smile because that missing piece reminds me of the love, happiness, and joy that I was blessed to have, and the world keeps moving. I can drive down Main Street and once again feel that I belong. I know in my heart that many of those people I see on Main Street also have a missing puzzle piece. I can't see it, but it's there for them just as it is for me.

I guess that's life. We're born and we die. It's what we do to create the puzzle that matters. It's the pieces of our life that we gather as we go along that create the final picture. I've learned to cherish the missing pieces as much as those that still exist.

OCTOBER 28

A Drastic Change

The day my spouse died; my grief journey started. It was too much change. I spent the first few years just trying to survive. I lost all my passion for living and got stuck in a routine of feeling sorry for myself. My fear of the future was keeping me stuck in one place, a bad place.

I went from loving my life to hating my life.

I was jealous of every couple I would see imagining their perfect life. I was bitter, angry, and not really proud of the person I was becoming. I was letting my loss and my pain change me and not in a good way.

The routine of my everyday life wasn't the same, and it wasn't enough. I wanted what I had, and I wanted answers to bigger questions than I ever asked before. I wanted the future that was stolen from me.

Because of my deep grief, I lost sight of who I really wanted to be and what I wanted to accomplish with the time I had left. I realized that it wasn't my life that suffered the most drastic change, it was my spouse's life.

I stopped feeling sorry for myself and decided that I would make the life after my loss the most extraordinary chapter of my story. It was time to live my life in ways I never dreamed possible.

To do the things I was always afraid to do.

The worst imaginable thing had happened to me, so the way I saw it, what did I have to lose?

I'm here, and I'm a survivor. I made it this far so I can keep going. I can step out of the edge of my comfort zone. I can live my life as if it's being lived for two, one for me and one for the person I love and lost.

If I can do it, so can you.

OCTOBER 29

Mindfulness

Sometimes you can get stuck in your head thinking about all the negative stuff that's gone wrong or could go wrong. It contributes to so many sad feelings. That's why getting unstuck is an important first step to getting through sadness and grief.

Try to imagine a bright future not a gloomy one.

When you suffer a loss, you become sadness prone, only thinking about the worst things that could happen. It's common because you feel like if you think through these bad outcomes, you can better prepare. But it just makes you feel worse in the long run. Your sadness can snowball into feeling all sorts of other negative emotions.

Practicing mindfulness can help you gain awareness and acceptance of your thoughts and emotions. Mindfulness can undo the negative thinking that generates excess sadness. Pay attention to your negative emotions and approach them with curiosity instead of judgment.

Bad things happen, but life is still full of happy things too. Think about what's good in your life. What are you grateful for? What small things are actually good? Feeling sad sucks.

But you can't allow yourself to obsess about it. If you focus too much on your lack of happiness and worry about being stuck in your sadness, you just make things worse. So, try to focus on actions you can take and things you can do to feel better rather than focusing specifically on your sadness.

Doing things to create more positive emotions is so important for reducing your sadness and getting unstuck. There are so many ways to create positive emotions. You can do things you enjoy like spending time with friends, going outside, or reading. Whatever makes you happy...do those things.

OCTOBER 30

When the Story Ends

You've probably heard that when a person you love dies, a part of you dies too. I used to think that was just a simple figure of speech, a touching way to express the sadness of a profound loss.

Then my spouse died, and that simple figure of speech became a reality. A part of me also left for good on that same day. The life we had together was over. The end.

Suddenly, I was walking a lonely journey of sadness, alone.

I still have a lot of memories of all our special times together, but I also have so much I'm starting to forget. That's the thing about losing part of yourself, the part of you only they knew.

You lose some of your story, and it's gone forever.

My spouse was the only one there with me during those special times together, so there's no one to help me relive them. There's no one to remind me about the details I forgot. No one to help me relive those moments that belonged only to us.

I hate that.

As much as you miss the person you love, you also miss the 'you' that they knew. You grieve your shared story.

When the story ends, you grieve that part of you that ends with it.

OCTOBER 31

Grief on Halloween, It's Spooky

I'm just going to say it, I don't like Halloween. Please don't be mad at me and TP my house or anything. I know many of you love Halloween, and I support you in that, but it's just not for me, not anymore.

Holidays can be difficult after the death of a loved one. Though we often think of major holidays as being the most difficult, we shouldn't underestimate the potential impact of traditions and grief triggers surrounding days like Halloween.

If Halloween is difficult for you, it's probably for reasons specific to you and your loved one. However, I'd like to discuss a few general reasons why Halloween might be tough if you're grieving a loss.

You may have bittersweet memories. Holidays are full of memories of the past. This year might remind you of last year and years before that. You may find yourself reflecting on years when your loved one was alive, years when things seemed happier, or simpler, or even years when things were really difficult.

After a loss, memories of the past gain new dimensions. A memory that at one point was remembered as purely happy can take on shades of sadness when it includes a person, place, or time that's gone from your physical reality. So, whether the memory is happy or sad, both can cause you to feel pain.

Does this mean you should avoid all memories of the past? No, definitely not. You lose far too much when you lock away all your memories, whether they're happy or sad. Memory can be a huge source of comfort and connection. Happiness with a side of sadness is just something you have to get used to after a loved one dies.

Gary Sturgis

Spirits, ghosts, tombstones, skeletons, and other reminders of death are everywhere during October. You might find it difficult to look at these symbols in the harmless and playful way you did as a child.

Halloween is a playful holiday. Some people really get into it. Maybe you even used to get into it, but this year you're not feeling it. Grief takes a lot out of you, and you may find you need to conserve your limited amounts of energy and enthusiasm. If so, just skip it if you can.

Leave the decorations in their boxes and go to a movie. Take comfort in the thought that maybe next year you'll feel more up to it (or maybe not, and that's okay).

NOVEMBER

NOVEMBER 1

A Season of Change

I looked in my garden one day and saw one lonely, shriveled tomato hanging on a broken stem, and it reminded me that the summer was over.

The change of seasons can be difficult if you're grieving the loss of someone you love. Especially the Autumn season when the days are getting shorter, and the early evening darkness can bring lonely quiet times that can make you feel painfully aware of the person you're missing.

Then on the horizon is the holidays.

I always loved the Autumn season before my loss, but after my loss, my perspective changed. It seemed like everything withered and died, and all that was left was the cold reality that the world is full of grief.

But then in time, I realized that nature is compassionate. The season of dying is also the season of new life.

Those trees that shed their leaves will grow again in the Spring, fresh and new. The days will become warmer and bright. Nature is supportive in its message to prepare us to have gratitude and hope.

The lonely early nights can also reveal stars like diamonds in the sky and the silence to reflect on what once was and what will come. Memories unfold. I know those I love and lost live within those stars.

You can actually find comfort in the changing of the seasons because nature can remind you of rebirth and a place where you can experience a connection to those you miss.

Autumn can be a warning of what to expect of your grief, how it will ebb and flow, ever changing, ever shifting, ever present, and never ending.

But what may be dark today, may be bright tomorrow. So, I'll wait.

NOVEMBER 2

Loved and Lost

The heavy burden of grief can hold us captive if we let it. If we refuse to try to move forward, we can get stuck in a place of sadness and sorrow forever. I don't think the person we lost, that loved us so much, would want that to be the effect their death had on us.

After the loss of my spouse, I found it impossible to visit any place we had been together. The thought of it was just too painful. As time went on, I began to visit these places, and instead of making me sad, they brought me joy. The happy memories flooded back. (Yes, in many ways it was also bittersweet because I knew we would never be there together again.) I began to actually go to these places more often because they provided me with a strong connection to the person I loved and lost. They were still 'our' places.

Find a photograph of yourself with your lost loved one. Return to the location of the original photograph. Go alone or take a trusted friend or family member that's supportive to your loss.

It's a chance to think back and remember, to tell the story of that day and of the person that you lost. Sometimes imagery allows for expression beyond what you can speak. It's an experience that contributes to the restorative process in overcoming the painful impact of the loss.

By doing this exercise, your loved one can be remembered, and memories can be relived. Even though the pain of the loss may remain, this often helps in relieving the hurt and the stigma of death and acts as a public declaration that death has lost its sting.

We all have a different experience of loss that can reveal itself in many ways. Sometimes it's a response that's quite clear for those around you to see. Perhaps there are lots of emotions that you just don't know how to let out, or you're not sure how you should be feeling, or whether it's right to be having certain angry or complicated thoughts.

If you decide to do this exercise, it's not about saying the right thing or having the answers. I just want to give you a chance to speak about your experience of loss. Maybe even recapture (or at least remember) the magic of the relationship.

I still go to places my spouse and I visited together, but instead of crying, I think of my spouse, and the memories we made, and I smile.

So, what this exercise does is allows you to embrace your memories, not only of your loved one, but for places you loved to visit. Instead of fearing these places and memories, you can actually learn to find comfort in them.

NOVEMBER 3

A Step Forward

When you suffer a major loss, it can be very difficult to even have the desire to live again and seek out ways to be happy. When the time is right, you might find yourself wanting to take a step forward, and it very likely won't be easy. Some days will be better than others, and the best way to do it is to take very small steps.

It's very important to let the grief process run its course before even expecting to be truly happy again. All the emotions and feelings associated with your grief must all be worked through before living again can be a reality.

Focus on what's important, like yourself. Think about what you can do to be happy again and spend your time and energy on living and loving those that are remaining.

It's all about redefining happiness. The relationship you had with the one who died may have been your definition of happiness, but perhaps something new (not necessarily a person) can help ease the pain.

It might not be feasible to try and fill the void but finding new things that make you happy. Whether it's the personal fulfillment of accomplishing goals or spending more time with remaining family and friends.

Learning to live, love, and be happy again might sometimes require an adjustment in your outlook and thinking.

Living again after loss isn't easy. It takes the courage to change your thoughts from negative to positive. To realize that life doesn't always work out the way you planned, but if you continue to have faith in the goodness that still exists, you can find joy again in living.

Sometimes you can't find happiness, it finds you.

So never give up. This one bad event is not what defines your entire life. Take that step forward. You're here for a reason, and that's good.

NOVEMBER 4

Recovered

People always ask me how my work and my life relate to my loss. They want to know if I'm recovered.

Recovered is such a strange word. I mean, I can talk all day about grief and about why this work matters. And my voice still cracks when I tell my story. Our story. That I've told the story a million times, doesn't matter. It's not just a story. It still matters. It still hurts.

Honestly, I can't believe I survived. In those early days (months, years), the thought of a good life, any life, was inconceivable to me. And yet, here I am. Happy. Despite the gaping hole in my life. Despite missing that person, I was back then. Life grew in and around that crater in ways I could not have imagined in those early days.

When I look at my life now, I'm such a different person than I was before my loss. Sometimes I don't even recognize myself. The guy that got nervous just walking into a crowded room, now gets up in front of large groups of people and talks for two hours. The guy who never cried, yet now cries at every sad movie I see or story I hear. The guy who knew next to nothing about grief or loss and is now an expert. Seriously?

So, to answer the question about my recovery, my answer would be this, I didn't die back then, much as I may have wanted to. In the early days, I was convinced that I would never be 'okay,' let alone happy again. I couldn't see any way that could happen and not diminish my memories of the life I once had.

The fact that it did happen, sort of on its own, still shocks me. I'm not complaining. I'm so thankful for it, but it's still a little strange.

I'm telling you this because it's important for you to hear it. You may not be capable of believing it now (just like I wasn't in the beginning of my journey), but however long it takes, your heart and your mind will find a new life among the ashes of your loss. Little by little, pain and love will find a way to live in harmony.

Being happy now doesn't negate the pain of my loss. They don't cancel each other out. I carry both of them. Those two realities share the same space, side by side. They most likely always will.

If you're wrestling with the idea (from inside yourself or from others around you) that at some point you'll be 'okay,' please know that it's absolutely normal to feel freaked out by the idea.
It won't feel wrong or bad to have survived. It will just be a life of your own making, the most beautiful life it can be given what's yours to live.

NOVEMBER 5

New Friends

Friendships change after a loss. It's like you're in a boat with all your friends, and when your loss happens, the boat starts rocking and some of them fall out.

Sometimes the friends you believe will be there for you are suddenly nowhere to be found. They don't call to ask how you're doing, and they don't come over to see you.

This friend is usually the one that's actually more concerned about the fact you've been neglecting them during your grief.

These friends are more than willing to stay in the boat as long as the water is calm. If you do see them, they probably won't bring up your loss, but they'll tell you how you've hurt them by not being there for them.

All you can do is find it in your heart to forgive these friends because they have no idea what you're going through, and they'll never understand it until it happens to them.

Your true friends are the people that know your boat is rocking and still get in and sit right beside you. These are the friends that call and aren't afraid to listen to your story over and over again. They listen and reassure you that you're 'normal' and your feelings are valid. They help you relive memories of your loved one when you're ready. They love you before and after the loss, unconditionally.

Sometimes the very best friends are new friends. These friends bring a smile to your face in the midst of your grief, and they give you hope for the future. They encourage you to do positive things that will help you through this journey, and they even offer to do it with you. They stay in your boat regardless of the weather.

Be open to allowing new friends into your life after loss. They can help you steer your boat along the way.

NOVEMBER 6

A Cruel Teacher

You might be wondering why just when you're feeling a bit better, you suddenly feel worse again. How can this be? With more time to process, more time to experience life without your loved one, and more time to re-learn what your new life looks like, why would it suddenly feel like it's harder to cope? Is this normal?

I don't need to tell you that losing a loved one is unlike any other experience. While there's nothing that can ever prepare you for it, you can't help but to expect all the same rules of life to apply.

Grief can be a cruel teacher, and one thing you quickly learn is that everything changes after loss. Life changes, and all the rules have changed too.

Prior to your loss, you probably experienced the healing nature of time. After a surgery or illness, after a fight with a friend, following a traumatic event, in almost every one of those cases you can say that while other things may have contributed to the recovery, it was time itself that ultimately made the difference.

But the rules are different in grief. Rather than experiencing improvement as a steady climb that can be charted on a graph, you probably feel that your emotions and coping skills are predictable only in that they are totally unpredictable.

While there's no predictable path for coping after loss, you still may find yourself asking, "Why am I having a harder time coping now than I was before?" And why not?

It's easy to feel like there's nothing to do about grief. Put it in the closet, stuff it under the bed, hide it away and forget about it. If you're too busy with other things that need your immediate attention, it may just feel like mourning is a luxury you can't afford.

But here's the bottom line: grief is very patient and will wait for you until every part of it has been fully realized. The grief you're feeling now may just be the grief that was there before, only now you have more time to sit with it.

Grief that's avoided will always be waiting for you. Because it was always there all along, but you may have just been too busy or too distracted or simply too unable to face it.

Sit with it. Realize it. Acknowledge it but don't label it. Experience it without judging it. Throw the timeline away and don't worry how many days, months, or years it's been. Don't let the calendar decide how you should be feeling.

NOVEMBER 7

Love Is Stronger Than Death

I wasn't ready, and grief sucker punched me in the face. Then it grabbed me by the throat and choked me until I couldn't breathe. This is what it always does and always when I least expect it.

I lost my spouse at 52 years old. I wasn't prepared, and sometimes I'm still not prepared now. No. I definitely wasn't prepared for grief to grab me by the throat three years later at my parent's 65th wedding anniversary.

We organized a big party with over 200 people in attendance. My niece made a video of their life over the years. Almost 70 years together. (I only got less than a quarter of that time.) I was happy for them.

Sad for me.

Then there was a video of their life. A video that also included my life, the one I lost. As the video began to run, I could already feel grief's grip tightening on my heart. As the first set of photos popped up, I reviewed all our years together in a flash, all the while feeling grief's grip getting tighter. I could feel all the eyes in the room focused on me, and the tears began to trickle down my face. Then another picture flashed on the screen. It was our wedding picture. I began to sob. Grief was choking me now. There was our honeymoon cruise. I could barely breathe.

So just when I least expected it, at what was supposed to be a joyous occasion, grief had caught me off-guard. I didn't want to upset my parents; it wasn't their fault my spouse died. Why ruin their good time? I was determined to get my feelings under control.

I was so tired of fighting with grief. Although I was caught off guard when grief attacked me, I wasn't going to let it win. I knew on a conscious level that grief feelings come from love, and that was something to celebrate. I knew I had the strength to fight grief and I had to act fast. I didn't want to make anyone feel bad. I was happy for my parents. Grief wasn't going to ruin my day or their day.

Grief lost the fight that day. But I learned that I'm not safe from grief's attacks. Grief can be quiet for months or even years and still grab me by the throat when I least expect it.

If you find yourself caught off-guard like I was, remember that you also have the power to fight grief. You just have to replace the negative thoughts with positive ones. Don't let grief steal your focus from the happy memories. Think about the love you still have in your heart.

You have the courage inside to fight back, and you can win. Why? Because love will always be stronger than death, and it will always outlive it.

NOVEMBER 8

You Have To Die To Be Perfect

I recently bumped into a friend from my old neighborhood that I haven't seen in years. She told me her husband died a few months ago, and that she was really struggling with her grief. She spent a long time telling me all the wonderful things she missed about him. She told me how he was so kind, generous, easy-going, compassionate, and perfect. She was surprised by the fact that not many people in the neighborhood were being very supportive given what an amazing and beloved guy he had always been.

I extended my sympathy to her, gave her some resources for dealing with her grief, and told her to contact me if she needed any additional support.

I'm sorry he died, but I have to be honest, her husband was a jerk. He was a miserable person that didn't get along with anyone in the neighborhood, and he was a terrible neighbor.

I understand why people put their loved one on a pedestal after they die. I did the same thing. I think my spouse was wonderful. After my loss I was acting like nobody in the world could ever come close to being as perfect. I for sure would never love anyone else again because nobody could be as good, wonderful, and absolutely perfect for me.

I'm not 'perfect' and I don't think anyone else is perfect. I think part of being human is being 'imperfect.' After someone you love dies, it's only natural to think about that person in a very positive way. But sometimes we can go too far, and if we do, we end up with unrealistic memories.

We're all human, and if we put someone who has left us that far up on a pedestal, it can cause problems in many different ways.

An acquaintance called me and gave me that same advice. She said after her husband died, she turned him into such a perfect person, that no one else could ever measure up to those high standards. She was a very young widow, and in her case, she said she wasted a lot of years ignoring "some really wonderful men who were right in front of me."

Not everyone wants or needs to get married again after the death of a spouse, but her point was well taken. To really move on, no matter what direction your new life takes you, you can't create unrealistic memories.

It's great to remember someone's wonderful qualities. But it's even better to remember everything that made that person unique. After all, flaws, quirks and even odd or unusual habits are just part of who we are. I believe our loved ones would want us to remember them the way they really were, not perfect like all the rest of us.

NOVEMBER 9

Building a Sandcastle

I believe grief is all about surviving. I've seen too many people that gave up and didn't survive, and I think that's tragic. Sometimes you just have to hold on for one more day.

Sometimes you just have to build a sandcastle.

Grief is hard, so you have to collect all your energy and strength and build on it. Feel the sand in your hands and feel the connection to something.

If you've suffered the loss of someone you love, you know the pain associated with that. I don't wish it on anybody, and I'm sorry if you know that pain. So how do you survive it, and what the heck does it have to do with building a sandcastle?

Like collecting sand in your hands to build a sandcastle, you're building up something to distract you. Concentrate on work, a project, family, something new, something old, something that feeds your soul. Be good to yourself.

Don't isolate yourself for too long. Like patting the sand, take care of you, do what you need to do. There's no shame in your tears, anger, or sadness. Like the grains of sand on the beach, there are so many others that have faced the pain of grief before you.

Creating something, anything, even a sandcastle can give you purpose.

Every time you go to bed at night remind yourself that you made it through another day.

You can do this. Step back and look at your sandcastle, what you've created, what you still have in the midst of your loss.

You have you, and you're worth the fight to survive, so sometimes you just have to build a sandcastle to remind yourself that you can do one more day.

449

NOVEMBER 10

It's Not Your Fault

Grieving the loss of someone you love is one of the worst experiences in life. (That's just my opinion, not a proven fact.)

But I think it's even worse when the person you love died due to suicide or from a drug overdose. Then the grief journey can be even more intense. It's tough to imagine that their life light went out so suddenly,

If you're reading this, and you're suffering from the loss of a child, friend, parent, or anyone else due to suicide or a drug overdose, I'm truly sorry for your loss. I can't take away your pain, but I can give you some tips on how to handle your grief in a healthy way. It's not your fault!

Remind yourself that what happened was not your choice and not your fault. You most likely had no attachment to outcome, and no control over the situation. You can't blame yourself for their actions. If you try to make sense of a sudden death, it will most likely leave you searching for a place to direct the blame. It might even be yourself you blame, but suicide and overdose is no one's fault. It's likely that the person you love had been struggling for a long period of time. You may have had no clue that this was even happening.

You're probably experiencing a wide range of emotions, and that's completely normal under the circumstances. There will be times when you may feel like the pain will never subside, but it will. It will take time, support, patience, and effort. It takes time to absorb the impact of a loss.

Surround yourself with supportive people who can help lift you back up. Don't give up on the things you enjoy and take care of your health. Focus on 'you!

Most of all, be patient with yourself. Everyone grieves differently and moves at their own pace. You might see that others move on more quickly than you do, and that's okay. It's not your fault!

NOVEMBER 11

Suffering of the Worst Kind

Losing someone you love is the hardest thing in the world to experience. It's a kind of pain that you physically and emotionally feel for a long time.

Its suffering of the worst kind.

Sometimes it seems like no one else understands how you're feeling. In the first few weeks and months people gather round, cry with you, listen to your stories, bring over food, check in on you, and help with all those little things you can't bring yourself to think about.

But after a while these people seem to disappear into thin air. They go back to their normal lives and expect that you'll do the same, leaving you alone in your grief.

Suddenly you're trying to survive the first birthday, anniversary, vacation, and holidays since the person you love died. Then the real suffering begins, the suffering of the worst kind. You realize that you have to keep doing it.

No one can tell you how to deal with your grief. Don't let anyone tell you when it's time to get rid of your loved one's things, or when it's time to stop crying or visiting the cemetery. You have to figure it out for yourself when you're ready. Your grief belongs to you.

Every time you cry it's a way of honoring who they are in your life and what you've lost. It lets the world know someone you love is gone, and that they still matter.

Surround yourself with people who will listen to you, that will let you feel sad, or will just sit quietly with you.

These people can't make the grief go away, but they can support you while you learn to walk through it.

NOVEMBER 12

You Don't Recover

I can tell you that you will always grieve the loss of the person you love, but that doesn't mean that you won't recover from the intense pain of that loss. It's so important that you understand that despite your loss, you still have the hope of healing. Even though it doesn't feel like it right now, you will not live with the acute anguish of grief forever.

What I'm saying is that you will recover from the pain, but you won't recover from the grief. Grief is forever. But just because you don't recover from the grief doesn't mean you're always going to feel as horrible as you do now. I promise!

There are millions and millions of people out there (including myself) living normal and purposeful lives while also experiencing ongoing grief. It would be a pretty amazing thing to find someone who lives a long life here on Earth and never experiences some kind of a loss. I've never met one.

The reason I don't believe we ever 'recover' from grief is because to recover from something means you return to normal. But when someone you love dies you never go back to normal. Everything changes.

People talk about 'closure,' and I hate that word. I never use that word unless I'm saying something negative about it. The problem with closure is it doesn't change anything. The person is still dead.

Here's what happens. The loss, the person who died, and your grief all get integrated into your life, and they profoundly change how you live and experience the world. My point is, although you will recover from the intense distress of grief, you won't ever recover from the grief itself.

Grief is one of those experiences you just can't understand until you actually experience it yourself. It comes into your life the second your loved one dies (sometimes even before) and as long as you continue to love that person, grief will remain.

NOVEMBER 13

When the Sympathy Stops

After your loss you have a lot of support, people seem to be all around you. They show up in the early days to show you how sorry they are and how much they care. But then as time goes on, they move on. Suddenly there are only a few people who seem to remember.

People seem to expect that after losing a loved one, you should be on some kind of steady track to getting better. But what people who haven't been through grief don't understand is, so often in the midst of that loss, you feel so supported by others, and that can provide a burst of strength to get through the early days. But then things get really quiet, and everybody seems to disappear, slowly one by one, and if you're lucky, a select few still remember.

The reality is people just go on with life, and they stop asking about it. That can really hurt because for a while, for you, it gets worse. The reality is just sinking in. There are all of these firsts that you don't get to experience with the person you lost, and all of the reminders seem so relentless.

Usually, it gets worse before it gets better, and just before you're at your lowest, that's when people really start to forget. You do have some options when that happens.

One option is that you can get really bitter and resentful toward people who aren't bringing it up anymore. You might have a sense of entitlement to everyone's attention and sympathy, and you might start 'keeping score.' What I mean by this is you won't write it down or anything, but you'll keep track of it in your heart and mind. You'll make a mental list of those that let you down.

It's so easy to be resentful in the midst of grief when you feel that people are forgetting you. But going down the path of choosing to take offense and become bitter leads to a loss of more people, and then your loneliness just grows.

The other option is to be realistic about people and their ability to enter into your suffering, to stay, and to remember. I hope if you're grieving you at least have a few people who still remember and still have the courage to ask you about your grief. Maybe it's a bit unrealistic to expect that everybody should continue to focus on it.

You can't help thinking about your loss because it's like a veil through which you see everything. But many people are going on with life and they do forget, and if they haven't been there, they don't understand that it might be getting harder for you instead of easier.

So, try to remember that someone who hasn't been there, isn't going to get it, and if they haven't been there, then they really don't know.

NOVEMBER 14

Still

On some days, I still can't seem to function the way normal adults do, my heart pulls me back in time. I think it's because although the person I love died, my love never died. On some days, grief still just seems to sit there in the back of my throat, like a storm gathered behind my eyes. I don't let on to this fact, others can't see it, but I feel it.

I don't share how I'm feeling almost as a rule now. I don't want to talk about it. I simply function, and never want to burden the people around me with how I'm actually feeling. I try not to let myself even think about how I wish I had hugged him more. Told him I loved him more. How I wish I worked less and took more time for us. How I really hope he knew I was there with him at the end.

This is the kind of behavior I keep to myself because I don't want to make anybody else feel awkward. When I don't want to feel like anyone is looking at me thinking, "Geez.......still?"

I plague myself with thoughts like this even though I actually have no idea how anyone else will feel about it. I've decided to not talk about it because I don't think I could stand to find out. But, yes, still.

When your world cracks in half, it causes you to question everything, even your own existence. It can take a great deal of time to figure out how you're going to move ahead, especially when it feels like you're fumbling around for a light switch in the dark.

It's taken me quite a while to accept that, yes, I still hurt sometimes. As long as I love, I grieve, and grief and love go hand-in-hand. My grief reminds me that love is worth it.

Yes, sometimes it still hurts, and what I really want, and need is one more hug or to call his name and hear him answer, but I can't. Still.

NOVEMBER 15

Braving the Storm

After losing my spouse, and then my father (and several other significant losses), my faith in life's goodness and purpose has been severely tested. Many times it's been difficult to find my way out of the darkness.

It's not just the loss of these people I love but also the loss of blissful ignorance of what can happen in life. When I was a child, I believed in the Tooth Fairy and Santa Claus, then one day I didn't.

When I was young and bad things didn't happen yet, I thought I was going to live forever. I thought the people I loved would also live forever. Then the bad things happened and, well, I learned what can happen. Once that information existed for me, I couldn't erase it.

Maybe I'm just old and cynical now? I might look like I'm functioning and even having fun, but sometimes I think I'm just going through the motions. But I've never given up, and I'm proud of that.

We all have an expiration date. Sometimes I feel like I'm hurtling towards that date too fast. When I was young, life was all about my dreams for the future. It was about birth and life. Then as I grew older, life became more about death and loss.

Life sometimes feels like a storm, and I'm standing right in the middle of it. But I'll still never give up. I'm always going to brace myself for what's coming next. I'm going to challenge it and embrace it.

I'm going to celebrate who and what I love in spite of the threat of them being taken away. If they're taken away, I'll celebrate that I had something that life itself can't claim, LOVE.

I'm still here, and I'm doing my best. I'm taking life one moment at a time.

I'm braving the storm, and for me that means HOPE.

NOVEMBER 16

On the Top Shelf

When my dad recently died, I had spent so many years grieving a spouse I feel like I'm a pro at it, but grieving my dad left me feeling like a rookie. It's a very different kind of grief.

My spouse died young, and I still don't think that was fair, but my father lived a long life. I feel grateful for having had him in my life for so long, which also makes me miss him that much more.

He was the keeper of my history. He remembered my first word, he taught me how to swim, fish, and love the ocean. He was always so proud of everything I did, and he was my biggest fan. He was always there when I needed him, and his advice always pointed me in the right direction.

I remember when my dad's father died, he said to me, "Well, now I'm on the top shelf." What he was saying was as long as our parents are alive, our mortality is a generation away. When my father died, with his death came the sobering realization that there's no longer anything standing between me and death. I know that there really never was because anything can happen to anyone at any time, but it still left me feeling like I was next.

Even if it was just symbolically, as long as my father was alive, I was somebody's child. His death has now left me 'on the top shelf.' His death is forcing me to face my own mortality and has made me acutely aware of the inescapable transition from this world to the next.

When my spouse died, his parents were still alive, so that kind of blew a hole in my father's theory about the 'top shelf.' That's the thing about life, there are just no guarantees. I know I'm going to die; I just don't know when, nobody does.

But if unconditional love means loving you no matter what, my father was as close as it gets, and I'm going to miss that. It's lonely on the top shelf.

NOVEMBER 17

The Longest Year

"Wow, I can't believe it's been a year" is the most frequent phrase I hear from those that have lost a loved one. When my spouse died, the year after my loss was the longest year of my life.

He was battling cancer and by the end of his life, I was wishing for him to be free of the endless mess of doctors' appointments, glimmers of hope that always faded, bad news and physical limitations that had overtaken our life together.

Our relationship was rooted in mutual respect. We navigated all of life's challenges together. He was my anchor, and life with him was fun, stable, and constant. Things were all in place until they weren't.

The difficulty with navigating the first year after the loss of a loved one can't be minimized. It's not only facing alone all of the milestones such as birthdays, the wedding anniversary, and the holidays but the shedding of your entire sense of self. You have to learn to deal with all the emotions, change routines, and experience social situations as an entirely new person.

Your grief is going to overtake your body, mind, and emotions and won't be controlled no matter how hard you try. Once you become comfortable with a deep fog or racing mind, mood swings and emotions that seem to arrive out of nowhere, you'll be in a better place. Just be with it. It's going to take time for your brain to work correctly again.

Ask for help. This is the time to do that. It might be hard but take offers for anything that comes your way. Don't just say, "I can handle this on my own." People are genuine in wanting to do something for you, so let them do it.

Stay in the present. You're in your new life now, and it takes time to adjust. Replaying many past experiences causes profound sadness and thinking about the unknown future causes intense anxiety. It sounds so simple, but once you can train your mind to do this, it makes each day easier.

Take care of yourself. This means being mindful of everything that can affect your health. Eat well, exercise, get enough sleep. While things like alcohol and medications to help you sleep may be tempting, they dull and delay the process of feeling better.

Find the support you need. It could be a therapist, counselor, or a support group. Social media is also a tremendous help in locating others sharing similar experiences.

Change forced upon you can be tremendously difficult, but the end result of that change is growth, strength, and resilience.

NOVEMBER 18

No Easy Way Out

I wish I could tell you there's five easy steps to get through grief. Unfortunately, there are no easy steps and no predictable timetable. Pure and simple, grief is just a difficult and painful experience.

The focus of grief always seems to be on the desire to find hope and healing in the aftermath. The problem with finding hope and healing is these things can't be found until the hurting happens. First you hurt then you heal.

Each loss is unique just as each relationship is unique. When you lose a significant person from your life, whatever the relationship, it hurts, and nothing takes away from your right to feel the loss and grieve the absence of that person.

Every individual is unique. Every individual takes their grief journey at their own personal pace. Some fast. Some slow. Some cry. Some don't cry. Some do it this way. Some do it that way.

There's no set rules. Everyone goes through it in the way that's right for them, and there's a reason for every behavior. While some reactions may seem strange to other people, there's a reason why they're reacting that way even though they may not be able to explain it. So, how can you find hope and healing? First feel the hurt.

There's no easy way out. Grief is the cost of caring. The best thing you can do is allow yourself to grieve. Seek out caring people and express your feelings. Take care of yourself and accept that life is for the living. Be patient with yourself. Finding hope and healing after a major loss takes time. If your grief seems like it's too much to handle, seek professional assistance. It's not a sign of weakness to ask for help.

With support, patience, and some effort, you will survive your grief, and someday the pain will lessen leaving you with cherished memories of the one you love.

NOVEMBER 19

A Light in the Darkness

If you're just beginning your grief journey, I'm here to reassure you and tell you I've been through loss and the grief that follows, and I want you to know it will get easier.

I know this might sound untrue and it feels wrong, but at the end of the tunnel of grief, there can be light. If you feel like you're spiraling down and nobody will catch you, I want you to know you're not alone. I've been through this tunnel of darkness and crawled out into the light on my knees. I'm so thankful I made it out.

Grief can crush you. It can cause you to cry uncontrollably and struggle to catch your breath. This is how your body reacts to the terrible thing that happened.

I was lost in the darkness of grief, but I found the light in the darkness. It took many months and even years of doing the grief work to make my way towards it.

If you want to talk about the person you lost, talk. Then talk some more. Cry, scream, and do what you need to do to get your emotions out. Remaining silent can be like letting a wound fester. As painful as it can be to speak about the person who died, it can also help with healing.

Grieving the loss of the person you love can last the rest of your life. The hurt can be there for a long time. This is loss. This is love.

But there will come a time when you can think of your person and smile. Perhaps with that smile you'll still shed some tears, but you'll have made it through a hard part of your grief journey.

In the darkness of grief, you'll spend long periods of time missing the one you love, but the love left behind can illuminate your soul. It's this eternal love that pulls you out of the darkness and into the light.

NOVEMBER 20

You Can't Avoid It

I think the reason we're here is all about 'happiness.' We spend all of our life trying to achieve it. We do anything we can to avoid being sad. Let's be honest, nobody wants to be sad.

But then someone you love dies and that all goes out the window. All of a sudden happiness seems so far out of reach. Then you spend a lot of your time trying to avoid grief.

You see, it's not just about losing someone you love, it's sometimes also about losing someone you counted on. It's the person that stood by your side, helped you make decisions, got you through all the bad times, and celebrated with you all the good times. No matter what happened they were there. This person was a huge part of your life and loved you unconditionally. Am I right? Then they were gone. Their life ended, and your life ended too.

It's no fun thinking about that. It makes sense that all you want to do is avoid the grief and pain. But the dangerous part of all that is when you become a prisoner of that practice. That's when you want desperately to have a break from your grief.

There's one problem with avoiding grief, you can't. Grief will sit and wait, and it will never just go away without being acknowledged. You have to find a balance. Healthy distraction is good; avoiding grief is bad.

Learning to adjust to living alone can be one of the most difficult tasks to learn (especially if you lived with the loved one you lost), so you need time to do it. It takes time to figure out what your new life is going to look like.

Find the balance when you can. Ask for help when you need it. Get the rest you need. And finally, remember that grief is patient, so you need to be patient too. Whenever you think that giving up and avoiding grief would be so much easier, be patient with those around you, and most of all, be patient with yourself.

NOVEMBER 21

Loving Again

I've been asked why I don't talk much about finding love after loss. I'm certainly not opposed to it, in fact, I encourage it. But, unfortunately, not many people grieving the loss of a partner or spouse want to hear it.

No one recovers easily from overwhelming grief. I think it's particularly painful after the loss of a partner or spouse. That's not the kind of relationship you can re-create overnight or would want to. It's just harder after a loss to open yourself up to that kind of vulnerability.

No wonder you feel overwhelmed or even repulsed by the prospect of seeking out a new companion. Feeling this way is completely normal. It takes a very long time to process the sudden death of your best friend, spouse, lover, co-parent, and all-around go-to person.

In fact, you're perhaps at even more of a disadvantage because you had something so very wonderful and rare; 'love of my life' is an extraordinary turn of phrase that few on this planet ever have occasion to use.

Let's get a few things straight, you might not be ready for loving again, even though you're lonely. Of course, you are. But maybe you are thinking about loving again, well, that's okay too!

Your mind might just be protecting your wounded heart right now by coming up with all sorts of thoughts like, "Am I cheating on the love of my life?" "Will a new love be replacing my first love?" "How will the kids react?" "Am I settling?" All these thoughts will most likely stop you from sailing into the dangerous currents of loving again.

It's completely okay to say, "Nobody can replace the one I loved and lost." Because nobody can! And if friends and family are nudging you to date again, tell those well-meaning folks that it's going to take time. End of story!

But I think the unspoken question is, perhaps, "Will I ever be ready to love again?"

And here's what I think about that: Yes. I think you will because you have a soul who knows how to love, knows how to be present for numerous loved ones, knows how to be responsible and caring and committed and kind.

Are you ready right now? I think if you were, you'd be less concerned about everyone else's feelings and all the circumstantial details.

And when you are ready? The noise in your head will drop from jet-engine levels to a soft hum, quiet enough for you to hear your heart finally saying, "Yes, maybe now, maybe this person, maybe loving again."

NOVEMBER 22

Remembering the Past

It's been many years since my spouse's death, and I find I'm not only grieving him but also my memory of him. I mean that literally, as in, I'm grieving the loss of actual memories as I struggle to really remember him in any tangible way. I want to feel his presence and see him clearly in my mind, but he's impossible to recreate. He's more abstract to me now than anything, and that's gutting.

We always say our grief evolves and grows with us as time goes on. Sometimes that means finding new points of comfort and connection, and sometimes it means stumbling upon new losses.

I guess I've stumbled again.

As time goes by, I feel so far away and disconnected from the past that I suddenly have an intense yearning to go back. To fill in my spotty memory with the smallest of things, like the smell of his cologne or the sound of his voice.

I like many things about my life in the present. But if I could turn around and walk into the past, knowing I'd find my way back here again to the people I love, I'd do it in a heartbeat. No one tells you when you're young that life can change so much. That one day you may realize the people and places of your past feel like they're from a completely different story.

I'm suddenly almost angry that I can't go back to before. I accept that my spouse is dead, but I must not fully accept that the past is the past because I keep reaching for it and finding over and over again that it's gone. It's a repetitive ache, like the chronic pain of a once broken bone.

People have shared with me that they struggle to remember the past and their loved ones, which is a troubling secondary loss. They connect to an idea of their loved one but struggle to access specific memories of them. Sometimes this is because their memories faded over time and sometimes because they had limited memories in the first place.

I recognize that many people early on in their grief fear this will eventually happen, so I'm sorry if this conversation exacerbates your worry.

Remember, there's no guarantee you will ever feel any particular way in grief. And if you struggle to remember the past someday, know there are many ways to feel psychologically connected to your loved one that can bring you comfort.

Take a few moments today to really think about all the memories you have of the one you love and lost. By doing this maybe you can remember the past while preserving the present.

NOVEMBER 23

The Greatest Gift

The only thing worse than not listening to someone is pretending to listen.

Giving the vague murmur of agreement or a quick nod to communicate, "Yes, I'm listening, totally," when really they're not.

After my loss I realized none of my friends wanted to hear about my grief. At first I was angry, but then I realized I was really angry with myself. I was equally guilty, and people in glass houses shouldn't throw stones.

Sometimes when people were talking to me, I wasn't always listening closely. Instead, I was thinking, "Did I buy milk?", "I wonder what I should have for lunch?", so why should I expect people to listen to me?

I've made a vow to get better at this, to be more present with friends and family, anyone I'm communicating with. I didn't want to make anyone feel how I felt after my loss, unheard and unimportant. I'm much better at it, but far from perfect.

Technology certainly is a huge barrier to presence, but it's not the main culprit. The main culprit lives between our ears, the mind. So much goes on in there! I think about so much stuff. Thoughts can pop up at any moment, pulling my focus away from the person in front of me.

Luckily, people can't always be certain when I'm not being fully present with them. But I've discovered that when someone is really listening to us, fully present with us in the moment, we know, without a doubt, because we can 'feel' it. It's tough to put such moments into words, but you just know.

Moments when we're fully present with someone who's grieving, it's like magic, like the rest of the world fades into the background. That's it. This, for me, is what presence is all about. It's the greatest gift you can give or receive.

NOVEMBER 24

Turkey With a Side of Grief

Looking back on the Thanksgiving after my spouse died, I don't regret spending that time with my family, but I do regret how we spent it.

There was of course the turkey and all the other food, none of which I felt like eating. The table was all couples except me.

I looked up from my plate to see my brother put his arm around his wife and felt a tightening in my throat. He told her how thankful he was for her being by his side, and I escaped to the bathroom to cry alone. It's hard to accept a reality that you didn't choose.

The holiday marketing machine has already roared to life; a new slew of holiday commercials and movies featuring a city girl or guy trying to save a small-town business during the holidays, only to fall in love and live happily ever after. But what about those of us that didn't get the 'happily ever after'?

You see, the need for joy and celebration can't erase or replace your sorrow, and your expression of gratitude or happiness isn't confined to specific dates.

I believe the pain of grief hurts just as much on the holidays as it does every other day, the holidays just highlight it.

Here I am eight years after that horrible Thanksgiving, my holiday spirit has begun to realign, even though it's still inextricably laced with grief and loss for me, like it is for so many people.

Remember this year that your grief and your gratitude are not in competition with one another. They don't cancel each other out.

You need to make space for each of them, especially during the holidays.

May you find some peace and comfort today.

NOVEMBER 25

Am I Going Crazy?

I'm afraid I have some bad news for you, grief makes you feel like you're going crazy.

But I also have some good news, it's perfectly normal!

It may be different for everyone because we all experience grief in a different way, but on some level, we all struggle to understand ourselves and the world around us after facing a major loss. Whether the loss was sudden, or you were able to anticipate it as soon as you understood and accepted that someone you love was dead or dying, you began the horrific journey through grief. There is shock, sadness, loneliness, isolation, forgetfulness, numbness, fatigue, guilt, anger, crying, worry, fear, oh heck, this could go on forever, but you get the point.

In the first few weeks, you are literally in a total fog. You wake up each morning thinking maybe it was all just a bad dream, and you try to get through the day trying to live without your loved one. Just when you think you're moving forward, you step right back into thinking about your life before your loved one died. It seems odd that the whole world keeps moving on in a normal fashion when this tragic event has occurred. Life is forever changed for you, and everything feels meaningless, gray, and empty.

This is when you really start to feel that you're going crazy. Friends and family don't know what to say anymore. You have to get back to work or school. But you don't feel the same. You worry that you are talking too much about your loved one and people don't really want to listen. You question your faith and life's meaning. You wonder if you should be getting better even though the world is no longer in color. Everything just seems black and white.

But don't worry. Honestly! You're not going crazy. You're grieving. These are all normal feelings.

Take comfort in knowing that, at some point, things will get easier. The intense and unrelenting distress of acute grief will be replaced by less frequent moments of sadness, anger, and frustration. You will still have bad days, but you will know things are getting better when those days are outnumbered by good days.

This doesn't mean that you're 'getting over it,' moving on, or forgetting. An important part of healing is discovering the role your loved one will play in your life after their death.

Very slowly things will begin to get brighter again. The colors come back into the world. Your journey through grief has left you weary but much stronger. You know you will never be the same, and you begin to accept that you must integrate your loved one and your experiences and continue to live. You will be a little bit tired, a little bit crazy, and a little bit wiser as you move forward keeping your loved one locked in your heart.

NOVEMBER 26

A Reason To Live Again

Some people never get to the stage that involves hope and a willingness to be happy again. If this is how you feel, I want you to know that it's possible to move forward without dishonoring the person you love and lost. Getting to this stage can be really hard.

Grief consists of so many emotions, especially the feelings of loneliness and helplessness. The only way to get through them is to let the feelings happen as they come. You can't go around them, under them, or over them, you have to go right through them.

But allowing yourself to feel, live, and even love again, can be really difficult. Time doesn't heal all wounds, especially grief, but it is a key element in the healing process. Once you get through all the emotions of the loss, you can start to rebuild your life and find a meaningful way to keep moving forward.

Human life is a gift, and the relationship you have with someone you love should be cherished. Holding on to fond memories of that life is important, and the memories remain long after the person is gone.

The best way to honor the person you lost is to live and to remember those who still remain that love you. This isn't always easy to do when you're grieving a loss, but it can be easier to do if you reach out and bring happiness to someone else that you love and care about.

The person you lost gave you the gift of love and that felt good, that's why you grieve the loss of it. A great way to heal your broken heart is to reach out to other people with love and kindness. This allows them to be the recipient of the gift you were fortunate enough to receive.

Do one thing today that touches another life and makes the world a better place. By doing that, you honor the one you love and lost while giving yourself a reason to live again.

NOVEMBER 27

Spreading the Love Around

Sometimes my grief feels like my companion for life, but it doesn't take over anymore. It's lost its control and intensity because I've acknowledged it, and I keep living.

Okay, so maybe I don't laugh as loud, act as carefree, and my heart is still cracked, but I function, I live, and I look for ways to help other people. I've reconciled to this new life.

Once I allowed myself to feel my grief and face it every day for as long as it took to understand it, there came a time when it stopped defining how I lived.

This doesn't mean that a memory won't be a trigger and I take up some part of that grief again, but that's okay. It's all part of my process of dealing with a loss. The loss never goes away, but my ability to understand and live with it improves over time. Sometimes, in order to survive a loss, you have to take all that love you have for the person that died and spread it around.

Volunteer your time, visit a sick friend, or donate the clothes of the person who died.

I was holding onto my spouse's winter coat not wanting to let it go, but then one day I gave it to a homeless man. I think that's what he would have wanted me to do.

I also didn't want to hide my grief and hiding myself away from everyone wasn't the answer either. I took a walk on the beach every day, I greeted people with a smile and kind words, and I volunteered at the local hospital.

The point was to get out there and be among others. By doing this, I found my way of being a part of the flow of life again, giving myself hope and a reason to get out of bed each morning.

I hope that you'll take all the love you feel for the person who died and spread that love around. The world sure needs it!

NOVEMBER 28

Ruminating

Do you ever find yourself constantly yearning for the one you love and lost? This is a very normal reaction to a significant loss, but if it's been a long time on your grief journey and you're still doing it, you may feel that something is wrong.

Ruminating is the psychological term used for describing how you may constantly think about the circumstances of the death or stories about the person who died. It's 'telling your story,' over and over again either in your mind or out loud.

This normal process of yearning helps bring your head and your heart together. Don't be angry with yourself if you can't seem to stop wanting to repeat your story. Although not always talked about, rumination and yearning are powerful and necessary parts of the hard work of mourning. But what happens when the yearning goes on too long?

If you find yourself experiencing intensely distressing yearning in an ongoing way and it negatively impacts your day-to-day functioning, then you should consider seeking professional help. This very long-term ruminating can lead to complicated grief that will keep you from moving forward in life in a healthy way.

It hurts to constantly think and talk about the person you loved so much. But when it comes to grief, it often gets worse before it gets better. Be compassionate with yourself and try to surround yourself with people who allow and encourage you to repeat whatever you need to say.

If you're worried about your constant yearning, it's important to acknowledge that it's a common experience. It's also important to understand that your feelings toward yearning may be ambivalent and change over time. Grief is about the loss of someone you love, so yearning and many other grief-related experiences are always going to be a mix of happy and sad.

The problem with yearning that never ends is you can get forever stuck trying to fill the void of your loss.

If you feel like your yearning is going on too long, seek out an understanding friend, support group, or counselor who can be supportive and understand your search for meaning. Having someone that will listen can help you to explore your reasons for being unable to move forward.

If your loss is recent, you might not believe your yearning is negative, and that's okay. Yearning can provide comfort and bring you closer to memories of your loved one, but if your loss was many years ago, it may be time to find the help you need to move forward. The one you love and lost wouldn't want you to spend the rest of your life feeling sad forever, especially on their account.

NOVEMBER 29

"Just Give It Time"

Something I heard a lot from friends and family after my loss was, "Just give it time." Those words frustrated me. What did they mean? Was there a certain day in the future that suddenly my grief would come to an end? I had a hard time believing that.

If your loved one recently died, your grief is probably extremely fresh and raw. It's probably so painful you can't even imagine that you will ever recover or heal from the overwhelming pain and sorrow. I can tell you with all surety that it's going to take a long time. No doubt about it. I can also tell you that it will get easier. Not better. Just easier. There will be brighter days coming. You will survive.

There is literally no good way to shorten the process. (Depressing, I know!)

But you must experience the pain of grief to get to the healing.

There's also no 'normal' amount of time for the grieving process. Everyone heals in their own time and way. Some more quickly than others. The only length of time that can be set is the best length of time for 'you'. It can't be based on anyone else's experience. Your grief is unique and exclusively your own. Take all the time you need.

Even after you're 'done,' you'll most likely experience grief feelings from time to time, especially during special dates like anniversaries or holidays.

You can count on that!

The end of grief doesn't mean that you forget your loved one or stop loving them. It just means you let go of the pain. The grief will always stay, but your heart will mend. You'll never forget them, and they'll always have a special place in your heart.

Time heals the pain not the grief.

NOVEMBER 30

A Letter to Heaven

A great way to find healing from your grief is to write your loved one a letter to Heaven. What would you tell them about how you feel and what you miss about them? What would you say that you wish they could hear?

Doing this can be very difficult but also very comforting. Maybe, just maybe, they know how you feel, and these words will bring you a much-needed connection. Here's my letter to Heaven…

"I hope this letter makes it up to you in Heaven. I imagine it has a long way to go.

I try not to dwell on how much you are missed here on Earth, but that can be easier said than done. I am often told how you are happier in Heaven, but honestly, that never makes me feel better.

Actually, if I'm completely honest, that thought makes me a bit angry. I don't want you to be happier in Heaven, I want you to be here with me. I want to talk to you, I want to see you, and I want you to be there for all the events in my life and the milestones no matter if they are big or small.

I hate that you left me so soon, and even more so when I think about how I never got the chance to say goodbye. Maybe I'm being selfish, but I don't care, I think in this situation I am allowed to be unreasonable and selfish. I just want to have you back in my life again. Today and every day.

You used to be the first person I would go to when I was upset, scared, confused, or happy. I miss your advice, your jokes, and even your bad days.

I know that things got hard in the end and that I was often frustrated with you. I'm sorry for that. It was really never you but the circumstances. I know you were just as frustrated at being trapped in a body that no longer worked as your mind did, and that is my only silver lining in knowing that you are no longer in your earthly body.

I miss you every day, and I pray you are able to see my accomplishments and even my sorrows. To feel that you are still present in my life and supporting me from Heaven helps.

You taught me what it felt like to be not only loved but cherished. You were always my biggest cheerleader and fan. You were the first to teach me the concept of unconditional love which is the best gift you gave me in life.

I love you and hope I'll continue to make you proud as I celebrate your life, and honor you by being the very best 'me' that I can be."

DECEMBER

DECEMBER 1

Grief Sneaks In

It surprises me every time it happens. I feel like I'm finally settling into a routine. I've hit my stride with finding ways to create a life after my loss. I'm doing all the things I feel I should be doing to 'move on.'

There always just seems to be so much going on. I figure that must be a good sign that I'm healing. Then out of nowhere I start to get this slow ache deep in my soul.

Grief sneaks in, and somehow my body and my soul know before my brain that this is going to be a bad day. One of those days where my memory skids and careens and bumps over the memories. The call to hospice. The oxygen tank. The way my bedroom was turned into a hospital room. The desperate prayers whispered in the kitchen or the bathroom in the darkest hours.

I prayed a prayer I never believed I could. I begged God to take him, to release him from his pain. I looked into his blue eyes and told him I would be okay. I lied.

Such beautiful, sweet redemption for him after an intense cancer battle. And unexpected relief for me. I didn't have to watch him suffer anymore. I had confidence he was running the streets of gold with a new body in Heaven.

It's days like today that my soul still knows. My body still remembers.

One thing I've learned is that I need to be intentional about carving out time and finding ways to practice 'remembrance.' I also always need extra courage to survive the day.

My mind is often still triggered by memories of him. He appears in my dreams, or I find myself saying something the way he used to say it. These make me pause. The grief never goes away, but the path somehow grows easier. Tomorrow I'll mark off another day on the calendar and I'll laugh, cry, and celebrate.

DECEMBER 2

Pity Party for One

The winter often brings snow, warm cups of tea, and fires in the fireplace. But for those who have experienced a loss, navigating grief during winter can be a challenging time. The shorter days, grey skies, and cold weather can reflect our feelings of grief. The holidays coming and going, the stillness of winter, and more time spent home alone because of the weather can make grief difficult to bear. What do you do to get through the winter?

Allowing yourself to experience your grief, even amid the stillness of winter, is an important part of healing. It's also important to create in your home a place of comfort and retreat, a place of safety and light in the darkness.

Start by finding ways to bring in the light. Open the blinds and take advantage of every bit of daylight. Get outside, even for a little while, as sunlight can be helpful both psychologically and physically.

Breathe. It sounds so simple, and yet you don't always realize how difficult it can be. Take deep breaths in, slowly letting them out. Take the time to concentrate on each breath. This helps you to be more present and can release tension within your body.

Ask for help. Don't try to brave your grief alone. Your loved ones are feeling helpless and are eager to be useful. Let them. It will benefit you both.

Keep track in a journal of what you have to be grateful for and challenge yourself to find at least one very specific thing to be grateful for each day.

Most of all, be kind to yourself. Don't be so hard on yourself; you may be expecting too much. Don't worry that at the end of the day you feel you've completed nothing. Lack of motivation is very common in grief, especially during the winter months. Sometimes when the winter gets you down you have to have what I call a 'pity-party for one,' so allow yourself days when nothing seems to be accomplished knowing that tomorrow you can try again.

DECEMBER 3

Caught Between Two Worlds

The death of a child is the worst trauma that a parent can endure. I say this not from personal experience, but from those I have worked closely with that have lost a child. One of the questions I hear the most from grieving parents is, "What do I do with the feeling that I want to die to be with my child?"

Your feelings of wanting to die to be with your child are normal and natural after his or her death. Of course, you want to be with your child. Many parents express these same desires. It's not uncommon to want to go to your child, to join your child in death so you can be together.
When you feel that you also want to die, it's actually because you want to be with your child and to feel no pain. These feelings represent your powerful resistance to being separated from your child.

Right now, you're caught between two worlds. Yet somewhere within you, there's the smallest, tiniest place of hope even though you may not know it's there. You have so much to live for here with those who love and still need you. Eventually, with time, the feeling of wanting to die fades as life here becomes more tolerable.

Your tears are important and necessary and will always be there. They come from your very soul. And they're really difficult to control. They come unbidden, and they're really intense.
But the torturous physical and emotional pain you feel now will soften.

Although it feels like time stops the moment your child dies, and there's a terrible grief you fear is forever, you'll be able to breathe freely one day, to appreciate the beauty surrounding you, and to live again.

We all have a great capacity to heal and transform our grief over time. As life goes on and the years pass, pain is altered, even disappears for large periods of time. It's surprising how and when that happens, but it does. It's possible to again feel joy and a renewed sense of purpose in life. It's even possible to thrive, though for you, at this point in time, this may seem impossible to believe.

I have never had the opportunity and gift of experiencing the joy of having a child. I only know my own experiences with grief and loss and that of the parents I counsel. They're my teachers in the grief of child loss.

I admit I don't have the words to help ease your pain. I can only listen and be present. But when your child's absence is more than you can bear, you can keep your child with you. You can hold them close forever. You hold them through your continued love, and you keep them with you through your memories. They'll forever be your child and an important and cherished part of your world.

DECEMBER 4

Resolution

We all know grief in our own unique way. Each of our relationships is unique, and it's not helpful for anyone to assume they really understand what you're going through.

There are no rules for losing and grieving. Sometimes you have to make up the script as you go along. Your script may include some things experienced by others, but it will be based on you and that unique relationship with the person or people you've lost.

The things most of us were taught about what to do and what not to do don't work. Often though, we must work at the job of completing our losses because they interfere with our going on to shape a new life.

Working at loss completion is pretty alien to our society. Most people automatically assume that just the passage of time will heal us, and that after a certain time, people are all right and can just put their losses and pain behind them.

It's true that death may end a physical relationship, but the spiritual and emotional aspects of that relationship stay with us.

There are also many other types of losses, aside from death that have a major impact on how we live. Every loss, hurt, and disappointment engenders feelings within us. Every change we undergo creates responses.

You may be encouraged to use short-term fixes to make your 'bad feelings' go away. You may be told not to feel bad, to get control of yourself, and to move on when you don't know how to do that. After a time, you find that others don't want to hear about your sadness and your feelings.

The difficult feelings end up getting pushed back and tucked away, at least part of the time, causing you to retreat more and more into a state of aloneness and sometimes into behaviors that may harm you or others around you.

It's never too soon and it's never too late to address your grief and to move on to a place of resolution and completion. Miracles in life do happen if you permit your heart to open, but in order for that to occur, you have to do the work of completing your grief first. I call this doing the 'grief work.'

When you're heartbroken, your heart needs to be fixed just as much as a broken bone in your body would need attention. Those who cared about you want you to move forward. Not let go, not forget, but take a step toward healing.

DECEMBER 5

Old Enough To Grieve

Most young children are aware of death, even if they don't understand it. Death is a common theme in cartoons and television.

But experiencing grief firsthand is a different and often confusing process for kids. As a parent, you can't protect a child from the pain of loss, but you can help them feel safe. And by allowing and encouraging them to express their feelings, you can help them build healthy coping skills that will serve them well in the future.

I always tell parents in my support groups that children grieve differently than adults. After losing a loved one, a child may go from crying one minute to playing the next. Their changeable moods don't mean that they aren't sad or that they have finished grieving. Children feel depressed, guilty, anxious, or angry at the person who has died or at someone else entirely, and this is all normal.

You should encourage a child grieving to express their feelings. It's good for kids to express whatever emotions they're feeling. There are many good children's books about death and reading these books together can be a great way to start a conversation with your child.

But be sure to be developmentally appropriate. It's hard to know how a child will react to death, or even if they can grasp the concept. Don't volunteer too much information as this may be overwhelming. Instead, try to answer their questions.

Very young children often don't realize that death is permanent, and they may think that a dead loved one will come back if they do their chores and eat their vegetables. Children understand that death is bad, and they don't like separation, but the concept of 'forever' is just not present.

Be direct and honest with them. When discussing death, never use euphemisms. Kids are extremely literal. When I was very small my grandmother died, and my mother told me she 'went to sleep.' After that I stayed awake every night fearing if I went to sleep, I would die too!

Although my mother's intentions were good, it made me afraid of bedtime. Euphemisms like my mother used can interfere with a child's opportunity to develop healthy coping skills that they'll need in the future.

Keep in mind that even the best-prepared child might get upset, and his behavior can be unpredictable. Kids will not behave in a way that you might want or expect.

Remember, if you're old enough to love, you're old enough to grieve.

DECEMBER 6

Tears in Heaven

Do our loved ones see us cry from Heaven?

I want to answer this question with all honesty. I have to admit I have never been to Heaven. I do hope very much to travel there one day, but as of now, it's still a mystery to me. I'm not 100% sure there is a Heaven. I have no actual proof. I'm not sure anybody does.

I prefer to spend my whole life believing there's a Heaven only to find out in the end there isn't, then to spend my whole life believing there's no Heaven only in the end to find out there is.

I do, however, believe that there's something after this life and be it Heaven or whatever you want to call it, I think I will be reunited with those I love and lost.

Here's what I believe: the tears you cry for your loved one are filled with one thing. Those tears are not filled with pain that you're handing over to your loved one. Your tears don't house hate, anger, guilt, frustration, or any other negative emotion. Your tears are purely made of LOVE.

Do they see you cry those tears? I believe the answer to that question is YES. Your loved ones absolutely see your tears upon your face. I think there's not a moment of your life that they miss from Heaven, all the way down to the little tears upon your face.

They're at your side as you cry those tears, and they are encouraging your beautiful smile through those tears. They know that your tears are made of love. They know how much you miss them. They don't want you to be sad. They're at peace.

Think about it, what kind of Heaven would Heaven be if we spent all of our eternity missing the ones that we love the most once we get there? Instead of missing you, I think they love you. I believe they have pure, unconditional, unwavering love for you from Heaven. They know without a doubt that they'll see you again when you get to Heaven someday.

I think they see you cry from Heaven, and they know you cry out of love. They hear your words to them as you speak with them. They hear you think to them in moments of silence. There's nothing in this world that you could do to make them anything other than proud of you.

You see, you're living, and they know that living is not an easy thing to do. Life is filled with lessons of love and strength. We grow the most through our struggles. Their passing was one of the biggest lessons of love and strength that you've ever worked through in life.

So, be proud of who you are. Cry your tears when they're needed. Above all, remember your worth, and know that they love you completely for all that you are.

DECEMBER 7

Staying Connected

It's been many years now since my loss. Sometimes it's difficult for me to comprehend that; there are times it feels just like yesterday. Working as a Grief Specialist, I help people every day who are struggling with their grief and loss. I'm able to do this because regardless of where they are on their journey, I still remember.

Sure, the rawness and pure gut-wrenching emptiness that I felt in the months immediately after my loss have lessened. I can write about my grief, speak in front of large groups of people, facilitate grief support groups, and still hold onto my memories in ways that are much easier now since so many years have passed.

But similar to the ways many other life experiences still form my sense of being, so too has the death of the person I love. I'm not the same person I was before my loss. I've been changed by it and by what I call my grief, and I'm OK with that.

I no longer feel the shame of being a grieving widower. I can both laugh and cry. In my grief I can get depressed, and I can jump with joy. My grief is me and I am my grief. It's all part of who I am, complicated for sure, but no more or less than others who have known trauma or loss, which is if you think about it, most of us.

Grief is the pain we cause ourselves when we want to be with someone we cannot be with. Love, rather than being grief, is actually the antidote to grief. What I mean is my wanting my spouse not to have died, to still have his life, is refusing to accept what's happened. So, to want my spouse to still be alive is almost the same as not accepting his death. But by continuing to love, I have survived my grief. My grief is not a passing phase. It's a part of my ongoing journey. I've just learned to let go of the pain, but not the grief. I am my grief. It's a part of me forever.

Acknowledging that reality is painful but living with it is something I've gotten used to, like walking with a pebble in my shoe.

In my opinion there's nothing at all problematic about holding onto pain as a way of staying connected. But continuing to love the person I lost is what keeps me connected.

But to live with the pain too long is another matter. If you're tormented by your grief to the extent it stops you from functioning or it drives you to drink or worse to thoughts of suicide, then in a way you've allowed the pain of loss to stay in control.

Grief for me is very much about living with the pain and finding a way to integrate it into my life. Only those who have never known love, escape the grief of loss. I'm my grief because I was loved.

DECEMBER 8

Keep Doing It

Grief is the painful process of dealing with loss. People die, and the closer we are to people, the harder it is when we lose them. Even though grief is something we'll all experience, no one can tell you exactly how you should grieve. Grieving after loss is a very personal thing. And there's no single right way to grieve.

However, understanding how grief works will prepare you better for coping with loss.

The process of grieving is far from straightforward. It's messy and, at times, it may feel like you're losing your mind. You're not. There's no standard pattern for grief.

Try not to pretend you're okay. Be real. Attempting to ignore the pain of grief by 'being strong' won't work. It will only eat you up inside. When you don't grieve, you stop yourself from healing.

It's important for you to accept the reality that someone you love has been lost. Call it what it is. If you've lost someone, tell people, and let them know how you feel about it. Don't bottle it up. Be honest about how you feel.

I can give you all kinds of advice in the world, but it's up to you to take it. I can tell you that life will feel normal again. It will just be different. Different doesn't mean 'bad'; it can also be very good. The pain will go away. Not the grief, that just softens, but the pain will go away.

There are no instructions for how to go through a loss, but if there were they would look like this:
1) Take a deep breath.
2) Hold it for a second.
3) Let the breath out.

You just moved forward.

DECEMBER 9

Crushed

I find it encouraging that people are recognizing so early on that they need support. In the past few years, the world has become a very strange and confusing place, then add to that a major loss, and I just don't expect anyone to be able to cope on their own nor should they.

If you just lost someone recently, there's so much you learn about grief, and very quickly! Welcome to the world of new grief.

I think you'll probably agree with me that just falling asleep at night (if you even can) is a nice break from the thoughts bouncing around in your head, the worries, and the pain. Everyone knows what it feels like to wake up from a nightmare, but if you've lost someone you love, only you know what it feels like to wake up into a nightmare.

You might still be getting up every day and taking a shower, getting dressed, and doing all the things you've always done to start your day, and this seems to be enough to fool those around you into thinking that you're okay. They'll say things like, "You look good!" This is probably well-intentioned, but when they say it, you're most likely thinking, "If only you knew just how crushed I really feel."

Then there are those same well-intentioned people that say, "If there's anything I can do for you." Your response will probably be, "I don't know what I need or how you or anyone else can help." They for sure can't offer the one thing you want and need, your loved one back.

You'll notice people will try to cheer you up. Maybe you were one of those happy people that smiled and laughed all the time. Well, now you're not. You don't feel like it anymore. All you can do now is function on autopilot. They don't understand that you're too preoccupied with loss and grief, that there just isn't room for anything else.

There will also be that person that compares your loss to the loss of their neighbor's sister's friend's brother. Which is just not the same as your spouse, child, sibling, or parent. These people want to connect with you and prove they understand your loss. They don't.

New grief leaves you crushed. It won't be the same for everyone, but the thoughts and feelings that go with it tend to be the same. My advice to you is to try not to pay too much attention to the calendar when deciding how you should feel.

It's different for everyone. This is where you fellow veterans can back me up.

DECEMBER 10

Loving a Little More

Loss can change you in some unexpected ways. Grief can bring you to your knees, but it can also change you for the better.

After my spouse died, I found myself saying goodbye to people I love, and then becoming afraid that it would be the last time I saw them. If the person I loved the most in the world could be ripped out of my life, then surely other people I love could be taken away as well. But instead of letting that fear make me sad, I started to focus on loving these people a little more because I now realize how sacred life is and how brief.

I began to embrace things in my life I never thought about before, like how just waking up in the morning and having the opportunity to live another day was a gift. I would walk on the beach each day and appreciate being able to see the ocean and the beauty of a sunrise or a sunset.

My priorities all shifted. If you lost someone you love you'll understand what I mean by this, that all the little things that used to bother me didn't seem important anymore. I lost what was most important to me, so how could anything else bother me?

Instead of focusing on what I lost, I started to focus on the love. By keeping the love alive, I no longer feel lonely. These are all ways that my loss changed me for the better. I know life is short, so I live it the best I can.

As a survivor, if you ask me how to get through your own grieving process, I encourage you not to run away from the hurt, but rather seek out the experiences that made your loved one special.

You're also a survivor, and because you have all this knowledge, you can now be the person who encourages a newly bereaved person on their grief journey. You have the compassion and empathy to understand what they're going through. This change alone has made you a better person.

DECEMBER 11

The Forgotten Loss

The death of a sibling is really hard. Sometimes you feel guilty because you're the sibling that survived. You probably knew your sibling inside and out and feel like you weren't able to protect them. You may miss your sibling because that was the one person you could confide in or who knew you the best.

I could go on, but the important thing is to understand that your feelings are unique and important. Good, bad, or anywhere in-between, your relationship with your brother or sister was different than anyone else's, and so you'll experience hurdles, triggers, and hardships that others may not.

Your parents, siblings, and other family members may grieve in many of the same ways that you do, but in many ways their grief may differ. It's important to remember this because misunderstandings can arise among family members when people react differently in response to a death.

This is just a guess, but I suspect a lack of sibling grief resources exists because sibling grief is often overshadowed. People simply cannot fathom the out of order aspect of a parent having to bury a child, so when this is the case their thoughts and concerns often immediately go to the parent's grief (not the sibling).

Shifting family dynamics can lead to the weakening of support systems. Parents and siblings who are grieving may be of less, little, or no help. If a person's support system largely consists of family (which is often the case for children and teens), they may find they're facing one of the hardest periods of their life without a safety net.

So, I'm going to say to you, "You're special and you're wonderful (come on, you know you are!). You have no one to live up to besides yourself, your goals, and your own potential."

Okay, I just wanted to say that as a reminder to anyone who feels like they're living in the shadow of a deceased sibling. Feeling compared or overshadowed is common after the death of a sibling, and (although you may be hesitant to admit it) this experience can result in feelings of resentment or anger towards family and/or the person who died.

If this sounds like you, the first thing I recommend you do is to ask yourself, "Who's making me feel this way?" If the answer is your parents or other family members, then the next thing you might do is try to communicate with your family about how you feel.

Siblings are our ties to family bonds. They've known us the longest. They understand our history and are the people with whom we have the longest running jokes. When they're gone, we miss them.

DECEMBER 12

Respect the Journey

When you're grieving the loss of someone you love, you have to respect the journey and be honest with yourself about how you're feeling. Don't compare your experience with anyone else's and ignore anyone who judges how you're doing it.

As time goes on, your thoughts will likely change and evolve while you process your loss. You may have questions that stay in the back of your mind or even facts that you wish you could forget.

It's so tempting to push these moments aside and bury the discomfort but learning to accept your new reality is a better plan.

It won't be easy, and you'll find that your grief seems to come in waves. You might feel calm and at peace one minute and then completely overwhelmed the next.

Learn to breathe through the difficult times and allow yourself to feel the pain of your loss. Postponing it won't make it go away.

Go easy on yourself when these emotions arise. Be honest about your experience with those around you. Lean on your friends and family as you work towards healing.

If you start feeling overwhelmed by your grief and are struggling to get through the day, you should consider reaching out for professional help. Speak to your primary care physician, a counselor, or check out a local support group. Talking to someone that understands what you're going through can help you feel more grounded.

Most of all be kind to yourself. Take a few minutes every day to be alone and do something you enjoy. Take a deep breath, and as you reflect on all that you're experiencing, let it serve as a reminder of how much you want and deserve to live your very best life.

DECEMBER 13

Eliminate the Negative

When I was caring for my spouse, the hospice team gave me the task to administer morphine. At the time I wasn't a medical professional, and I certainly wasn't prepared to be giving the person I loved narcotics.

In the days following his death I would spend so many days wondering if I had given him too much or too little. The feelings of regret and guilt added to my already broken heart. I even wondered at times if I had been responsible for his death.

These feelings can be so destructive and overwhelming that it sometimes feels like we'll never recover from them. But, by understanding the grieving process and the emotional fallout that can occur, we can be better prepared to deal with these feelings.

Society tends to believe that grief makes us 'sad.' If it were only that simple! The reality is that when you lose someone you love, the grief can drag you through a huge expanse of feelings. If these feelings aren't acknowledged and eventually worked through, they can pull you down like a weight attached to your ankle. Often, you'll push these feelings away because they're too painful, but that isn't the answer.

You can't ignore your feelings about the loss of your loved one; all you can do is try and move through them. You shouldn't be so hard on yourself or let society make you feel a certain way. It's your loss and your feelings and you shouldn't be ashamed of them.

So how do you process these feelings?

One way is to not push them aside.

Your emotions are actually trying to help you heal.

You're different because of your loss. You need to experience these feelings and let them help you move forward by accepting them. As you work through your feelings, you can hold tight to the love you had for the person you lost, and that love will help to heal your heart. You can allow all the negative feelings to move through you while holding onto the love and positive memories. This doesn't mean that you'll forget the person you love.

The love is forever and can never be lost.

You know your loved one loved you and wouldn't want you to hold onto all those negative feelings. Love and loss can walk side by side, and you can experience joy in life again if you can learn to let go of the negative feelings and find the joy that your loved one would want for you.

Instead of focusing on all the negative aspects of your loss, learn to focus on the love and happy times you shared.

DECEMBER 14

Forgiving Yourself

Do you feel guilty your loved one died?

Guilt is actually a normal response to death. You may have the perception that you somehow failed in your duties and obligations, or that you've done something wrong. It creates a mixture of feelings including doubt, shame, inadequacy, insecurity, failure, unworthiness, self-judgment, anxiety, fear, and blame.

Maybe your loved one was diagnosed with a terminal illness, and as a caregiver you may feel guilty that you hadn't noticed symptoms sooner, waited too long to seek treatment, or didn't do enough to comfort them.

If death came suddenly or unexpectedly, you may feel guilty for not being present when it happened. Maybe you feel like you could have prevented it.

You may even feel guilty that you are the one who survived or uncomfortable that you received an insurance settlement or inheritance following the death of your loved one.

Unfortunately, guilt is a natural and common reaction to the death of a loved one. When someone you love dies, it's only human to search for an explanation, to look at what you did or did not do, to dwell on the 'what ifs.' You agonize and tell yourself, "If only I'd done something differently, this never would've happened."

Sometimes, though, there simply isn't anything you could have done differently. When your loved one's illness or death occurred, chances are that whatever happened beforehand was not intentional on your part.

You most likely did the best you could with what you knew at the time. You basically gave your best effort, and you should be proud of that. Instead of beating yourself up about what you did or didn't do, remind yourself that when you know better, you do better. You were doing whatever you did on what you knew given the information available to you then.

Harsh as it may seem, consider that even if you had done things differently, your loved one still could have died in some other way at some other time. Death is a fact of life, and you have no control over when people die including your loved one.

Maybe you did make mistakes, and that's okay too. You need to forgive yourself for what you believe you could have done differently. Healthy guilt allows you to own up to and learn from your mistakes. It gives you a chance to make amends, to do things differently next time, and to come to a better understanding of yourself, to forgive yourself and move forward.

DECEMBER 15

I Still Think of You

I want you to know I still think of you. Just because I don't talk about you as much, doesn't mean I've forgotten you. You see, it's just that other people don't want to hear it. They don't understand. It makes them uncomfortable.

I still experience flashbacks of that day I held you in my arms, and you took your last breath. You whispered, "I love you", and then you were gone.

What other people don't understand is there's really no way to forget something like that. I still dream of you now and then. I still drive past that beach where we first met, and sometimes the tears start falling out of my eyes. I still wear the shirt you bought me, and I still carry your picture in my wallet. I still see your smile and hear your laugh.

And when it gets very hard, when the memories jumble and force themselves to splash out of my head, I sit silent. I think about how much I miss you. I think about how much I want to see you. I think about how much I want to feel your presence beside me.

The other thing people don't understand is that thinking about you is what reminds me that I'm going to be okay. Your memory is what reminds me that life goes on. That even when you died, it's still your memory that makes me feel alive.

Just because I don't talk about you as much, doesn't imply that you're forgotten because I still love you. No matter what happens, you're still a part of my life. A very important part.

So don't you worry because I'm okay. I'm happy. I've let the pain go. I've finally learned how to embrace loss and happiness all at the same time.

Thank you for stopping by my life.

I'll see you again when it's time.

DECEMBER 16

Fearing the Future

After a loss the fear of a future without a loved one is a common emotion. Been there. Done that. I get it. I really do. When your planned future is no longer your reality and the fear of your new reality is staring you in the face, what do you do?

Fear of the future is facing you head on with no answers, direction, guidance, or alternatives. You can't make it go away. You can't stop wondering why. You can't pretend it isn't happening. You might even go into denial for a short period of time. But then, you realize that life is continuing on while you're still stuck. So, what do you do?

Pick a quiet time to be alone. Light a candle in honor of your loved one and take a picture of them with you to a comfortable and quiet space and CRY! Tears are cleansing and healing. But give yourself a time limit for this exercise so that you don't stay in your grief too long. Grief is a place to go when you need to, just don't stay there.

Accept that life will never be the same; I totally know that this is easier said than done. There are steps to get to the place of acceptance; however, when you accept that your life will never be the same again, you can begin to plan your new life going forward. Your fear will diminish as you accept that this new life can be meaningful, and you can find peace and joy.

Find your purpose for the future. You have two choices in this one. As you work through the grief process, continue on your path to fulfill the purpose you had before the loss or use the experience of loss to find meaning and purpose in life going forward.

Fear is normal, and everyone experiences it at some point in life.

I know it's scary, but I encourage you to move from a place of grief to gratitude. You're loved one would want you to live your life for the rest of your life.

DECEMBER 17

Living In a Different Way

Your loved one's memory does not live in the pain of your grief. Then where does your loved one's memory live? It lives in YOU.

It lives in the stories that you tell people about your loved one. It lives in the memories you share together with friends and family. It lives in the things you do that your loved one taught you. It lives in the things you do in their honor and memory. It lives in every little thing you do to stay connected to them, from listening to music they loved to cooking their favorite food to anything else you do to continue the bond.

Now, it's easy to see why this reality might be confusing because in the beginning many of the above things might have caused you pain or maybe they still do. Reminders can make you sad, so sometimes you might think that if the pain starts to go away, things mean less to you, or if your loved one's memory is disappearing, your love for them is diminishing. This is NOT what is happening! I promise.

As time passes your brain learns to manage the emotional pain, and slowly you get a little more control over the memory. As you get further from your loss, the pain starts to ease just a bit.

What you should realize is that your loved one is not disappearing as your pain diminishes, you are just learning to live with the memory of your loved one in a different way.

You can let go of the pain and not let go of the love. Deciding to continue the bonds you had with your loved one is a way to do just that. Your connection to your loved one can be part of your daily life even as you move forward. Figure out what that looks like for you.

You may be surprised to see that as you find positive ways to continue bonds with the person you lost, you can let go of some of the pain without the fear that you're letting go of the person you love.

DECEMBER 18

I Survived

I can remember some parts of the first few weeks as a newly bereaved widower. Most of its foggy and distant, but some of it remains. My body was exhausted from the physical toll of being a caregiver for so long. My heart was broken that I had done all I could to save the person I love, and still he died.

I woke up each morning, and for a brief moment I thought I had dreamed up the whole thing. Maybe it was just a nightmare? But then I realized the nightmare was really happening. It wasn't a dream. The nightmare was real. The person I love was replaced by grief. I was consumed by sadness, and I felt like I couldn't breathe. I didn't know what I was doing or where I was going. It didn't matter anyway. Nothing did.

The days went by, and I took care of all the things I was now left alone to do all on my own. Even though all I wanted to do was stay in bed and hide under the covers, I had to start finding my way in this new unfamiliar world I was pushed into without the person I love by my side.

It was time to begin 'surviving,' and that was going to take every ounce of my strength and courage to accomplish. Each day I set a goal of doing one thing. That one thing most days was something as simple as going out to get food, picking the mail up at the post office, or paying the bills. These were all things I saw as part of my survival.

My focus on just surviving became my new normal for quite some time. I was doing just enough to take care of myself. Plenty of things got lost in the shuffle, but at least the most important things were done.

So here I am now. I can now say with all confidence that I survived. I get out of bed each morning, and I go about my life just like everyone else who has a 'normal' life. The only difference is grief is forever a part of who I am; it just no longer defines me.

But I didn't want to just survive anymore, I wanted to become a better person. My life now is full of wonderful things that have come out of the ashes of my loss. My passion for helping others has grown from the love I have for my spouse; helping others is what allows me to honor his life, love, and legacy.

I feel an intense connection to those who are suffering, and I seek out opportunities to be with them. It gives me a purpose for moving forward.

I want you to know that surviving is about living in the fullness of a life where grief and joy coexist. They can both become a part of who you are and occupy the same space in your heart.

So don't give up, you are surviving!

DECEMBER 19

It's Not for Wimps

Some people think grief is linear, but it's not. There's not a defined path from devastation to moving on. Grief is also not straight-forward. It's difficult. More like a squiggly line.

Because it's not linear, the first days, weeks, months are unimaginable, and just because it starts to get better doesn't mean it stays better.

Time moves on so people expect that you also do. But grief doesn't care that your friends and family think you should be doing better than you're actually doing. They don't care how long it's been. It didn't happen to them. They're confused. They don't even think that it could still be grief that's bothering you because how could you still be crippled by grief? Still?

So, you try to act like you're not dying inside until the moment when it starts coming back to the surface. Like it just happened yesterday. This usually happens in the time leading up to anniversaries, birthdays, and holidays. But other times, it comes out of nowhere for no reason.

Sometimes just when you think you're finally feeling better, BAM!

All of a sudden, you're crying every day again. Then all those people will look at you funny and ask you how you're feeling. (Isn't it obvious?) So, you answer, "I don't know" when they ask what is wrong with you. Because you won't know. This isn't still grief, is it? Still?

Yes, still. That's the problem with trying to measure your healing according to timelines. Grief isn't linear. It's not an experience you go through before moving on and getting back to your life.

There's no moving on. There's no getting back to life because now your life is changed. You have to learn to create a new life, and that takes time. It may take six months, but it may also take six years. Forget what everyone says, and don't let them rush you.

Most importantly, don't rush yourself. Take all the time you need. Pull close those who are trying to help you, especially those that are going through the same thing. Let yourself heal on your own time, and in your own way.

Shortly after you lose someone you love, especially at the beginning of your grief journey, your main goal is just to stay alive. And if you're reading this, then you've succeeded.

Yes, it gets better. But it doesn't stay better. There will be bad days, weeks, months, even years. Expect them, and don't fight against them. Let them pass and know that the good days will be back. You're surviving (even if it's barely) and that takes strength and courage.

This whole grief thing, it's not for wimps!

DECEMBER 20

Staying Broken

When you keep your grief bottled up inside, it twists you out of shape and can make other people not want to be around you. That's the ugly truth about grief. But writing, talking, or finding any other activity that releases some of the pain does help.

Allowing yourself to break is probably the hardest thing you'll do because for most of us it's just not easy when we think others believe we're not coping. Our society expects us to be rational and over our loss in a few days or months. I found out that's not possible. You have to allow yourself to break, and stay broken, for as long as you need to be that way.

A common reaction of most adults upon hearing bad news is to reach for a bottle. I'm no exception. In the weeks following my husband's death, I'd describe my days as 'foggy' but not only from grief. I found that a glass (or four) of my good friend Chardonnay temporarily smoothed the edge off my grief only for it to return in the morning even worse. Now I not only felt flattened by my grief but also crushed with a hangover.

Where I did find comfort was in taking a walk on the beach. It was much more calming (and healthy) to take a walk on the beach and cry instead of trying to find peace at the bottom of a wine bottle.

Be honest with the people in your life that tend to complain about everything. Nothing is worse than when you're grieving a major loss, and someone is complaining to you about some random unimportant thing that happened to them. Tell them you're just not strong enough (right now) to listen to them. You have enough on your own plate.

I'm a big advocate of exercise because you can't deny its positive impact on your mood. If your heart is broken, you might as well try to strengthen it a bit.

Staying broken also includes trying to stop pushing everyone away. Why do we do that? Because grief is something you don't like to share, like secrets or a large pizza when you're hungry.

If there's one thing that I've learned on my grief journey, and I've learned a lot, it's that you have to stay broken for as long as that takes. When you suffer a loss, grief will take up residence in your life, and that's okay. It's there to be felt and experienced. That's how you work through it and learn to integrate it into the fabric of your life.

Surviving grief means allowing yourself to be broken and having the courage to heal.

DECEMBER 21

Those Left Behind

I've been to a lot of funerals in the past year. I have two best friends that lost their spouses. Then I lost several friends and family members. And unfortunately, several other funerals that had me stuffing myself into the same suit.

The problem with being a Grief Specialist and going to funerals is everyone thinks I have the answers to all their questions surrounding the death of their loved one. I don't.

My best friend lost her mother last year and then shortly after her spouse. I went to both funerals. I do know that the aftermath is going to be tough for her especially during all the holidays. Her mother was always her rock and now she isn't around. That's the thing when your parent dies, you feel like instead of going into every fight with backup, you're going into every fight alone. She also doesn't have her spouse to comfort her, so that makes it even more difficult.

I asked her how she was doing without her mother and her spouse, and her reply was, "It's not the same."

Four small words that encompass so much. I assume she was referring to life. It's not the same and never will be, at least not for her or anyone else that has lost a significant person that they love.

I don't go to funerals for the person that died but for those left behind. When they look to me for answers, I listen. I don't have all the answers. The only gift I have to give is my presence.

This coming year may hold in store for me more funerals. I wish that wasn't the case, but I know that's the way life is, and even though I hate funerals, I'll go and be present. I'll walk with those left behind and use the knowledge I've gained on my own journey to help guide them through their own.

DECEMBER 22

Secondary Losses

There's a piece of your identity that's defined by your relationships. After a loss, the secondary losses that happen, like dominoes falling, create far more to cope with than just the loss of the person that has just died.

You may notice a big change in your social status or that you have no purpose or reason to live. You may even feel that you lost a sense of yourself and loss of community and connection to your loved ones that are still living.

The most difficult part of all these losses of your identity is that your perspective on the world gets shaken. You may have believed that the world was a fair and just place. You may have been a happy person before your loss and felt the world was predictable and safe. Now you may be more negative, jaded, and pessimistic.

If you're thinking, "yes, this is me" you may also be thinking, "what do I do about it?" There's no easy answer, but the first thing to keep in mind is your identity will never be what it was before your loss.

We all have ideas about how life is supposed to look. When life doesn't work out that way, it can be easy to assume that no alternative will ever allow us to have a sense of well-being.

You can bring the past into the present. The person you lost, the person you were, those are all things that will still be a part of you as you go forward. The stupid notion of 'letting go' might leave you feeling like the healthy way to grieve is to shut the door to the past. It's not true!

A continued connection to your loved one, as well as a continued connection to the person you used to be, can be a very healthy part of moving forward. By acknowledging the pieces of your life that will never be the same, you can learn how to establish new pieces of yourself that are built on things that came before.

DECEMBER 23

Feel the Crack

Falling in love is awfully simple, but losing that love is simply awful. When someone you love dies, your heart gets broken and to stop loving them is NOT an option. But how do you get beyond the pain? How do you mend a broken heart?

First you have to feel the pain, and then you have to go through it. I realize the most difficult task for a person with a broken heart is to stand still and feel the crack. But that's exactly what you need to do.

There's no shortcut. Loss has its share of obstructions. One of them is grief. You have to grieve in order to move on. You have to go through it, you can't go around it, under it, or over it. Nope! You have to go right through it.

If you try to avoid some of the emotions and feelings that are tearing you apart inside, you'll find yourself bumping into them somewhere down the line, just like being caught in the center of a traffic circle. By going through the intense pain, you will eventually surface as a stronger person ready to tackle problems head on. Soon the pain will lose its hold over you.

Another way to mend a broken heart is to make a 'good and bad' list. You need to know which activities will make you feel good and which ones will make you feel bad. You won't really know which activity belongs on which list until you start trying. I suspect that some things like sitting in a chair a whole entire day looking at an old photograph and crying is not going to make you feel good. So put that on the 'bad' list. On the 'good' list you may want to put taking a walk or doing something in their honor. Basically, anything that brings you comfort should be added to your 'good' list.

There's one emotion that's stronger than fear and that's forgiveness. To mend your broken heart, you not only need to forgive yourself for any guilty feelings you have around your loss, but you also need to forgive your loved one for dying.

But forgiveness requires hope: believing that a better place exists, that the aching emptiness experienced in your every activity won't be with you forever, that one day you'll be excited to get up and start your day.

Hope is believing that the sadness can evaporate, that if you try like hell to move on with your life, your smile won't always be forced. Therefore, in order to forgive and to move past fear, you need to find hope and remember to love. Once your heart is broken you have two options: you can close off pieces of your heart so that one day love will never be able to get inside, or you can love again. It doesn't have to be a romantic love; it can simply be a renewed love for life.

DECEMBER 24

It's a Wonderful Life

You've most likely seen the Frank Capra holiday classic "It's A Wonderful Life."

If you haven't seen it, George Bailey, played by Jimmy Stewart, is an all-around nice guy who sacrifices his dreams to help others. One Christmas Eve, he finds himself in a lot of trouble. He's contemplating ending it all when Clarence, an angel-in-training, steps in to help. He listens as George rants about his litany of problems then states that he wishes he'd never been born at all. His wish is granted.

George is given an amazing gift that night. He's able to see all the ways he positively affected the world, and what things would be like if he had never been born. In the end, George is grateful for everything he has…including the painful and disappointing times.

The movie is about both acceptance and gratitude, something that can also be associated with grief and loss. Think for a moment what your life would look like if your loved one had never been born, never entered your life. What would you have missed? What memories would you now not be able to treasure?

You could choose to protect yourself from all this pain by removing these memories, or you can be courageous enough to face your grief head-on and fight through the pain that comes with taking ownership of these memories for the rest of your life. If you think of your loss in these terms, is your grief worth it?

Having gratitude for what you had is about accepting that you've earned your pain and your grief. You have a wonderful life because of the existence of the person you love. You can look back on so many amazing experiences.

Because this person existed, you really did, and still have, a wonderful life.

DECEMBER 25

Searching for Santa

I remember when I was a very young child, and I truly believed in Santa.

I remember that extreme feeling of excitement when I'd go to bed on Christmas Eve. I couldn't sleep because the anticipation was so great thinking about all the treasures that Santa would bring me.

But then came that first year when I was no longer quite sure Santa was real. I feared not believing because then maybe there would be no presents.

So, I went to bed with hope but a little less excitement, and that's how it feels after someone you love dies.

As young children we live in a world unaware that someday we'll learn unpleasant truths or experience unhappy events.

But our lives begin to change as we find out things like Santa isn't 'real' or doesn't exist.

As we grow older, we experience events that change us.

We don't want to know they'll happen, but they do, and some of them shatter our lives.

That's how losing someone you love feels, the blissful ignorance that you would be together forever is gone. Life goes on, but it's different, less exciting.

I'm a survivor of my loss, and this means I've gained a new sense of empathy and compassion for others who are experiencing it.

In many ways, I'm always searching for Santa because I still believe that there's beauty, joy, and happiness in the world, and it's my responsibility to find it and share it.

DECEMBER 26

Praying for a Way Out

The loss of anything can cause a certain amount of grief. The depth of our grief is related to our attachment to what we have lost. For example, if I lose my favorite hat, I'll be sad, but it's not a serious sorrow. All I have to do is buy a new hat to get over my feeling of loss. No more loss, and no problem.

But the death of a loved one is completely different. We can't undo a loss of that magnitude. We can't replace a person who was important to us, nor can we stop loving them. This brings on an overwhelming feeling of grief.

Grieving does not necessarily start with death. When death doesn't come suddenly, the grieving process may start with a terminal diagnosis.

Because I have experienced the death of a spouse, the grief of losing him was like me losing part of myself. The grief was far, far beyond any pain I had ever experienced. I wasn't prepared for it.

After a year of seeing me grieve, my family and friends started to think it was odd that I was still not recovered from my loss. So, for their benefit, I started to pretend that I was better.

It was all an act. No more did I break down in public, but I was nowhere near recovered. Being alone on our anniversary, my birthday, Thanksgiving, and Christmas was probably the worst. I couldn't celebrate anything.

After two years of grieving, I started to worry about my mental health. I thought I should have made some move toward acceptance by then, but I was still deeply grieving.

I decided I had to make a more active effort to somehow recover. I did some deep soul searching to find what was keeping me from moving forward with my life.

For months, I prayed for a way out. In a moment of clarity, I realized that I was afraid to let go of grief because that would mean I was letting go of my love for him.

It seems irrational that I was hanging on to grief in order to feel love, but extreme grief can throw common sense out the window.

I knew that he would always be in my heart whether he was alive or not. So, every time the sadness came, I reminded myself that nothing could diminish that love. I could never lose him completely.

The awareness that love transcends death was a turning point. The sadness lifted, and the grief ended. Yes, I did change. Grief broke me down and rebuilt me.

DECEMBER 27

Just Words

I've survived my grief, and I've healed, but I'm not the same person I was before my loss. I never will be again. Surviving my grief doesn't mean I've stopped grieving; I don't think I ever will. I can't be fixed. I don't want to be fixed.

Some people think surviving grief means being happy again, all the time. I don't. I'm happy, sad, angry, confused, lost, found, and many more things all at the same time. It's more important to me to be who I really am than to pretend things I don't feel.

If I get stuck in one emotion, I try to be present to what else is happening. I give myself time to feel the pain of loss and time to find things that bring me joy and happiness. I couldn't do that in the first months of grief or even years after my loss. That's how I know I've healed.

I'm just like everyone else. I have different emotions, always flowing through me, always shifting, always changing. No one knows my grief, it's mine and only mine. They see me smiling and laughing, and they ask, "How are you?" and I say, "Great, but of course the person I love is still dead."

I'd much rather other people acknowledge my pain because that frees me up to have a better time. If you only see my joy and my accomplishments and you don't see my pain, then you don't know me.

There's no time limit on grief, but there's also no limit on filling the empty space with happy moments when you can and when you're ready. I'm just like you. I suffered a terrible loss. But I'm still here.

Sure, I survived, but there's more to surviving than meets the eye.

If you ask me how I am, I'll tell you, but it will just be words, and words sometimes don't say very much at all.

DECEMBER 28

It Gets Different

I wish I could tell you this won't hurt. I wish I could tell you that you're in control of the situation. I wish I had all the right words to take away your pain.

It's difficult to even put into words how it feels to lose someone you love. It's almost impossible unless it's happened to you. If it has, you know!

When someone you love dies, life as you know it dramatically changes. Watching your loved die is absolute hell. When you watch them die, you die right alongside them.

When you're grieving a loss, it's exhausting. You try your best to go through the motions of life, but it's next to impossible to not think of your loved one and desperately wanting them back.

The process of dying isn't only for the person that dies, it's also for those of us left behind. You have to learn how to process how you're going to live without them and how that's going to make you feel. Your brain tells you that you need to move forward with your life, but your heart just wants to hold on forever.

If the person you loved was suffering, it might seem selfish to not have wanted to let them go, but even in that situation, you are still never ready to say goodbye. You might have hated to see them suffer, but the thought of never seeing them again is even more terrifying. Death makes you selfish sometimes.

You might be one of those people like me that has spent a lot of time thinking you could have 'saved' them. I realized in time that the problem with that kind of thinking is we are so focused on what we want, we don't stop for a moment to think about what we actually have control over and what we don't.

Then when they die, we discover they taught us so much and left us with so many memories. The only thing they didn't do was tell us how to survive without them.

I wish I could tell you it gets easier, but grief is messy and complicated. It takes time.
You'll never 'get over it' and it's okay to be sad. A piece of your heart will always be broken.

Always remember the greater the love, the greater the grief.

I wish I could tell you that in time it won't hurt as bad and it will get better, but I've learned that grief lasts a lifetime. I wish I could tell you that it gets better, but it really just gets different.

DECEMBER 29

Loving a Child That's Gone

How does a parent continue on after the loss of a child? I can't answer this question because I have never lost a child.

But I bet they can feel their unasked questions. I often wonder how they can still stand, still walk, still laugh. I don't ask. I can't ask that of a parent who has lost their child. Instead I ask, "How are you?" that pause, that inflection, tells them that's really what I want to know. I can only guess, assume, and try to imagine what it is they feel.

But when I do grief coaching with parents who lost a child, they tell me all about it, and I listen, and I learn, and I care.

They're lost without them. They search for them, knowing they are nowhere on this earth. And still, it would not surprise them if their child were to appear by their side wearing their favorite shirt and eating a snack they loved. At times they can almost smell them and feel their breath on the back of their neck, but when they look over their shoulder, their child isn't there.

Their mind invents stories. That their child is not really dead. They are just at school or at work, soon to return. They are in their room watching TV, playing video games, getting dressed for the prom. They are away at college or planning their wedding.

Then these parents shout, "Where are you!?" They scream, "Why did you die!?" The answer they receive is silence.

These stories they invent don't always heal the pain, for them nothing will heal the pain. The cloud of grief that surrounds them doesn't block out that they know their child is dead.

They feel that the one instinct that runs through every parent, to protect their child, was something they couldn't do. Just the fact that their child is dead, while they still live, defies the natural order of life. This alone isn't fair.

These parents love their other children if they have them, but the love they have for their child that died can't be transferred to another living person. And so, for the longest time after their child's death, maybe forever, their heart remains broken.

So, they wonder what they will do with this love that has no place to go. Then they hear the whisper of their child's voice saying, "Just love me."

"But where are you?" They ask.

They answer, "I'm here, just love me."

DECEMBER 30

Being Okay Again

Sometimes it seems like he was here just yesterday, smiling at me, talking to me, and other times it seems like it has been ages since I saw his warm, comforting face.

He's always in the back of my mind. I still think about him on most days. Sometimes when I think of him, I get really sad, but I'm okay. Then other times I get really happy. He just kind of passes through my thoughts, and then I just continue on with what I'm doing. The missing him is always there, but sometimes my memory of him is calming. It's reassuring. It's safe and feels good.

More than anything, I wish I could see him. I wish I could talk to him. I wish I could ask him how's he's doing. I'd love to get a call or text from him. I wish I could give him a hug.

And this is why losing someone is so hard. Because the feeling of missing that person never ends. The ache never fully goes away. The pain lessens over time, and you learn to live with it. But the part where you miss them never really changes. It just doesn't hurt as much. It's becoming bearable.

It you're fresh in your grief, I want you to know that this is how grief changes over time. It doesn't end, and it doesn't go away. It just changes. You really do feel ALMOST normal again.

It's just different in a surreal kind of way.

You have to learn how to live in a world without the person you love. That's hard! But you do begin to learn how to live with it. I know this might be hard to believe now, but you even learn how to be okay again.

I think that those we lose never fully leave us. I believe they become a part of us, that they live on within us. They live in our heart and are by our side each step of the way. Even though you might heal from your grief, you will still carry some of it with you. It's just not as heavy a load.

You'll still miss your person because they are a part of who you were and of who you are. Your life has been permanently changed because of them. So, while you may have this hole in your heart forever, you can find comfort in knowing that because of the person you miss, your life has been changed for the better.

Don't you agree?

DECEMBER 31

Alone on New Year's Eve

Grief isn't pretty. It's loneliness at a primal level. Like some organ has been removed and you can't really breathe properly. It's waking up each morning where your first thought is this is another day without your person. And in that way, without the you that you were. It's going to bed alone each night without the one you love.

I can't offer any advice. It's been over eight years since my spouse died, and I haven't found any solutions. What I have done is found a way to move forward while taking him with me. So here are my modest suggestions:

Stay off of social media, it hurts more to see the celebrations of others. I, of course, can't seem to do this. Comparison may be the enemy of joy; Facebook rubs it in.

If you descend into the pit of decadent take out and binge-watching Netflix, set a specific date to get out or call someone you really trust to ask for help.

Don't order a large pizza when you're really depressed. You can only eat a small one by yourself. Really.

Don't make big, irrevocable resolutions during the holiday. Selling your house and moving to another country may be hard to reverse.

I don't have any easy answers. I wish I did. All I can tell you is to do what makes you feel better. Ask yourself this question before doing anything, "Will doing this make me feel better or will it make me feel worse?" I guarantee that the answer will make a big difference.

Remember this New Year's Eve that there's always tomorrow. Today you may be drowning, but tomorrow you'll float to the top again.

That's the way grief works. Moment by moment is the way through it.

My Letter To You

I commend you for using the precious little energy you have to read this book. I hope you found comfort within its pages. Doing anything when you're grieving is difficult, but I hope that by doing it one day at a time made it less daunting.

I know first-hand that grief lasts longer than 365 days, it lasts a lifetime. Just as life is full of love, appreciation, and fond memories, there will also be sadness, yearning, and pain. Even though these experiences seem in opposition to one another, you can experience them all at the same time. If the pain of losing someone you love always exists, it makes sense because there will never come a day when you won't wish for one more moment with the one you love.

Grief is ongoing. It's always there like a tender scar on your heart. But let me reassure you, experiencing pain doesn't negate the potential for healing. It evolves over time. You'll have days of ups and downs, days of good and bad, but eventually you'll reach a place where you may find that your bad days are few and far between.

This grief journey you're on may be scary, but in time, you'll find that you wouldn't have it any other way. This is because your grief is also an expression of your love. Grief is how you love a person despite their physical absence. It helps connect you to memories of the past; it bonds you with others, and it helps provide perspective on your immense capacity for finding strength and wisdom in a very difficult time.

I wrote this book for you and used what I've learned along the way on my own personal grief journey. A journey that continues to this day. I wanted to lead you through the days with as much comfort, security, and hope as is reasonably possible.

I know that this book can't take away your pain or hurt, but maybe it made you feel less alone to know that I, along with many others, have walked the road you're on and survived. If you remember nothing else, remember this: you're not alone.

I realize that not all the thoughts and reflections in this book have applied equally to your situation. Some might have fit better than others. Take the thoughts and suggestions that suited you best, hold them close to your heart, and share the others with someone else that may need them.

However long this pain of grief lasts for you, chances are it will seem too long. I know it's uncomfortable and some days it feels like you'll never survive, but your grief is actually serving a purpose. It's helping you heal.

I hope in some small way this book has made you feel less alone because I truly believe we're all just walking each other home.

Truly yours, Gary

Acknowledgements

I offer my sincere gratitude to the thousands of followers on my Facebook page, *Surviving Grief*. Those of you who have shared your stories and have allowed me to share mine. It's your continued support that encouraged me to write this book and share with others the daily struggle of grief and loss.

My mother, Barbara Sturgis, you are a constant source of love and support. Even in your own sorrow you have bravely found the courage to move forward with compassion, faith, and love for those that have the privilege to know you. Thank you for your support in making this book possible. You're not just my mother, you're also my friend.

My "Dahlin" sister-in-law Betsy Kinter. Without your love and support this book would not exist. You're truly the 'sister' I never had and always wanted. Thank you for reading my words, fixing my errors, and having the patience to do both. You are a gift in my life for which I'm forever grateful.

Zoe, my 'Pumpkin', you spend hours sitting by my side and no man has had a better four-legged best friend and secretary. You bring joy to every day of my life just by being a part of it.

I'm so thankful for the love I receive from my 'Southern Family,' Gerry, Woody, Betsy, John, Susan, Tom, T and T. I love y'all!

My husband, best friend, and raftmate, Scott. Without your love and support I wouldn't be where I am today. As we continue on our journey together, may we never forget the love and devotion of Rob, Dave, and all the others we still feel ever so present in our lives. I love you forever and for always, no matter what, pinky swear!

In loving memory of my father, Harry Sturgis. I love you and miss you more than words can express. Thank you for teaching me to be a good person and that life is more than just what we see here on Earth. I'll see you on the other side, somewhere over the rainbow.

Visit my *Surviving Grief* website at
www.sgrief.com

or

Follow me on Facebook at *Surviving Grief*

**https://www.facebook.com/SurvivingGrief
GarySturgis**

If you have any comments, questions, or
would like to share your own experiences
with grief and healing, you can email me
directly at: **gary@sgrief.com**

I look forward to hearing from you!

Gary Sturgis

CPSIA information can be obtained
at www.ICGtesting.com
Printed in the USA
LVHW081904220922
729063LV00014B/880